2011
YEAR BOOK OF
PSYCHIATRY AND
APPLIED MENTAL HEALTH®

The 2011 Year Book Series

Year Book of Anesthesiology and Pain Management™: Drs Chestnut, Abram, Black, Gravlee, Lien, Mathru, and Roizen

Year Book of Cardiology®: Drs Gersh, Cheitlin, Elliott, Gold, Graham, and Thourani

Year Book of Critical Care Medicine®: Drs Dellinger, Parrillo, Balk, Dorman, Dries, and Zanotti-Cavazzoni

Year Book of Dermatology and Dermatologic Surgery™: Dr Del Rosso

Year Book of Diagnostic Radiology®: Drs Osborn, Abbara, Birdwell, Elster, Manaster, Oestreich, Offiah, Rosado de Christenson, and Walker

Year Book of Emergency Medicine®: Drs Hamilton, Bruno, Handly, Mullin, Quintana, and Ramoska

Year Book of Endocrinology®: Drs Schott, Apovian, Clarke, Eugster, Ludlam, Meikle, Ovalle, Schinner, Schteingart, and Toth

Year Book of Gastroenterology™: Drs Talley, Ambikaipaker, Bollipo, DeVault, Harnois, Pearson, Picco, Rombeau, Scolapio, and Smith

Year Book of Hand and Upper Limb Surgery®: Drs Yao and Steinmann

Year Book of Medicine®: Drs Barker, Garrick, Gersh, Khardori, LeRoith, Seo, Talley, and Thigpen

Year Book of Neonatal and Perinatal Medicine®: Drs Fanaroff, Benitz, Donn, Neu, Papile, Polin, and van Marter

Year Book of Neurology and Neurosurgery®: Drs Klimo and Rabinstein

Year Book of Obstetrics, Gynecology, and Women's Health®: Drs Dungan and Shulman

Year Book of Oncology®: Drs Arceci, Bauer, Gordon, Lawton, and Thigpen

Year Book of Ophthalmology®: Drs Rapuano, Cohen, Flanders, Hammersmith, Milman, Myers, Nelson, Penne, Pyfer, Sergott, Shields, and Vander

Year Book of Orthopedics®: Drs Morrey, Beauchamp, Huddleston, Swiontkowski, and Trigg

Year Book of Otolaryngology-Head and Neck Surgery®: Drs Sindwani, Balough, Franco, Gapany, and Mitchell

Year Book of Pathology and Laboratory Medicine®: Drs Raab, Parwani, Bejarano, and Bissell

Year Book of Pediatrics®: Dr Stockman

Year Book of Plastic and Aesthetic Surgery™: Drs Miller, Gosain, Gurtner, Gutowski, Ruberg, Salisbury, and Smith

Year Book of Psychiatry and Applied Mental Health®: Drs Talbott, Ballenger, Buckley, Frances, Krupnick, and Mack

Year Book of Pulmonary Disease®: Drs Barker, Jones, Maurer, Raza, Tanoue, and Willsie

Year Book of Sports Medicine®: Drs Shephard, Cantu, Feldman, Jankowski, Khan, Lebrun, Nieman, Pierrynowski, and Rowland

Year Book of Surgery®: Drs Copeland, Behrns, Daly, Eberlein, Fahey, Huber, Jones, Mozingo, and Pruett

Year Book of Urology®: Drs Andriole and Coplen

Year Book of Vascular Surgery®: Drs Moneta, Gillespie, Starnes, and Watkins

2011

The Year Book of PSYCHIATRY AND APPLIED MENTAL HEALTH®

Editor in Chief
John A. Talbott, MD
Professor, Department of Psychiatry, University of Maryland School of Medicine, Baltimore, Maryland

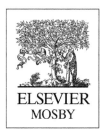

ELSEVIER
MOSBY

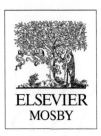

ELSEVIER
MOSBY

Vice President, Continuity: Kimberly Murphy
Developmental Editor: Sarah Barth
Production Supervisor, Electronic Year Books: Donna M. Skelton
Electronic Article Manager: Jennifer C. Pitts
Illustrations and Permissions Coordinator: Dawn Vohsen

2011 EDITION

Composition by TNQ Books and Journals Pvt Ltd, India

Editorial Office:
Elsevier
Suite 1800
1600 John F. Kennedy Blvd.
Philadelphia, PA 19103-2899

International Standard Serial Number: 0084-3970
International Standard Book Number: 978-0-323-08175-7

Printed and bound by CPI Group (UK) Ltd, Croydon, CR0 4YY

Transferred to Digital Print 2011

Editors

James C. Ballenger, MD
Retired Professor and Chairman, Department of Psychiatry and Behavioral Sciences; Director, Institute of Psychiatry, Medical University of South Carolina; Private Practice, Charleston, South Carolina

Peter F. Buckley, MD
Professor and Chairman, and Associate Dean for Leadership Development, Department of Psychiatry, Medical College of Georgia, Augusta, Georgia

Richard J. Frances, MD
Clinical Professor of Psychiatry, New York University Medical School, New York, New York; Director of Professional and Public Education, Silver Hill Hospital, New Canaan, Connecticut

Janice L. Krupnick, PhD
Professor of Psychiatry and Director of the Trauma and Loss Program, Department of Psychiatry, Georgetown University, Washington, District of Columbia; Private Practice, Chevy Chase, Maryland

Avram H. Mack, MD
Associate Professor of Psychiatry and Director of Medical Student Education, Department of Psychiatry, Georgetown University, Washington, District of Columbia

Table of Contents

Journals Represented

Journals represented in this YEAR BOOK are listed below.

Academic Emergency Medicine
Academic Psychiatry
American Journal of Clinical Nutrition
American Journal of Epidemiology
American Journal of Gastroenterology
American Journal of Human Genetics
American Journal of Preventive Medicine
American Journal of Psychiatry
American Journal of Public Health
American Journal on Addictions
Annals of Surgery
Archives of General Psychiatry
Archives of Pediatrics & Adolescent Medicine
Biological Psychiatry
Bipolar Disorders
BMC Biomedical Chromatography Psychiatry
Brain
Brain Research
British Journal of Psychiatry
British Journal of Sports Medicine
Canadian Journal of Psychiatry
Cancer Epidemiology, Biomarkers & Prevention
Circulation
Communications Mental Health Journal
Comprehensive Psychiatry
Critical Care Medicine
Diabetes Care
Endocrinology
European Journal of Pain
Injury
International Journal of Obesity
JAMA Journal of the American Medical Association
Journal of Adolescent Health
Journal of Affective Disorders
Journal of Behavior Therapy and Experimental Psychiatry
Journal of Clinical Endocrinology & Metabolism
Journal of Clinical Oncology
Journal of Clinical Psychiatry
Journal of Clinical Psychopharmacology
Journal of Consulting and Clinical Psychology
Journal of General Internal Medicine
Journal of Laryngology and Otology
Journal of Nervous and Mental Disease
Journal of Neurosurgery
Journal of Oral and Maxillofacial Surgery
Journal of Pain
Journal of Pharmacology and Experimental Therapeutics

Journal of the American Academy of Child & Adolescent Psychiatry
Journal of the American Geriatrics Society
Lancet
Medical Care
MMWR Morbidity and Mortality Weekly Report Surveillance Summaries
Neurology
New England Journal of Medicine
Pain
Pediatrics
Proceedings California Academy of Sciences
Proceedings of the National Academy of Sciences of the United States of America
Psychiatric Services
Psychologie Medicale
Schizophrenia Bulletin
Sleep
Transplantation Proceedings

STANDARD ABBREVIATIONS

The following terms are abbreviated in this edition: acquired immunodeficiency syndrome (AIDS), cardiopulmonary resuscitation (CPR), central nervous system (CNS), cerebrospinal fluid (CSF), computed tomography (CT), deoxyribonucleic acid (DNA), electrocardiography (ECG), health maintenance organization (HMO), human immunodeficiency virus (HIV), intensive care unit (ICU), intramuscular (IM), intravenous (IV), magnetic resonance (MR) imaging (MRI), ribonucleic acid (RNA).

NOTE

The YEAR BOOK OF PSYCHIATRY AND APPLIED MENTAL HEALTH® is a literature survey service providing abstracts of articles published in the professional literature. Every effort is made to assure the accuracy of the information presented in these pages. Neither the editors nor the publisher of the YEAR BOOK OF PSYCHIATRY AND APPLIED MENTAL HEALTH® can be responsible for errors in the original materials. The editors' comments are their own opinions. Mention of specific products within this publication does not constitute endorsement.

To facilitate the use of the YEAR BOOK OF PSYCHIATRY AND APPLIED MENTAL HEALTH® as a reference tool, all illustrations and tables included in this publication are now identified as they appear in the original article. This change is meant to help the reader recognize that any illustration or table appearing in the YEAR BOOK OF PSYCHIATRY AND APPLIED MENTAL HEALTH® may be only one of many in the original article. For this reason, figure and table numbers will often appear to be out of sequence within the YEAR BOOK OF PSYCHIATRY AND APPLIED MENTAL HEALTH®.

1 Child and Adolescent Psychiatry

Introduction

The past years have brought some remarkable advances in child and adolescent psychiatry and mental health, and this year's selections were made to capture this energy.

Advances were clearly made in the neurobiology of conduct disorder and the effects of bullying. In addition, major epidemiologic studies were published that will be helpful to us for years to come. The public was exposed to media reports on the possibility that environmental toxins, such as organophosphates, may be causative of attention-deficit/hyperactivity disorder (ADHD). Data from the Treatment for Adolescents with Depression Study (TADS) have been helpful in discerning the best treatment for depression.

Readers who have followed this text over the past few years will be unsurprised by the inclusion of articles on the very important literature on the excessive rates of diagnosis of bipolar disorder in youth, on the efforts to refine the diagnostic process for those misdiagnosed, and on the impact of overdiagnosis. Another frequent topic has been literature denying that extant data pointed to vaccine or preservatives as the cause of autism or the other pervasive developmental disorders. Instead, there continues to be a march of new literature on developmental and genetic theories as to the basis of those disorders.

And an intellectual breakthrough might be present in our view of the autoimmune theory behind Tourette syndrome and obsessive-compulsive disorder (OCD) (or pediatric autoimmune neuropsychiatric disorders associated with streptococcal infections [PANDAS]). The breakthrough is that infection with streptococcus may not necessarily produce an antibody that causes these symptoms, but that infection causes some stress that leads to the uncovering of symptoms and signs in a vulnerable individual. In the absence of having found an antibody that functions as in Sydenham chorea, this is a more plausible theory.

Finally, it is important to observe the research and clinical interest into the effects of military deployment on children and adolescents. The deleterious effects of deployment were shown in some elegant research studies. Of course, today's wars do differ in terms of the capacity for parents to be in contact with their families, which can have varying effects as well. As a whole, these studies and many other selections demonstrate real advances, and I hope you find them as interesting as I do.

Avram H. Mack, MD

Risk and Etiologic Factors

Sleep and the Transition to Adolescence: A Longitudinal Study

Sadeh A, Dahl RE, Shahar G, et al (Tel Aviv Univ, Israel; Univ of Pittsburgh, PA; Ben-Gurion Univ of the Negev, Beer-Sheva, Israel)
Sleep 32:1602-1609, 2009

Study Objectives.—To assess the links between sleep and pubertal development using a longitudinal design.

Design.—Three consecutive annual assessments of sleep and pubertal development. Sleep was assessed using a week of home actigraphy.

Setting.—Naturalistic sleep in the home setting of school children, Tel Aviv Area, Israel.

Participants.—A sample of 94 (41 boys) typically developing healthy school-age children (age range at first assessment: 9.9–11.2 years).

Intervention.—N/A.

Measurements and Results.—The Petersen's Pubertal Development Scale (PDS) and Sexual Maturation Scale (SMS) were used to assess pubertal development, and a week of actigraphy served to assess naturalistic sleep patterns. The results reflect expected developmental trends: an increase in signs of pubertal maturation, delayed sleep onset, and shorter sleep time. After controlling for age, significant relationships were found between sleep onset time, true sleep time, and number of night wakings at Time 1 and pubertal ratings at Time 2, and pubertal changes from Time 1 to Time 2. Delayed and disrupted sleep at Time 1 predicted faster pubertal changes from Time 1 to Time 2. These results were supported by structural equation modeling. These findings were similar in boys and girls.

Conclusions.—Based on these longitudinal data, it appears that pubertal changes in sleep (delayed sleep phase and disrupted sleep patterns) antedate bodily changes associated with puberty. The underlying mechanisms explaining these predictive links should be further explored.

▶ We all are confronted with adolescents who have sleep disturbances, and the concept of delayed sleep phase conditions has been an important finding that likely has helped many to understand patients or to educate parents. In addition, while neurodevelopment is assumed to be behind changes, few studies that come to the attention of mental health professionals take pains to solve questions about sleep disturbance. This is a longitudinal, rather than cross-sectional, study, and it is exquisitely planned—it reviews sleep according to pubertal stage, even going as far as to determine pubertal stage in its subjects. Fig 3 in the original article demonstrates the alterations according to Tanner stage movement. The questions of how or why adolescent sleep patterns are distorted remain, but the fact that a transition occurs as one enters puberty is a novel finding. While sleep remains poorly understood, the need for sleep is important, and given that adolescents' success depends on the ability to calmly sit in a classroom, future attention can have a real effect on patients and their relationship with their parents, teachers, and peers.

A. H. Mack, MD

The Stigma of Childhood Mental Disorders: A Conceptual Framework
Mukolo A, Heflinger CA, Wallston KA (Vanderbilt Univ Med Ctr, Nashville, TN; Vanderbilt Univ, Nashville, TN)
J Am Acad Child Adolesc Psychiatry 49:92-103, 2010

Objective.—To describe the state of the literature on stigma associated with children's mental disorders and highlight gaps in empirical work.

Method.—We reviewed child mental illness stigma articles in (English only) peer-reviewed journals available through Medline and PsychInfo. We augmented these with adult-oriented stigma articles that focus on theory and measurement. A total of 145 articles in PsychInfo and 77 articles in MEDLINE met search criteria. The review process involved identifying and appraising literature convergence on the definition of critical dimensions of stigma, antecedents, and outcomes reported in empirical studies.

Results.—We found concurrence on three dimensions of stigma (negative stereotypes, devaluation, and discrimination), two contexts of stigma (self, general public), and two targets of stigma (self/individual, family). Theory and empirics on institutional and self-stigma in child populations were sparse. Literature reports few theoretic frameworks and conceptualizations of child mental illness stigma. One model of help seeking (the FINIS) explicitly acknowledges the role of stigma in children's access and use of mental health services.

Conclusions.—Compared with adults, children are subject to unique stigmatizing contexts that have not been adequately studied. The field needs conceptual frameworks that get closer to stigma experiences that are causally linked to how parents/caregivers cope with children's emotional and behavioral problems, such as seeking professional help. To further research in child mental illness, we suggest an approach to adapting current theoretical frameworks and operationalizing stigma, highlighting three dimensions of stigma, three contexts of stigma (including institutions), and three targets of stigma (self/child, family, and services).

▶ Consideration of the stigma directed toward children and adolescents with mental disorders breaks new ground. This report tackles it in a thoughtful and comprehensive manner, particularly in terms of exploring the special facets of this issue. The authors gain credibility by using the work of Erving Goffman as a standard definition, and then they move further as they consider the internal devaluation that may come from external discrimination and devaluation. It is helpful that the authors review whether or not the more-extensive adult stigma literature is applicable to this more vulnerable population. What is not available is any measurement of the stigma or the effects of the stigma on the child and his or her family. But by creating a framework of stigma, they hope to provide the structure for further research. This is clearly an endeavor that would be worthwhile in improving the mental health of children and adolescents and their families.

A. H. Mack, MD

The Long War and Parental Combat Deployment: Effects on Military Children and At-Home Spouses

Lester P, Peterson K, Reeves J, et al (UCLA Semel Inst for Neuroscience and Human Behavior, Los Angeles, CA; Madigan Army Med Ctr, Tacoma, WA; Naval Med Ctr San Diego, CA; et al)
J Am Acad Child Adolesc Psychiatry 49:310-320, 2010

Objective.—Given the growing number of military service members with families and the multiple combat deployments characterizing current war time duties, the impact of deployments on military children requires clarification. Behavioral and emotional adjustment problems were examined in children (aged 6 through 12) of an active duty Army or Marine Corps parent currently deployed (CD) or recently returned (RR) from Afghanistan or Iraq.

Method.—Children (N = 272) and their at-home civilian (AHC) (N = 163) and/or recently returned active duty (AD) parent (N = 65) were interviewed. Child adjustment outcomes were examined in relation to parental psychological distress and months of combat deployment (of the AD) using mixed effects linear models.

Results.—Parental distress (AHC and AD) and cumulative length of parental combat–related deployments during the child's lifetime independently predicted increased child depression and externalizing symptoms. Although behavioral adjustment and depression levels were comparable to community norms, anxiety was significantly elevated in children in both deployment groups. In contrast, AHC parental distress was greater in those with a CD (vs. RR) spouse.

Conclusions.—Findings indicate that parental combat deployment has a cumulative effect on children that remains even after the deployed parent returns home, and that is predicted by psychological distress of both the AD and AHC parent. Such data may be informative for screening, prevention, and intervention strategies.

▶ A colleague related to me recently that while growing up during World War II, he once asked his mother, "What does Daddy look like?" But today's war is different, if for no other reason than the availability of real-time communication. And so this report is valuable not only for its important content but also for its methodology—it is a multisite evaluation of families of those who have been deployed in service in the 2 wars that have been ongoing for years. And it is accurate to emphasize that the report focuses on families because the effects of war, violence, separation, and grief are felt by loved ones on many levels. What affects the parent affects the child and vice versa, and this is one study that addresses these many relationships. This study specifically looked at the impact of cumulative length of deployments to Iraq and Afghanistan but only for those families experiencing combat-related separations. The study confirms long-held assumptions about the health of family members depending on the combat veteran, even linking them to length of deployment. Children who were assessed also manifested a cumulative wear and tear effect, showing depression and externalizing behaviors associated with total months deployed. When we have concerns that these combat experiences will last for many years, we must pay attention to this special article and consider future interventions and studies as a result. And we might ask: how do today's many forms of instant communication make children's experience in this wartime different from others? Or, does knowing what Daddy looks like make any difference?

A. H. Mack, MD

Clinical, Demographic, and Familial Correlates of Bipolar Spectrum Disorders Among Offspring of Parents With Bipolar Disorder
Goldstein BI, Shamseddeen W, Axelson DA, et al (Univ of Toronto Faculty of Medicine, Ontario, Canada; Univ of Pittsburgh School of Medicine, PA)
J Am Acad Child Adolesc Psychiatry 49:388-396, 2010

Objective.—Despite increased risk, most offspring of parents with bipolar disorder (BP) do not manifest BP. The identification of risk factors for BP among offspring could improve preventive and treatment strategies. We examined this topic in the Pittsburgh Bipolar Offspring Study (BIOS).

Method.—Subjects included 388 offspring, ages 7-17 years, of 233 parents with BP-I or BP-II (via the Structured Clinical Interview for DSM-IV). Offspring diagnoses were determined using the Schedule for Affective Disorders and Schizophrenia for School-Aged Children, Present and Lifetime version (KSADS-PL). Analyses focused on the 41 offspring who were diagnosed with BP-I (N = 9), BP-II (N = 5), or BP-NOS (N = 27).

Results.—Offspring with BP had proband parents who were significantly younger at the time of their birth, were more likely to be female, and had lower socio-economic status, versus proband parents of offspring without BP. Parental clinical variables and obstetric variables were not significantly associated with BP among offspring. History of physical and/or sexual abuse, exposure to antidepressants, and exposure to stimulants was significantly greater among offspring with versus without BP. There was significantly greater prevalence of attention-deficit/hyperactivity disorder

(ADHD), anxiety disorders, oppositional defiant disorder/conduct disorder (ODD/CD), and exposure to stimulants and antidepressants among offspring with versus without BP. Variables significantly associated with BP among offspring in regression analyses were as follows: older offspring age, younger parent age at birth, offspring anxiety disorders and ODD/CD, and biological coparent with BP.

Conclusion.—History of anxiety and/or disruptive behavior disorders, as well as presence of bi-lineal parental BP, is associated with elevated risk of bipolar spectrum disorders among offspring. If replicated prospectively, these findings could have implications for the diagnosis and treatment of psychopathology among BP offspring.

▶ One approach to the confusion around bipolar disorder in youth has been the continued linkage to relatives who definitely have bipolar disorder, and this well-planned study does just that, as it assesses relatives of index patients with bipolar disorder. Many others have been focusing on the psychiatric presentation of children and siblings of those with diagnosed bipolar disorder, as in the study by Duffy et al,[1] which focuses not only on phenomenology but also on the course. However, the Bipolar Offspring Study is singular in its size and scope and standardization methods. Of course, its findings are based on data that are yet unreplicated, and they cover a wide number of modifiable and unmodifiable risk factors. To the extent that the provision of a diagnosis of bipolar disorder during adulthood has become the gold standard, it is hoped that these linkages can provide insight into which children should be seen as at risk for bipolar disorder, needing the medication and psychosocial interventions for this serious condition.

A. H. Mack, MD

Reference

1. Duffy A, Alda M, Hajek T, Grof P. Early course of bipolar disorder in high-risk offspring: prospective study. *Br J Psychiatry.* 2009;195:457-458.

Streptococcal Upper Respiratory Tract Infections and Psychosocial Stress Predict Future Tic and Obsessive-Compulsive Symptom Severity in Children and Adolescents with Tourette Syndrome and Obsessive-Compulsive Disorder
Lin H, Williams KA, Katsovich L, et al (Yale Univ School of Medicine, New Haven, CT; et al)
Biol Psychiatry 67:684-691, 2010

Background.—One goal of this prospective longitudinal study was to identify new group A beta-hemolytic streptococcal infections (GABHS) in children and adolescents with Tourette syndrome (TS) and/or obsessive-compulsive disorder (OCD) compared with healthy control subjects. We then examined the power of GABHS infections and measures of psychosocial stress to predict future tic, obsessive-compulsive (OC), and depressive symptom severity.

Methods.—Consecutive ratings of tic, OC, and depressive symptom severity were obtained for 45 cases and 41 matched control subjects over a 2-year period. Clinical raters were blinded to the results of laboratory tests. Laboratory personnel were blinded to case or control status and clinical ratings. Structural equation modeling for unbalanced repeated measures was used to assess the sequence of new GABHS infections and psychosocial stress and their impact on future symptom severity.

Results.—Increases in tic and OC symptom severity did not occur after every new GABHS infection. However, the structural equation model found that these newly diagnosed infections were predictive of modest increases in future tic and OC symptom severity but did not predict future depressive symptom severity. In addition, the inclusion of new infections in the model greatly enhanced, by a factor of three, the power of psychosocial stress in predicting future tic and OC symptom severity.

Conclusions.—Our data suggest that a minority of children with TS and early-onset OCD were sensitive to antecedent GABHS infections. These infections also enhanced the predictive power of current psychosocial stress on future tic and OC symptom severity.

▶ When we think of PANDAS (pediatric autoimmune neuropsychiatric disorders associated with streptococcal infections), we sometimes minimize the import of the word "associated" as it is so very interesting to consider that there is some antibody that causes some psychiatric manifestation. With Sydenham's chorea as the model, there once was great interest in the antiribosomal P antibody as such a pathophysiologic agent in lupus psychosis; however, this mechanism has not been demonstrated with clarity. Perhaps such a direct link may not be the pathophysiology in cases of neuropsychiatric conditions following streptococcal infection. This report provides a new perspective in that it focuses not on the autoantibody but on the possibility that there is an underlying biological trait—a vulnerability—that is present in such individuals. They used running blood cultures with running assessments of tics and obsessive/compulsive symptoms to demonstrate that stress in and of itself is a common factor: perhaps this is a vulnerable group in which infection exacerbates tics or obsessive/compulsive symptoms. Further study is needed to refine this perspective. At the same time, other groups have continued to question whether there is any relationship at all.[1]

A. H. Mack, MD

Reference

1. Schrag A, Gilbert R, Giovannoni G, Robertson MM, Metcalfe C, Ben-Shlomo Y. Streptococcal infection, tourette syndrome, and OCD: is there a connection? *Neurology.* 2009;73:1256-1263.

Early Risk Factors and Developmental Pathways to Chronic High Inhibition and Social Anxiety Disorder in Adolescence

Essex MJ, Klein MH, Slattery MJ, et al (Univ of Wisconsin-Madison)
Am J Psychiatry 167:40-46, 2010

Objective.—Evidence suggests that chronic high levels of behavioral inhibition are a precursor of social anxiety disorder. The authors sought to identify early risk factors for, and developmental pathways to, chronic high inhibition among school-age children and the association of chronic high inhibition with social anxiety disorder by adolescence.

Method.—A community sample of 238 children was followed from birth to grade 9. Mothers, teachers, and children reported on the children's behavioral inhibition from grades 1 to 9. Lifetime history of psychiatric disorders was available for the subset of 60 (25%) children who participated in an intensive laboratory assessment at grade 9. Four early risk factors were assessed: female gender; exposure to maternal stress during infancy and the preschool period; and at age 4.5 years, early manifestation of behavioral inhibition and elevated afternoon salivary cortisol levels.

Results.—All four risk factors predicted greater and more chronic inhibition from grades 1 to 9, and together they defined two developmental pathways. The first pathway, in girls, was partially mediated by early evidence of behavioral inhibition and elevated cortisol levels at age 4.5 years. The second pathway began with exposure to early maternal stress and was also partially mediated by childhood cortisol levels. By grade 9, chronic high inhibition was associated with a lifetime history of social anxiety disorder.

Conclusions.—Chronic high levels of behavioral inhibition are associated with social anxiety disorder by adolescence. The identification of two developmental pathways suggests the potential importance of

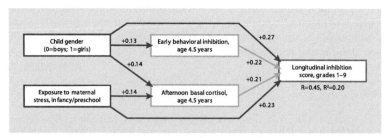

FIGURE 2.—Longitudinal Model of Inhibition in 238 Children Assessed From Grades 1 to 9. Coefficients are bivariate Spearman correlations (see Table 1 in the original article). All correlations are significant at p<0.05. (Reprinted from Essex MJ, Klein MH, Slattery MJ, et al. Early risk factors and developmental pathways to chronic high inhibition and social anxiety disorder in adolescence. *Am J Psychiatry.* 2010;167:40-46, with permission from the American Psychiatric Association, Copyright 2010.)

considering both sets of risk factors in developing preventive interventions for social anxiety disorder.

▶ Perhaps the finest feature of this report is its attention to both the potential psychological as well as physiological antecedents to the development of behavioral inhibition, a precursor to adolescent social anxiety disorder. Using a prospective cohort throughout Wisconsin, the authors were able to track the development of the condition, and they followed 4 variables over time—in terms of antecedents of the behavioral inhibition they discerned 2 developmental tracks (Fig 2). But the 4 variables included parental distress and salivary cortisol among others; these were empirical findings rather than setups toward a psychological or physiological perspective on anxiety. The authors really are demonstrating a novel approach here for the elucidation of the etiology of anxiety in children and adolescents, and ideally, they will continue to follow up. What is uncertain is the significance of behavioral inhibition and whether it is to be seen as a final common pathway or a state ripe for intervention itself? Obviously, more details will emerge over time.

A. H. Mack, MD

Neural Abnormalities in Early-Onset and Adolescence-Onset Conduct Disorder
Passamonti L, Fairchild G, Goodyer IM, et al (Univ of Cambridge, England)
Arch Gen Psychiatry 67:729-738, 2010

Context.—Conduct disorder (CD) is characterized by severe antisocial behavior that emerges in childhood (early-onset CD [EO-CD]) or adolescence (adolescence-onset CD [AO-CD]). Early-onset CD is proposed to have a neurodevelopmental basis, whereas AO-CD is thought to emerge owing to social mimicry of deviant peers. However, this developmental taxonomic theory is debated after reports of neuropsychological impairments in both CD subtypes. A critical, although unaddressed, issue is whether these subtypes present similar or distinct neurophysiological profiles. Hence, we investigated neurophysiological responses to emotional and neutral faces in regions associated with antisocial behavior (ie, the amygdala, ventromedial prefrontal cortex, insula, and orbitofrontal cortex) in individuals with EO-CD and AO-CD and in healthy control subjects.
Objective.—To investigate whether EO-CD and AO-CD subjects show neurophysiological abnormalities.
Design.—Case-control study.
Setting.—Government research institute, university department.
Participants.—Seventy-five male adolescents and young adults aged 16 to 21 years, including 27 with EO-CD, 25 with AO-CD, and 23 healthy controls.

Main Outcome Measure.—Neural activations measured by functional magnetic resonance imaging while participants viewed angry, sad, and neutral faces.

Results.—Comparing angry vs neutral faces, participants with both CD subtypes displayed reduced responses in regions associated with antisocial behavior compared with controls; differences between the CD sub-types were not significant. Comparing each expression with fixation baseline revealed an abnormal (increased) amygdala response to neutral but not angry faces in both groups of CD relative to controls. For sad vs neutral faces, reduced amygdala activation was observed in EO-CD relative to AO-CD and control participants. Comparing each expression with fixation revealed hypoactive amygdala responses to sadness in individuals with EO-CD relative to AO-CD participants and controls. These findings were not accounted for by attention-deficit/hyperactivity disorder symptoms.

Conclusions.—Neurophysiological abnormalities are observed in both CD subtypes, contrary to the developmental taxonomic theory of CD. Additional amygdala hypofunction in relation to sad expressions might indicate why EO-CD is more severe and persistent than AO-CD.

▶ This is a well-designed and well-executed study of the neuropsychological status of 2 different groups of children with conduct disorder: the early onset and the adolescence-onset groups. These groups are identified in the current classification system, but their validity has been questioned, and, similar to bipolar disorder, there is good research ongoing into any neurobiological basis for the distinction. Of course, the current *Diagnostic and Statistical Manual* disclaims that its categories correspond to underlying real entities, but it does promote its value as a descriptive system. In that case, then, could there be value to this distinction after all? To the extent that there are prognostic data that can come from this dichotomy, to me the answer is clear that there is a value. And, in addition, we need to use the leads we get from this study to continue to try to elucidate the development of conduct disorder—at least being mindful of the theory that conduct disorder is a final common pathway of antisocial behavior because of other factors. This is an important area of research for child mental health.

A. H. Mack, MD

Decreased Hippocampal Volume in Healthy Girls at Risk of Depression
Chen MC, Hamilton JP, Gotlib IH (Stanford Univ, CA)
Arch Gen Psychiatry 67:270-276, 2010

Context.—Researchers have documented that the hippocampus is smaller in individuals with depression than in those without. The temporal or causal association of this reduction in hippocampal volume in depression, however, is not known.

Objective.—To test the hypothesis that reduced hippocampal volume precedes and therefore may be implicated in the onset of depression.

Design. –We used magnetic resonance imaging to examine brain structure volume in individuals at high and low familial risk of depression. Anatomic images from magnetic resonance imaging were analyzed using both whole-brain voxel-based morphometry and manual tracing of the bilateral hippocampus.

Setting.—A research university.

Participants.—Fifty-five girls aged between 9 and 15 years: 23 daughters of mothers with recurrent episodes of depression in the daughter's lifetime (high risk) and 32 age-matched daughters of mothers with no history of psychopathology (low risk). None of the girls had any past or current Axis I psychopathology.

Main Outcome Measures.—Group differences in voxel-based morphometry brain matter density estimates and traced hippocampal volume.

Results.—Voxel-based morphometry analyses indicated that individuals at high risk of depression had significantly less gray matter density in clusters in the bilateral hippocampus ($P < .001$) than low-risk participants. Tracing yielded a volumetric reduction in the left hippocampus in the high-risk participants ($P < .05$).

Conclusions.—Compared with individuals at low familial risk of the development of depression, high-risk individuals have reduced hippocampal volume, indicating that neuroanatomic anomalies associated with depression may precede the onset of a depressive episode and influence the development and course of this disorder.

▶ This report is like many others of the time in that it addresses a psychiatric disorder through study of those at high risk of developing the disorder. In this case, the disorder is depression and those at high risk are a group of women. The findings prove the value of this endeavor, because group differences are found. And in particular, there are alterations of central nervous system structure, no less than in the hippocampus among those at high risk, and this finding was greater on the left hippocampus than in the right. This is a small study, but its findings may be stated with significance. The study uses imaging techniques that are able to provide continuous data, which can assist in making large-scale assessments. What we cannot know from this review is whether or not these findings represent illness or if they are precursors for later disease (and perhaps they connote severity of illness too). We shall look forward to further outcomes in this area.

A. H. Mack, MD

Gyrification brain abnormalities associated with adolescence and early-adulthood cannabis use

Mata I, Perez-Iglesias R, Roiz-Santiañez R, et al (Univ of Cantabria, Santander, Spain; et al)
Brain Res 1317:297-304, 2010

Although cannabis is the most widely used illicit drug in the world, the long-term effect of its use in the brain remains controversial. In order to determine whether adolescence and early-adulthood cannabis use is associated with gross volumetric and gyrification abnormalities in the brain, we set up a cross-sectional study using structural magnetic resonance imaging in a sample of general population subjects. Thirty cannabis-using subjects

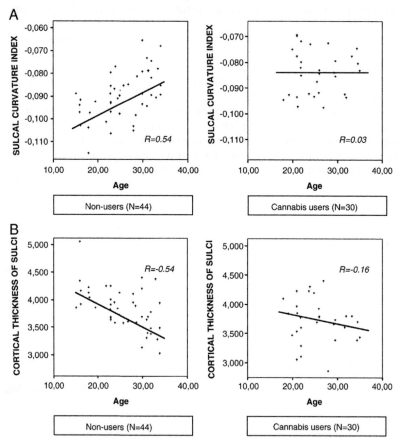

FIGURE 1.—Scatterplots illustrating the pairwise associations between age and, (A) sulcal curvature index among cannabis users and non-users, and (B) cortical thickness of sulci among cannabis users and non-users. (Reprinted from Mata I, Perez-Iglesias R, Roiz-Santiañez R, et al. Gyrification brain abnormalities associated with adolescence and early-adulthood cannabis use. *Brain Res.* 2010;1317:297-304, with permission from Elsevier.)

(mean age, 25.7 years; mean duration of regular use, 8.4 years, range: 3–21) with no history of polydrug use or neurologic/mental disorder and 44 non-using control subjects (mean age, 25.8 years) were included. Cannabis users showed bilaterally decreased concavity of the sulci and thinner sulci in the right frontal lobe. Among non-users, age was significantly correlated with decreased gyrification (i.e., less concave sulci and more convexe gyri) and decreased cortical thickness, supporting the notion of age-related gyrification changes. However, among cannabis users gyrification indices did not show significant dependency on age, age of regular cannabis use initiation, or cumulative exposure to cannabis. These results suggest that cannabis use in adolescence and early-adulthood might involve a premature alteration in cortical gyrification similar to what is normally observed at a later age, probably through disruption of normal neurodevelopment.

▶ The world's most widely used illicit substance needs to be better understood. By my experience, few clinicians or policymakers would claim that regular cannabis use is beneficial to mental health (not to mention other health measures), but few analyses have been performed on the neurobiological effects of the substance. In distinction with assessments of cognitive function[1] or gray/white matter volumetric analyses, even newer methods of imaging allow for many new assessments like this one regarding cortical gyrification and surface area. As seen in Fig 1, discernible differences were found between the group of users and nonusers. The authors cite as a limitation the lack of information, which would address the mechanism of this finding but that is of course a massive undertaking. In the meantime, while no differences were found based on sex, a further investigation might use males or females solely to maximize the power of the study, recognizing anatomic differences between the sexes.

A. H. Mack, MD

Reference

1. Jager G, Block R, Luitjen M, Ramsey NF. Cannabis use and memory brain function in adolescent boys: a cross-sectional multicenter functional magnetic resonance imaging study. *J Am Acad Child Adolesc Psychiatry.* 2010;49:561-572.

The Association of Suicide and Bullying in Childhood to Young Adulthood: A Review of Cross–Sectional and Longitudinal Research Findings
Klomek AB, Sourander A, Gould M (Columbia Univ, NY)
Can J Psychiatry 55:282-288, 2010

Objective.—To review the research addressing the association of suicide and bullying, from childhood to young adulthood, including cross-sectional and longitudinal research findings.

Method.—Relevant publications were identified via electronic searches of PsycNet and MEDLINE without date specification, in addition to perusing the reference lists of relevant articles.

Results.—Cross-sectional findings indicate that there is an increased risk of suicidal ideation and (or) suicide attempts associated with bullying behaviour and cyberbullying. The few longitudinal findings available indicate that bullying and peer victimization lead to suicidality but that this association varies by sex. Discrepancies between the studies available may be due to differences in the studies' participants and methods.

Conclusions.—Bullying and peer victimization constitute more than correlates of suicidality. Future research with long-term follow-up should continue to identify specific causal paths between bullying and suicide.

▶ This study is another among many by Dr Gould and coauthors on the characteristics of bullying. It is a systematic review that extends the findings on suicidality to young adulthood. Furthermore, this review uses longitudinal findings and demonstrates distinctions between sexes, particularly in terms of the psychopathological background of females who bully. We must not forget that bullying occurs in cyberspace as well.[1] It has become so pervasive that another study was able to document the morbidity associated with it in 3 different national studies of longitudinal health of youth.[2] Inherent in all of these studies and reports is the need for intervention in cases of bullying or peer victimization. While schools around the nation have begun to implement policies against the behavior, mental health clinicians who are involved with schools should ensure that systems of surveillance and reaction are in place.

A. H. Mack, MD

References

 1. Sourander A, Brunstein Klomek A, Ikonen M, et al. Psychosocial risk factors associated with cyberbullying among adolescents: a population-based study. *Arch Gen Psychiatry.* 2010;67:720-728.
 2. Kaminski JW, Fang X. Victimization by peers and adolescent suicide in three US samples. *J Pediatr.* 2009;155:683-688.

Basal Ganglia Shapes Predict Social, Communication, and Motor Dysfunctions in Boys With Autism Spectrum Disorder
Qiu A, Adler M, Crocetti D, et al (Division of Bioengineering and Clinical Imaging Res Ctr of Natl Univ of Singapore; Kennedy Krieger Inst, Baltimore, MD; et al)
J Am Acad Child Adolesc Psychiatry 49:539-551, 2010

Objective.—Basal ganglia abnormalities have been suggested as contributing to motor, social, and communicative impairments in autism spectrum disorder (ASD). Volumetric analyses offer limited ability to detect localized differences in basal ganglia structure. Our objective was to investigate basal ganglia shape abnormalities and their association with behavioral features of ASD, which may involve multiple frontal–subcortical circuits.

Method.—Basal ganglia were manually delineated from MR images of 32 boys with ASD and 45 typically developing (TD) boys. Large deformation diffeomorphic metric mapping (LDDMM) was used to assess between-group differences in basal ganglia shape and to examine associations with motor, praxis, and reciprocal social and communicative impairments in ASD.

Results.—Boys with ASD showed changes in right basal ganglia shape as compared with TD boys; surface deformation was present in the caudate, putamen, and globus pallidus but did not stand up to correction for multiple comparisons. Brain–behavior correlation findings were more robust; analyses accounting for multiple comparisons revealed, in boys with ASD, surface inward deformation of the right posterior putamen predicted poorer motor skill, whereas surface inward deformation of the bilateral anterior and posterior putamen predicted poorer praxis. Surface outward deformation in the bilateral medial caudate head predicted greater reciprocal social and communicative impairment.

Conclusions.—Motor, social, and communicative impairments in boys with ASD are associated with shape abnormalities in the basal ganglia. The findings suggest abnormalities within parallel frontal–subcortical circuits are differentially associated with impaired acquisition of motor and reciprocal social and communicative skills in ASD.

▶ This study provides the literature with something new: a new method for volumetric analysis. In this case, it has been applied to autism in a group of 32 boys with autism spectrum disorder. But the results are fascinating: that the large deformation diffeomorphic metric mapping is able to go beyond volume to assess shape. And it is all the more breathtaking as we realize that the different shapes may be correlated with specific human functions. It is important that the study used a comparison group, and the basal ganglia shapes of the patients were related to their psychomotor functions as well. While purely genetic approaches to autism have so far not yielded significant leads, the study of the brain in vivo is a promising approach; that this study highlights a new approach to those studies makes it exceptional, and its findings of differences will hopefully bring us closer to understanding the pathology, if not the etiology of this condition.

A. H. Mack, MD

The Moderating Role of Close Friends in the Relationship Between Conduct Problems and Adolescent Substance Use

Glaser B, Shelton KH, van den Bree MBM (Univ of Bristol, UK; Cardiff Univ, UK)

J Adolesc Health 47:35-42, 2010

Purpose.—Conduct problems and peer effects are among the strongest risk factors for adolescent substance use and problem use. However, it is unclear to what extent the effects of conduct problems and peer behavior interact, and whether adolescents' capacity to refuse the offer of substances may moderate such links. This study was conducted to examine relationships between conduct problems, close friends' substance use, and refusal assertiveness with adolescents' alcohol use problems, tobacco, and marijuana use.

Methods.—We studied a population-based sample of 1,237 individuals from the Cardiff Study of All Wales and North West of England Twins aged 11–18 years. Adolescent and mother-reported information was obtained. Statistical analyses included cross-sectional and prospective logistic regression models and family-based permutations.

Results.—Conduct problems and close friends' substance use were associated with increased adolescents' substance use, whereas refusal assertiveness was associated with lower use of cigarettes, alcohol, and marijuana. Peer substance use moderated the relationship between conduct problems and alcohol use problems, such that conduct problems were only related to increased risk for alcohol use problems in the presence of substance-using friends. This effect was found in both cross-sectional and prospective analyses and confirmed using the permutation approach.

Conclusions.—Reduced opportunities for interaction with alcohol-using peers may lower the risk of alcohol use problems in adolescents with conduct problems.

▶ We continue to attempt to tease out the components of risk of substance use among adolescents, and conduct disorder remains central to these efforts. This is a large study that reviewed various aspects of the relationships among users and index cases. It was also important that both youth and parent reports were obtained. What is not present in this report is attention to the presence of attention-deficit/hyperactivity disorder (ADHD); it is undoubtedly present in many of the youths studied in this report. Obviously, it is a complicating piece of the puzzle but an important one, as conduct disorderedness moderates the substance use in those with ADHD. The study ultimately confirms what has been assumed—that peers drive risk of substance use in this age group; treatment interventions that encourage new peer groups are an important portion of attention to substance abusing youth. What is new is the interest in what types of peer relationships and what forms they occur in; this new frontier, as explored here, can ultimately inform clinicians.

A. H. Mack, MD

Static and Dynamic Cognitive Deficits in Childhood Preceding Adult Schizophrenia: A 30-Year Study
Reichenberg A, Caspi A, Harrington H, et al (Duke Univ, Durham, NC; King's College London, UK; Univ of Otago, Dunedin, New Zealand)
Am J Psychiatry 167:160-169, 2010

Objective.—Premorbid cognitive deficits in schizophrenia are well documented and have been interpreted as supporting a neurodevelopmental etiological model. The authors investigated the following three unresolved questions about premorbid cognitive deficits: What is their developmental course? Do all premorbid cognitive deficits follow the same course? Are premorbid cognitive deficits specific to schizophrenia or shared by other psychiatric disorders?

Methods.—Participants were members of a representative cohort of 1,037 males and females born between 1972 and 1973 in Dunedin, New Zealand. Cohort members underwent follow-up evaluations at specific intervals from age 3 to 32 years, with a 96% retention rate. Cognitive development was analyzed and compared in children who later developed schizophrenia or recurrent depression as well as in healthy comparison subjects.

Results.—Children who developed adult schizophrenia exhibited developmental deficits (i.e., static cognitive impairments that emerge early and remain stable) on tests indexing verbal and visual knowledge acquisition, reasoning, and conceptualization. In addition, these children exhibited developmental lags (i.e., growth that is slower relative to healthy comparison subjects) on tests indexing processing speed, attention, visual-spatial problem solving ability, and working memory. These two premorbid cognitive patterns were not observed in children who later developed recurrent depression.

Conclusions.—These findings suggest that the origins of schizophrenia include two interrelated developmental processes evident from childhood to early adolescence (ages 7–13 years). Children who will grow up to develop adult schizophrenia enter primary school struggling with verbal reasoning and lag further behind their peers in working memory, attention, and processing speed as they get older.

▶ In the study of the premorbid presentation of those with schizophrenia, researchers have turned to analyzing cognition, particularly the trajectory of cognitive change. Various streams of information have dismantled the assumption that cognitive decline is universal in schizophrenia (but even Kraepelin accepted that schizophrenia might be a static encephalopathy in some cases).[1] This study makes use of a cohort of persons born in a specific time frame who have been followed over time up to age 32 years for whom IQ assessments at 4 time points (between ages 7 and 13 years) were available. Additional factors that improved the value of the study included comparison with cohort members who were eventually found to be either depressed or without diagnosis. And the IQ scores were broken down into the portions of intelligence.

The authors tried to fit the findings into assumptions about trajectory and found that those who developed schizophrenia later had different trajectories for different cognitive functions, with some having lags in development and others displaying deficits altogether. The important point is that these findings support that premorbid cognitive deficits in schizophrenia do represent early and enduring vulnerabilities to the disease. Yet, the extent to which these data provide implications for the early identification of children who might develop schizophrenia is unclear. Our ability to perform research in this area might indeed be enhanced by studies that use a standard definition of findings; but that concept is likely not yet ready for a diagnostic category and all its potential epidemiologic and clinical implications.

A. H. Mack, MD

Reference

1. Mack AH, Feldman JJ, Tsuang MT. A case of "pfropfschizophrenia": Kraepelin's bridge between neurodegenerative and neurodevelopmental conceptions of schizophrenia. *Am J Psychiatry.* 2002;159:1104-1110.

Policy Statement—Alcohol Use by Youth and Adolescents: A Pediatric Concern
Committee on Substance Abuse
Pediatrics 125:1078-1087, 2010

Alcohol use continues to be a major problem from preadolescence through young adulthood in the United States. Results of recent neuroscience research have substantiated the deleterious effects of alcohol on adolescent brain development and added even more evidence to support the call to prevent and reduce underaged drinking. Pediatricians should be knowledgeable about substance abuse to be able to recognize risk factors for alcohol and other substance abuse among youth, screen for use, provide appropriate brief interventions, and refer to treatment. The integration of alcohol use prevention programs in the community and our educational system from elementary school through college should be promoted by pediatricians and the health care community. Promotion of media responsibility to connect alcohol consumption with realistic consequences should be supported by pediatricians. Additional research into the prevention, screening and identification, brief intervention, and management and treatment of alcohol and other substance use by adolescents continues to be needed to improve evidence-based practices.

▶ Here is an excellent review of the entire picture of alcohol use by youth in the United States at this time. It is important not only because it communicates the magnitude and importance of this problem to pediatricians but also because it provides a succinct update of a topic that unfortunately is undercovered as a topic of focus by physicians. The medical consequences of alcohol misuse differ from those of adult alcohol abusers/dependents, and this unique perspective is welcome—consequences at the bodily, neural, and behavioral levels are discussed. One specific point to be made is that the policy statement reminds pediatricians that parents should not provide alcohol to their children or host parties with alcohol among their friends.

A. H. Mack, MD

Prenatal Organochlorine Exposure and Behaviors Associated With Attention Deficit Hyperactivity Disorder in School-Aged Children
Sagiv SK, Thurston SW, Bellinger DC, et al (Harvard School of Public Health, Boston, MA; Univ of Rochester, NY; et al)
Am J Epidemiol 171:593-601, 2010

Organochlorines are environmentally persistent contaminants that readily cross the placenta, posing a potential risk to the developing fetus. Evidence for neurodevelopmental effects at low levels of these compounds is growing, though few studies have focused on behavioral outcomes. The authors investigated the association between prenatal polychlorinated biphenyl (PCB) and p,p'-dichlorodiphenyl dichloroethylene (p,p'-DDE) levels and behaviors associated with attention deficit hyperactivity disorder (ADHD), measured with the Conners' Rating Scale for Teachers (CRS-T), in a cohort of 607 children aged 7–11 years (median age, 8.2 years) born in 1993–1998 to mothers residing near a PCB-contaminated harbor in New Bedford, Massachusetts. The median umbilical cord serum level of the sum of 4 prevalent PCB congeners (118, 138, 153, and 180) was 0.19 ng/g serum (range, 0.01–4.41 ng/g serum). The authors found higher risk for ADHD-like behaviors assessed with the CRS-T at higher levels of PCBs and p,p'-DDE. For example, the authors found higher risk of atypical behavior on the Conners' ADHD Index for the highest quartile of the sum of 4 PCB congeners versus the lowest quartile (risk ratio = 1.76, 95% confidence interval: 1.06, 2.92) and a similar relation for p,p'-DDE. These results support an association between low-level prenatal organochlorine exposure and ADHD-like behaviors in childhood.

▶ Here is a report of the association between attention-deficit/hyperactivity disorder (ADHD) and a number of toxic compounds—organochlorines (which include polychlorinated biphenyls). The authors studied the disaster that is the pollution in a southeastern Massachusetts fishing hub and provided empirical evidence of an association. Sagiv et al investigated a discrete set of children and had special access to their cord blood. They were able to determine exposure of different children to these chemicals and compare that with results of a standard assessment of ADHD behaviors. As noted in Fig 1, greater exposure is associated with greater risk of ADHD behaviors using criteria from a Conners' scale and those of *Diagnostic and Statistical Manual of Mental Disorders*, Fourth Edition.

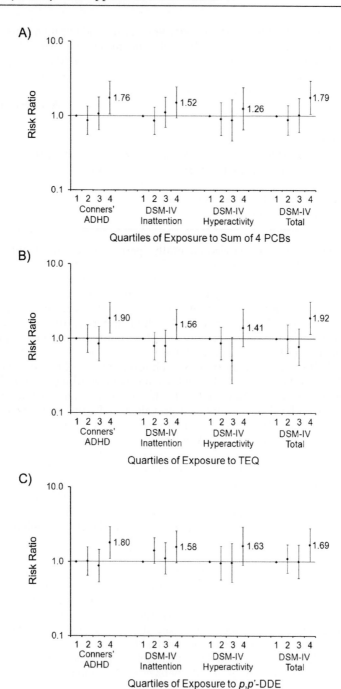

The authors are careful in stating that the chemical exposure is associated not with ADHD itself but with behaviors associated with ADHD. This statement is important not only because they have not established causality but also because they have not established that the subjects actually have ADHD. But, on the other hand, a valuable facet of this report is that it helps to focus concern on the effects of organochlorines, from neurobehavioral effects to behaviors associated with ADHD and that moves the literature 1 step toward greater detail and clarity.

At the same time there is new urgency to associate ADHD with other prenatal metabolic problems: low folate[1] or caffeine in soft drinks.[2] In both of these areas there should continue to be refinement of studies that use instruments with clarity and specificity.

A. H. Mack, MD

References

1. Schlotz W, Jones A, Phillips DI, Gale CR, Robinson SM, Godfrey KM. Lower maternal folate status in early pregnancy is associated with childhood hyperactivity and peer problems in offspring. *J Child Psychol Psychiatry.* 2010;51: 594-602.
2. Bekkhus M, Skjøthaug T, Nordhagen R, Borge AI. Intrauterine exposure to caffeine and inattention/overactivity in children. *Acta Paediatr.* 2010;99:925-928.

Outcomes of occasional cannabis use in adolescence: 10-year follow-up study in Victoria, Australia
Degenhardt L, Coffey C, Carlin JB, et al (Univ of New South Wales, Sydney, Australia; Murdoch Children's Res Inst, Melbourne, Victoria, Australia; et al)
Br J Psychiatry 196:290-295, 2010

Background.—Regular adolescent cannabis use predicts a range of later drug use and psychosocial problems. Little is known about whether occasional cannabis use carries similar risks.

FIGURE 1.—Adjusted risk ratios for behaviors associated with attention-deficit/hyperactivity disorder (ADHD) among school-aged children ($n = 573$) born in New Bedford, Massachusetts, in 1993–1998, according to umbilical cord serum levels of A) the sum of 4 polychlorinated biphenyl (PCB) congeners (118, 138, 153, 180), B) the sum of monoortho toxic equivalency factor-weighted PCB congeners (TEQ), and C) p,p'-dichlorodiphenyl dichloroethylene (p,p'-DDE). Behaviors associated with ADHD were assessed using 4 subscales of the Conners' Rating Scale for Teachers: Conners' ADHD Index, *Diagnostic and Statistical Manual of Mental Disorders*, Fourth Edition (DSM-IV) Inattention, DSM-IV Impulsive-Hyperactive, and DSM-IV Total. Values were dichotomized at the 86th percentile. Results for Conners' ADHD Index were adjusted for child's age and sex and for maternal age, marital status, smoking during pregnancy, alcohol consumption during pregnancy, local fish consumption during pregnancy, and illicit drug use. All DSM-IV outcomes were adjusted for child's age and sex and for maternal age, marital status, smoking during pregnancy, and Home Observation for Measurement of the Environment score. A statistically significant P value for trend ($P < 0.05$) was detected for A) the sum of 4 PCBs and all outcomes, except for DSM-IV Hyperactivity; B) TEQ and all outcomes; and C) p,p'-DDE and Conners' ADHD Index and DSM-IV Total. Bars, 95% confidence interval. (Reprinted from Sagiv SK, Thurston SW, Bellinger DC, et al. Prenatal organochlorine exposure and behaviors associated with attention deficit hyperactivity disorder in school-aged children. *Am J Epidemiol.* 2010;171:593-601. Copyright 2010. Published by Oxford University Press on behalf of the Johns Hopkins Bloomberg School of Public Health. All rights reserved.)

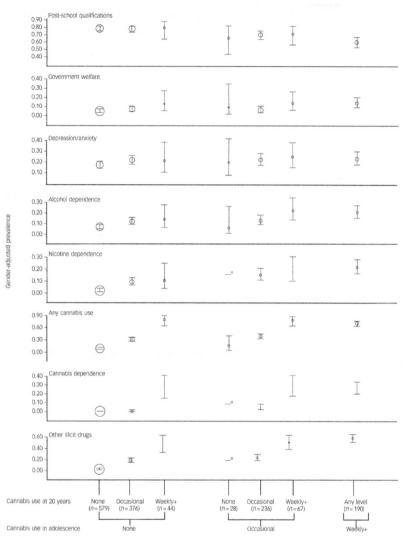

FIGURE 2.—Gender-adjusted prevalence of each outcome at age 24 years according to level of cannabis use during adolescence, and then by level of cannabis use at age 20 years. The diameter of the circle reflects the precision of the estimate (essentially the size of the subgroup); the vertical lines represent the 95% confidence interval around the estimate. a. Cell frequencies were too small to allow for sensible estimation of proportion and standard errors. (Reprinted from Degenhardt L, Coffey C, Carlin JB, et al. Outcomes of occasional cannabis use in adolescence: 10-year follow-up study in Victoria, Australia. *Br J Psychiatry*. 2010;196:290-295, with permission from the Royal College of Psychiatry.)

Aims.—To examine associations between occasional cannabis use during adolescence and psychosocial and drug use outcomes in young adulthood; and modification of these associations according to the trajectory of cannabis use between adolescence and age 20 years, and other potential risk factors.

Method.—A 10-year eight-wave cohort study of a representative sample of 1943 secondary school students followed from 14.9 years to 24 years.

Results.—Occasional adolescent cannabis users who continued occasional use into early adulthood had higher risks of later alcohol and tobacco dependence and illicit drug use, as well as being less likely to complete a post-secondary qualification than non-users. Those using cannabis at least weekly either during adolescence or at age 20 were at highest risk of drug use problems in young adulthood. Adjustment for smoking in adolescence reduced the association with later educational achievement, but associations with drug use problems remained.

Conclusions.—Occasional adolescent cannabis use predicts later drug use and educational problems. Partial mediation by tobacco use raises a possibility that differential peer affiliation may play a role.

▶ Rare is the adolescent who does not at lease consider experimental or recreational use of substances. Great energy and resources have been put into the study of the risks and effects of heavy use (with or without a substance dependence diagnosis), but here is a focus on occasional use of cannabis. In addition, it is a significant study, as it is longitudinal and large, and it is of a representative sample of students. The authors remark that a limitation is that the data are based on self-report, but the information is nonetheless of great value as a means to describe trajectories of a wide range of negative psychological and social outcomes. As seen in Fig 2, the group is broken down by degree of usage of cannabis and then by several measures of outcomes—educational status, reliance on government assistance, and depressed mood. It demonstrates the relationship with use of other substances and nicotine as well. One can see that the relationships are not simply linear according to use. This is a very interesting study whose results should be readily applied to clinical practice as well as prevention.

A. H. Mack, MD

Attention-Deficit/Hyperactivity Disorder and Urinary Metabolites of Organophosphate Pesticides
Bouchard MF, Bellinger DC, Wright RO, et al (Harvard Univ, Boston, MA)
Pediatrics 125:e1270-e1277, 2010

Objective.—The goal was to examine the association between urinary concentrations of dialkyl phosphate metabolites of organophosphates and attention-deficit/hyperactivity disorder (ADHD) in children 8 to 15 years of age.

Methods.—Cross-sectional data from the National Health and Nutrition Examination Survey (2000–2004) were available for 1139 children, who were representative of the general US population. A structured interview with a parent was used to ascertain ADHD diagnostic status, on the basis of slightly modified criteria from the *Diagnostic and Statistical Manual of Mental Disorders, Fourth Edition.*

Results.—One hundred nineteen children met the diagnostic criteria for ADHD. Children with higher urinary dialkyl phosphate concentrations, especially dimethyl alkylphosphate (DMAP) concentrations, were more likely to be diagnosed as having ADHD. A 10-fold increase in DMAP concentration was associated with an odds ratio of 1.55 (95% confidence interval: 1.14–2.10), with adjustment for gender, age, race/ethnicity, poverty/income ratio, fasting duration, and urinary creatinine concentration. For the most-commonly detected DMAP metabolite, dimethyl thiophosphate, children with levels higher than the median of detectable concentrations had twice the odds of ADHD (adjusted odds ratio: 1.93 [95% confidence interval: 1.23–3.02]), compared with children with undetectable levels.

Conclusions.—These findings support the hypothesis that organophosphate exposure, at levels common among US children, may contribute to ADHD prevalence. Prospective studies are needed to establish whether this association is causal.

▶ As its authors state, this report provides support for a hypothesis about a potential causative relationship between organophosphates, which are widely ingested because of their use in pesticides, and attention-deficit/hyperactivity disorder (ADHD). In this case, at issue is the intake of an individual during his or her life. Ostensibly, this is a modifiable risk factor, yet it is an exposure we all face in the food we all eat—the relatively smaller hepatic size in some periods of childhood makes their exposure even more significant. This report is notable for its prescient mixing of The National Health and Nutrition Examination Survey data with biological sampling and psychiatric diagnosis (using The Diagnostic Interview Schedule for Children IV) when warranted. It uses a large N and is a help to our field not only in helping to refocus attention on environmental toxins but also in contributing to the elucidation of ADHD. Like other studies referenced in this year's selections, there are many new ideas being analyzed regarding ADHD or altered behavior following exposures to substances, and this is an important contribution.

A. H. Mack, MD

Unraveling the Nature of Hyperactivity in Children With Attention-Deficit/Hyperactivity Disorder
Ohashi K, Vitaliano G, Polcari A, et al (McLean Hosp, Belmont, MA)
Arch Gen Psychiatry 67:388-396, 2010

Context.—Seated hyperactivity is a defining feature of the combined and predominantly hyperactive-impulsive subtypes of attention-deficit/hyeractivity disorder (ADHD), but its underlying nature is unknown.

Objective.—To determine whether hyperactivity is a consequence of an impaired ability to inhibit activity to low levels or to maintain positional stability.

Design.—Case-control study.

Setting.—Academic research center and school.

Participants.—Sixty-two boys 9 to 12 years of age (of 73 screened), recruited from the community by advertisement, who met *DSM-IV* criteria for ADHD combined subtype on structured interview. Sixty-two controls were selected by matching for age and sex from a community sample of 1168 subjects in 3 participating school districts. Pupils with Conners' Teacher Rating Scores Revised within ±1 SD of the mean for age were eligible for randomized matching.

Intervention.—Infrared motion analysis of headmarker movements (50 Hz) during performance of a 15-minute cognitive control task. Subjects with ADHD were tested at least 18 hours following their last dose of methylphenidate and again 120 minutes after a 0.4-mg/kg probe dose.

Main Outcome Measures.—Inhibitory control (spike and basal amplitude) and head-marker stability (approximate entropy, Lyapunov, and spectral exponents).

Results.—Inhibitory control measures were 2-fold higher in subjects with ADHD ($d' = 0.63$-0.95). Group differences in head-marker stability were even greater ($d' = 2.204.71$; receiver operating characteristic area $= 0.956$-1.0). Methylphenidate restored inhibitory ability to control levels but only partially corrected stability deficits, which still distinguished subjects with ADHD from controls (receiver operating characteristic area $= 0.722$-0.995).

Conclusions.—Children with ADHD have a deficient ability to inhibit activity to low levels and unstable control of head-marker position characterized by deterministic chaos (sensitivity to initial conditions). These deficits differed in degree of correctability by methylphenidate, suggesting that they may be mediated by different neural circuits (eg, corticostriatal vs cerebrovestibular).

▶ Here is a much-needed report from a group of researchers who typically tend to address problems creatively or "out of the box." Consumers of the literature on attention-deficit/hyperactivity disorder (ADHD) are invariably exposed to theories about the relationship between the prefrontal cortex and ADHD. But here is a perspective that considers ADHD, and hyperactivity especially, from the standpoint of movement. As a result, the cerebellum is one area of the central nervous system too often ignored in this arena. The group analyzed "seated hyperactivity" and even used infrared visualization to determine exactly how much movement actually occurred. Furthermore, the use of methylphenidate led to improvement in some and not others. As in schizophrenia, we may consider that perhaps there are many ADHDs: some that are based on different circuits versus others, some due to toxins, some not. ADHD research continues;

further new ideas such as this will be important leads in furthering our state of the literature.

A. H. Mack, MD

Prediction of Psychosis in Adolescents and Young Adults at High Risk: Results From the Prospective European Prediction of Psychosis Study

Ruhrmann S, Schultze-Lutter F, Salokangas RKR, et al (Univ of Cologne, German; Univ of Turku, Finland; et al)
Arch Gen Psychiatry 67:241-251, 2010

Context.—Indicated prevention is currently regarded as the most promising strategy to attenuate, delay, or even avert psychosis. Existing criteria need improvement in terms of specificity and individual risk assessment to allow for better targeted and earlier interventions.

Objective.—To develop a differential predictive clinical model of transition to first-episode psychosis.

Design.—Prospective multicenter, naturalistic field study with a total follow-up time of 18 months.

Setting.—Six early-detection outpatient centers in Germany, Finland, the Netherlands, and England.

Participants.—Two hundred forty-five help-seeking patients in a putatively prodromal state of psychosis according to either ultra-high-risk (UHR) criteria or the basic symptom–based criterion cognitive disturbances (COGDIS).

Main Outcome Measure.—Incidence of transition to psychosis.

Results.—At 18-month follow-up, the incidence rate for transition to psychosis was 19%. Combining UHR and COGDIS yielded the best sensitivity. A prediction model was developed and included positive symptoms, bizarre thinking, sleep disturbances, a schizotypal disorder, level of functioning in the past year, and years of education. With a positive likelihood ratio of 19.9, an area under the curve of 80.8%, and a positive predictive value of 83.3%, diagnostic accuracy was excellent. A 4-level prognostic index further classifying the general risk of the whole sample predicted instantaneous incidence rates of up to 85% and allowed for an estimation of time to transition.

Conclusions.—The prediction model identified an increased risk of psychosis with appropriate prognostic accuracy in our sample. A 2-step risk assessment is proposed, with UHR and cognitive disturbance criteria serving as first-step criteria for general risk and the prognostic index as a second-step tool for further risk classification of each patient. This strategy will allow clinicians to target preventive measures and will support efforts to unveil the biological and environmental mechanisms underlying progression to psychosis.

▶ No one would disagree with the authors' main premise, as noted in the first words of the report, that prevention "is most important in psychiatry today."

And this has been perhaps most appropriate in the identification of schizophrenia or other severe psychotic disorders; especially given the severe, often-unremediable, social effects of the illness, not to mention the ostensible neuropathology that results from active psychosis or the serious psychological and cognitive effects of the condition. This study provides a meager, but valuable, step toward a system of the prediction of the development of schizophrenia. It is a prospective study of persons at risk of schizophrenia and assesses the value of an instrument in demonstrating the rate of development of schizophrenia based on previously made assessments of risk. However, it should be recalled that the subjects were not only those at risk but also those at ultra-high-risk (or UHR, as the authors call it.)

Having a usable tool for the assessment of risk is highly desirable. At the same time, there is concern that the information contained in this report and others is to be used in justifying a psychosis risk syndrome in the next diagnostic classification system. That there is a prodrome or that there are some who are at risk of schizophrenia is not in question; but whether a new category that defines "risk" rather than "diagnosis" should be a sobering thought for those who have watched today's classificatory system built methodically and carefully. This study's use of those in ultra high risk suggests that application to a general population is not currently in the cards—at least for now.

A. H. Mack, MD

Assessment and Diagnosis

Prevalence and Treatment of Mental Disorders Among US Children in the 2001–2004 NHANES

Merikangas KR, He J-P, Brody D, et al (Natl Inst of Mental Health, Bethesda, MD; Natl Ctr for Health Statistics, Hyattsville, MD; et al)
Pediatrics 125:75-81, 2010

Objective.—This article presents the 12-month prevalence estimates of specific mental disorders, their social and demographic correlates, and service use patterns in children and adolescents from the National Health and Nutrition Examination Survey, a nationally representative probability sample of noninstitutionalized US civilians.

Methods.—The sample includes 3042 participants 8 to 15 years of age from cross-sectional surveys conducted from 2001 to 2004. Data on *Diagnostic and Statistical Manual of Mental Disorders, Fourth Edition* criteria for mental disorders were derived from administration of selected modules of the National Institute of Mental Health Diagnostic Interview Schedule for Children, version IV, a structured diagnostic interview administered by lay interviewers to assess psychiatric diagnoses of children and adolescents.

Results.—Twelve-month prevalence rates of Diagnostic and Statistical Manual of Mental Disorders, Fourth Edition–defined disorders in this sample were 8.6% for attention-deficit/hyperactivity disorder, 3.7% for mood disorders, 2.1% for conduct disorder, 0.7% for panic disorder or generalized anxiety disorder, and 0.1% for eating disorders. Boys had 2.1 times greater prevalence of attention-deficit/hyperactivity disorder than girls, girls had twofold higher rates of mood disorders than boys, and there were no gender differences in the rates of anxiety disorders or conduct disorder. Only approximately one half of those with one of the disorders assessed had sought treatment with a mental health professional.

Conclusion.—These data constitute a first step in building a national database on mental health in children and adolescents.

▶ Here is a 12-month prevalence study over a 3-year time period as studied by the NIMH. It strives to assess a representative sample of the United States and includes 3085 US youths aged 8 to 15 years. Diagnoses were made using the Diagnostic Interview Schedule for Children (DISC). It is also important that this is a US sample, not regional sample. Of course, any study that utilizes a common validated instrument provides a great advance; however, one reasonably may question whether findings from the DISC are generalizable to everyday practice. That concern notwithstanding, this is an epidemiological report rather than one on clinical cases and its value is high. Another point is why the National Health and Nutrition Examination Survey chose to oversample low socioeconomic individuals, but their weighting system seems to have overcome any problems because of that. Findings included attention-deficit/hyperactivity disorder, conduct disorder, and mood disorders at 8.7%, 2.1%, and 3.7%, respectively. These findings are seen in the light of a similar study performed in the past year in Israel[1]; of 957 Israelis whose diagnoses were confirmed by a psychiatrist following the gathering of other information (of note, in that sample the rate of posttraumatic stress disorder was only 0.8).

A. H. Mack, MD

Reference

1. Farbstein I, Mansbach-Kleinfeld I, Levison D, et al. Prevalence and correlates of mental disorders in Israeli adolescents: results from a national mental health survey. *J Child Psychol Psychiatry.* 2010;51:630-639.

National Comorbidity Survey Replication Adolescent Supplement (NCS-A): III. Concordance of *DSM-IV*/CIDI Diagnoses With Clinical Reassessments
Kessler RC, Avenevoli S, Green J, et al (Harvard Med School, Boston, MA; Natl Inst of Mental Health, Bethesda, MD; et al)
J Am Acad Child Adolesc Psychiatry 48:386-399, 2009

Objective.—To report results of the clinical reappraisal study of lifetime *DSM-IV* diagnoses based on the fully structured lay-administered World Health Organization Composite International Diagnostic Interview (CIDI) Version 3.0 in the U.S. National Comorbidity Survey Replication Adolescent Supplement (NCS-A).

Method.—Blinded clinical reappraisal interviews with a probability subsample of 347 NCS-A respondents were administered using the Schedule for Affective Disorders and Schizophrenia for School-Age Children (K-SADS) as the gold standard. The *DSM-IV/CIDI* cases were oversampled, and the clinical reappraisal sample was weighted to adjust for this oversampling.

Results.—Good aggregate consistency was found between CIDI and K-SADS prevalence estimates, although CIDI estimates were meaningfully higher than K-SADS estimates for specific phobia (51.2%) and oppositional defiant disorder (38.7%). Estimated prevalence of any disorder, in comparison, was only slightly higher in the CIDI than K-SADS (8.3%). Strong individual-level CIDI versus K-SADS concordance was found for most diagnoses. Area under the receiver operating characteristic curve, a measure of classification accuracy not influenced by prevalence, was 0.88 for any anxiety disorder, 0.89 for any mood disorder, 0.84 for any disruptive behavior disorder, 0.94 for any substance disorder, and 0.87 for any disorder. Although area under the receiver operating characteristic curve was unacceptably low for alcohol dependence and bipolar I and II disorders, these problems were resolved by aggregation with alcohol abuse and bipolar I disorder, respectively. Logistic regression analysis documented that consideration of CIDI symptom-level data significantly improved prediction of some K-SADS diagnoses.

Conclusions.—These results document that the diagnoses made in the NCS-A based on the CIDI have generally good concordance with blinded clinical diagnoses (Table 1).

▶ There is a need for continual refinement of our epidemiological understanding of those who seek care and of the public generally, but how can large-scale studies assess actual diagnoses? The National Comorbidity Study, initiated decades ago, has proven to be the most valuable instrument for doing this, and the results of the current effort at replication are vital as well. This particular report, the third of many reports from the replication, focuses on the reliability of the *Diagnostic and Statistic Manual (DSM)-IV* diagnoses through the Schedule for Affective Disorders and Schizophrenia for School-Age Children (K-SADS) and the World Health Organization's Composite International Diagnostic Interview (CIDI), which was the instrument used in the National Comorbidity Survey Adolescent Supplement. The K-SADS is presented as a semistructured interview performed by a clinician, viewed as the gold standard in contrast to interviews that are highly structured and which can be performed by lay interviewers, such as the Diagnostic Interview Schedule for Children or the CIDI, which uses parent and child responses. Previously, the Structured Clinical Interview for DSM-III-R was used to compare CIDI and results were congruent in adults. Here, a nationally representative sample was used to undergo blinded clinical interviews using a modified version of the K-SADS. As the authors point out, the K-SADS interviews were done by telephone, and they were focused on diagnosis rather than severity. Concordance at the individual level and the group level were, in their words,

TABLE 1.—Consistency of Lifetime Prevalence Estimates of *DSM-IV* Disorders Based on the CIDI and the K-SADS in the NCS-A Clinical Reappraisal Sample ($n = 347$)

	CIDI		K-SADS		McNemar
	%	SE	%	SE	χ^2_1
Anxiety disorders					
Panic disorder	2.4	0.5	2.1	0.7	1.0
Agoraphobia without panic disorder	2.6	0.6	1.5	0.7	8.0*
Specific phobia	19.2	3.1	12.7	2.4	41.6*
Social phobia	9.8	1.4	9.2	1.7	1.5
Generalized anxiety disorder	2.6	0.8	3.3	1.0	3.3*
Posttraumatic stress disorder	4.4	1.0	4.2	1.2	0.9
Any anxiety disorder	31.4	3.3	25.0	3.0	40.5*
Mood disorders					
Major depressive episode	17.7	2.1	17.5	2.4	1.4
Major depressive episode or dysthymic disorder	18.0	2.2	19.8	2.5	8.3*
Bipolar spectrum disorder[a]	6.6	1.7	6.2	1.7	3.7
Any mood disorder	21.9	2.6	23.7	2.8	10.2*
Disruptive behavior disorders					
Attention-deficit/hyperactivity disorder	7.9	1.6	7.8	1.6	0.1
Conduct disorder	8.8	3.6	7.8	3.5	2.5
Oppositional defiant disorder	14.7	4.1	10.6	4.0	112.0*
Any disruptive behavior disorder	20.8	2.7	17.0	2.5	55.5*
Substance disorders[b]					
Alcohol abuse with or without dependence	6.7	1.6	6.4	1.7	0.8
Alcohol dependence with abuse	1.2	0.5	0.5	0.4	24.9*
Illicit drug abuse with or without dependence	8.4	1.7	8.9	1.8	1.9
Illicit drug dependence with abuse	1.9	0.7	0.9	0.5	62.8*
Any substance disorder	11.1	2.1	11.1	2.2	2.1
Any					
Any lifetime diagnosis	56.9	4.5	52.5	4.0	27.1*
Two or more lifetime diagnoses	22.5	2.7	21.5	2.7	2.4
Three or more lifetime diagnoses	9.5	1.4	9.7	1.5	0.9

Note: CIDI = Composite International Diagnostic Interview; K-SADS = Schedule for Affective Disorders and Schizophrenia for School-Age Children; NCS-A = National Comorbidity Survey Replication Adolescent Supplement.

Editor's Note: Please refer to original journal article for full references.

[a]Bipolar spectrum disorder includes bipolar I and II and subthreshold bipolar spectrum disorder. See "Disorder Assessment" for our operation definition of subthreshold bipolar spectrum disorder.

[b]Substance abuse was diagnosed in both the CIDI and K-SADS with or without dependence. The CIDI assessment of substance dependence was made only among respondents who met lifetime criteria for abuse based on the finding in an early study that the prevalence of dependence without abuse is uncommon.[12] This result has recently been called into question.[45] The K-SADS assessment of substance dependence was made with or without a history of abuse. The fact that the estimated prevalence of any substance disorder in the CIDI is identical to the estimate in the K-SADS confirms the assumption that dependence seldom occurred in the absence of a history of abuse in this sample.

*Significant at the .05 level, two-sided test.

good, but they were not perfect, and this is seen in Table 1. Why? There was not as good concordance when it came to bipolar disorder as well as alcohol dependence and other substances of abuse. In the former, it is unclear whether any source is being received as authoritative. Moreover, the study found information that may help the CIDI in the future for the planned replication. Diagnostic reliability and its sibling—generalizability—are keys to the future of psychiatric progress. This study's determination of differences among large-scale assessment studies simply points out new directions for refinement.

A. H. Mack, MD

Posttraumatic growth and reduced suicidal ideation among adolescents at month 1 after the Sichuan Earthquake
Yu X-N, Lau JTF, Zhang J, et al (The Chinese Univ of Hong Kong, China; Sichuan Univ, Chengdu, China; et al)
J Affective Disord 123:327-331, 2010

Background.—This study investigated posttraumatic growth (PTG) and reduced suicidal ideation among Chinese adolescents at one month after the occurrence of the Sichuan Earthquake.

Methods.—A cross-sectional survey was administered to 3324 high school students in Chengdu, Sichuan. The revised Posttraumatic Growth Inventory for Children and the Children's Revised Impact of Event Scale assessed PTG and posttraumatic stress disorder (PTSD), respectively.

Results.—Multivariate analysis showed that being in junior high grade 2, having probable PTSD, visiting affected areas, possessing a perceived sense of security from teachers, and being exposed to touching news reports and encouraging news reports were associated with probable PTG; the reverse was true for students in senior high grade 1 or senior high grade 2 who had experienced prior adversities.

Among the 623 students (19.3% of all students) who had suicidal ideation prior to the earthquake, 57.4% self-reported reduced suicidal ideation when the pre-earthquake and post-earthquake situations were compared. Among these 623 students, the multivariate results showed that being females, perceived sense of security obtained from teachers and exposure to encouraging news reports were factors associated with reduced suicidal ideation; the reverse was true for experience of pre-earthquake corporal punishment and worry about severe earthquakes in the future.

Limitations.—The study population was not directly hit by the earthquake. This study is cross-sectional and no baseline data were collected prior to the occurrence of the earthquake.

Conclusions.—The earthquake resulted in PTG and reduced suicidal ideation among adolescents. PTSD was associated with PTG. Special attention should be paid to teachers' support, contents of media reports, and students' experience of prior adversities.

▶ And now for something completely different: the concept that we might measure growth and other positive effects that follow a traumatic event. Regardless of our understanding of posttraumatic stress disorder, here posttraumatic growth (PTG) is a state that has been observed and described empirically, in this case after a natural disaster. The rates do vary, and the measures are all self-reported, including predisaster and postdisaster suicidal ideation (which did reduce after the earthquake in more than half of respondents). The authors emphasize also that this is the first study of this phenomenon in China. To that extent, its generalizability is increased. We should all watch for further studies on this topic and consider it as a finding in patients that one sees in everyday practice. In addition, it is important to be aware of studies that have provided support for the current structure of posttraumatic stress disorder in the *Diagnostic and Statistical Manual of Mental Disorders.*[1]

A. H. Mack, MD

Reference

1. Kassam-Adams N, Marsac M, Cirilli C. Posttraumatic stress disorder symptom structure in injured children: functional impairment and depression symptoms in a confirmatory factor analysis. *J Am Acad Child Adolesc Psychiatry.* 2010;49: 616-625.

Trends in Antipsychotic Drug Use by Very Young, Privately Insured Children

Olfson M, Crystal S, Huang C, et al (Columbia Univ and the New York State Psychiatric Inst; Health Care Policy & Aging Res of Rutgers Univ, NJ; et al)
J Am Acad Child Adolesc Psychiatry 49:13-23, 2010

Objective.—This study describes recent trends and patterns in antipsychotic treatment of privately insured children aged 2 through 5 years.

Method.—A trend analysis is presented of antipsychotic medication use (1999–2001 versus 2007) stratified by patient characteristics. Data are analyzed from a large administrative database of privately insured individuals. Participants were privately insured children, aged 2 through 5 years, with 12 months of continuous service enrollment in 1999–2001 (N = 400,196) or 2007 (N = 755,793). The main outcomes are annualized rates of antipsychotic use and adjusted rate ratios (ARR) of year effect on rate of antipsychotic use adjusted for age, sex, and treated mental disorder.

Results.—The annualized rate of any antipsychotic use per 1,000 children increased from 0.78 (95% confidence interval [CI] 0.69–0.88) (1999–2001) to 1.59 (95% CI 1.50–1.68) (2007) (ARR 1.76, 95% CI 1.56–2.00). Significant increases in antipsychotic drug use were evident for boys (ARR 1.66, 95% CI 1.44–1.90) and girls (ARR 2.26, 95% CI 1.70–3.01) and for children diagnosed with several different psychiatric disorders. Among antipsychotic-treated children in the 2007 sample, pervasive developmental disorder or mental retardation (28.2%), attention deficit/hyperactivity disorder (ADHD) (23.7%), and disruptive behavior disorder (12.9%) were the most common clinical diagnoses. Fewer than one-half of antipsychotic-treated young children received a mental health assessment (40.8%), a psychotherapy visit (41.4%), or a visit with a psychiatrist (42.6%) during the year of antipsychotic use.

Conclusions.—Despite increasing rates of antipsychotic use by very young children, provision of formal mental health services remains sparse. These service patterns highlight a critical need to improve the availability

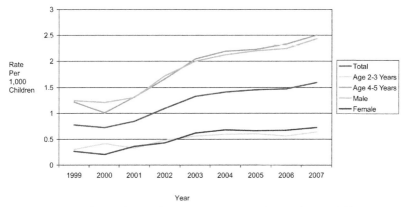

FIGURE 1.—Annual rates of antipsychotic use per 1,000 privately insured young children by age and sex. (Reprinted from Olfson M, Crystal S, Huang C, et al. Trends in antipsychotic drug use by very young, privately insured children. *J Am Acad Child Adolesc Psychiatry.* 2010;49:13-23.)

of specialized and well integrated mental health care for very young children with serious mental health problems (Fig 1).

▶ The findings of this study are encapsulated in its figure (Fig 1)—this is stark in several ways: first, the sheer fact of antipsychotic prescription in the preschool age range; second, that the use is rising; and third, that there was an acceleration in use in 2006-2007. Olfson, a leading psychiatric epidemiologist, and other groups have reviewed the use of antipsychotic medications in other patient population groups. especially disadvantaged groups such as those in the foster system or Medicaid recipients, but here are data from a group of insured patients. It is important for practitioners to bear in mind that all psychotropic medications are not created equal for this age group; some medications are known to be safe and effective for certain indications, such as stimulants for attention-deficit/hyperactivity disorder or even antipsychotics for tics, but antipsychotics for aggression or other behavioral dyscontrol disorders pose major concerns about whether they are the appropriate treatments, with the risks of serious side effects and potential adverse effects that remain unknown. Practitioners would do well to be wary of any wish, by primary care providers, other mental health clinicians, or guardians, for prescription of antipsychotics among preschoolers. This report excellently captures the imminence of the problem.

A. H. Mack, MD

Psychiatric Disorders in Preschool Offspring of Parents With Bipolar Disorder: The Pittsburgh Bipolar Offspring Study (BIOS)
Birmaher B, Axelson D, Goldstein B, et al (Western Psychiatric Inst and Clinic, PA; Univ of Pittsburgh Med Ctr, PA; Univ of Pittsburgh, PA; et al)
Am J Psychiatry 167:321-330, 2010

Objective.—The authors evaluated lifetime prevalence and specificity of DSM-IV psychiatric disorders and severity of depressive and manic symptoms at intake in preschool offspring of parents with bipolar I and II disorders.

Method.—A total of 121 offspring ages 2–5 years from 83 parents with bipolar disorder and 102 offspring of 65 demographically matched comparison parents (29 with non-bipolar psychiatric disorders and 36 without any lifetime psychopathology) were recruited for the study. Parents with bipolar disorder were recruited through advertisements and adult outpatient clinics, and comparison parents were ascertained at random from the community. Participants were evaluated with standardized instruments. All staff were blind to parental diagnoses.

Results.—After adjustment for within-family correlations and both biological parents' non-bipolar psychopathology, offspring of parents with bipolar disorder, particularly those older than age 4, showed an eightfold greater lifetime prevalence of attention deficit hyperactivity disorder (ADHD) and significantly higher rates of having two or more psychiatric disorders compared to the offspring of the comparison parents. While only three offspring of parents with bipolar disorder had mood disorders, offspring of parents with bipolar disorder, especially those with ADHD and oppositional defiant disorder, had significantly more severe current manic and depressive symptoms than comparison offspring.

Conclusions.—Preschool offspring of parents with bipolar disorder have an elevated risk for ADHD and have greater levels of subthreshold manic and depressive symptoms than children of comparison parents. Longitudinal follow-up is warranted to evaluate whether these children are at high risk for developing mood and other psychiatric disorders.

▶ The consideration of the psychopathology of bipolar disorder remains one of active interest. The avenue being taken of the study of the development of the disorder and other disorders among children of persons with bipolar disorder seems likely to bear significant fruit over the long term. At the moment, however, it is unclear what to make of the findings that this study adds to, that youth of parents with bipolar disorder tend to have a variety of psychiatric syndromes. Actually, the authors are to be commended for many reasons; one of them is their exploration of the limitations of the study, especially in terms of the potential for biased self-reports and their effect of the study's diagnoses of the children, even among those who were assessed by mental health clinicians. But this highlights concern over reliability of psychiatric diagnosis in children generally. Is it possible that the various diagnoses being given are prodromal to bipolar disorder, rather than unrelated? Longitudinal studies are needed to answer these questions.

A. H. Mack, MD

The association of visuospatial working memory with dysthymic disorder in pre-pubertal children
Franklin T, Lee A, Hall N, et al (Univ of Melbourne, Parkville, Victoria, Australia)
Psychol Med 40:253-261, 2010

Background.—Visuospatial working memory (VSWM) deficits have not been investigated specifically in children with dysthymic disorder (DD), although they are associated with impairments in attention that commonly occur in DD. This study investigates VSWM impairment in children with DD.

Method.—A cross-sectional study of VSWM in 6- to 12-year-old children with medication-naive DD ($n = 26$) compared to an age-, gender- and 'performance IQ' (PIQ)-matched healthy control group ($n = 28$) was completed.

Results.—The DD group demonstrated impairment in VSWM, including impairment in the spatial span and strategy components of VSWM. Furthermore, the VSWM impairment remained after controlling for spatial span. Inattentive symptoms were significantly associated with the VSWM impairment.

Conclusions.—This study of children with DD found deficits in performance on VSWM tasks, suggesting that fronto-striatal–parietal neural networks that underlie processes of attention and the executive component of VSWM are dysfunctional in children with DD. These findings further our understanding of DD and suggest more specific interventions that might improve functioning.

▶ All too often, our trainees in medicine and mental health, and even some practicitioners, are misled to think that dysthymic disorder is a depressive disorder of lesser severity, but, by definition, there is nothing to specify this bias. And in fact, we may need to ensure that peers and trainees understand that the effects of dysthymic disorder can be greater than other types of depressive disorder, and, furthermore, that subtle effects may cause serious problems in younger age groups. Perhaps depressive conditions affect different circuits in these 2 age groups. In any event, these empirically derived data show specific areas of deficit and it is incumbent on us to practice with as much concern over dysthymic disorder as any other disorder of mood. Furthermore, the effects of cognitive deficits can be devastating in this age group, making its understanding more pressing. And, of course, perhaps then we could move toward evidence of medications that are helpful in this condition as well.

A. H. Mack, MD

Mental Health Treatment Received by Youths in the Year Before and After a New Diagnosis of Bipolar Disorder

Olfson M, Crystal S, Gerhard T, et al (Columbia Univ, NY; Rutgers Univ, NJ; et al)
Psychiatr Serv 60:1098-1106, 2009

Objective.—Despite a marked increase in treatment for bipolar disorder among youths, little is known about their pattern of service use. This article describes mental health service use in the year before and after a new clinical diagnosis of bipolar disorder.

Methods.—Claims were reviewed between April 1, 2004, and March 31, 2005, for 1,274,726 privately insured youths (17 years and younger) who were eligible for services at least one year before and after a service claim; 2,907 youths had new diagnosis of bipolar disorder during this period. Diagnoses of other mental disorders and prescriptions filled for psychotropic drugs were assessed in the year before and after the initial diagnosis of bipolar disorder.

Results.—The one-year rate of a new diagnosis of bipolar disorder was .23%. During the year before the new diagnosis of bipolar disorder, youths were commonly diagnosed as having depressive disorder (46.5%) or disruptive behavior disorder (36.7%) and had often filled a prescription for an antidepressant (48.5%), stimulant (33.0%), mood stabilizer (31.8%), or antipsychotic (29.1%). Most youths with a new diagnosis of bipolar disorder had only one (28.8%) or two to four (28.7%) insurance claims for bipolar disorder in the year starting with the index diagnosis. The proportion starting mood stabilizers after the index diagnosis was highest for youths with five or more insurance claims for bipolar disorder (42.1%), intermediate for those with two to four claims (24.2%), and lowest for those with one claim (13.8%).

Conclusions.—Most youths with a new diagnosis of bipolar disorder had recently received treatment for depressive or disruptive behavior disorders, and many had no claims listing a diagnosis of bipolar disorder after the initial diagnosis. The service pattern suggests that a diagnosis of bipolar disorder is often given tentatively to youths treated for mental disorders with overlapping symptom profiles and is subsequently reconsidered.

▶ The bipolar epidemic continues, but studies such as this provide hope! As the authors remind readers, there is great concern not only about misdiagnosis, but also the resultant effects in terms of stigma and, dangerously, excess use of antipsychotic medications. An important feature of this study is its use of an informative, yet often-overlooked, population set: persons with health insurance other than public sector systems. Studies suggesting that antipsychotic use is excessive according to lower socioeconomic status will need to incorporate samples such as this one to ensure that the conclusions are generalizable. The authors are clear in proposing a distinction between diagnoses given in the community versus specialized or academic clinics; no one should be offended by such a town/gown dichotomy, especially if it helps to foster our understanding of this epidemic. Both community as well as academic/specialist psychiatrists will need to have better understanding of the meaning of *DSM-IV* and of *DSM-V*'s definition of bipolar disorder.

A. H. Mack, MD

Prevalence of Autism Spectrum Disorders — Autism and Developmental Disabilities Monitoring Network, United States, 2006
Autism and Developmental Disabilities Monitoring Network Surveillance Year 2006 Principal Investigators (Univ of Alabama, Birmingham; Univ of South Florida, Tampa, FL; et al)
MMWR Surveill Summ 58:1-20, 2009

Problem/Condition.—Autism spectrum disorders (ASDs) are a group of developmental disabilities characterized by atypical development in socialization, communication, and behavior. ASDs typically are apparent before age 3 years, with associated impairments affecting multiple areas of a person's life. Because no biologic marker exists for ASDs, identification is made by professionals who evaluate a child's developmental progress to identify the presence of developmental disorders.

Reporting Period.—2006.

Methods.—Earlier surveillance efforts indicated that age 8 years is a reasonable index age at which to monitor peak prevalence. The identified prevalence of ASDs in U.S. children aged 8 years was estimated through a systematic retrospective review of evaluation records in multiple sites participating in the Autism and Developmental Disabilities Monitoring (ADDM) Network. Data were collected from existing records in 11 ADDM Network sites (areas of Alabama, Arizona, Colorado, Florida, Georgia, Maryland, Missouri, North Carolina, Pennsylvania, South Carolina, and Wisconsin) for 2006. To analyze changes in identified ASD prevalence, CDC compared the 2006 data with data collected from 10 sites (all sites noted above except Florida) in 2002. Children aged 8 years with a notation of an ASD or descriptions consistent with an ASD were identified through screening and abstraction of existing health and education records containing professional assessments of the child's developmental progress at health-care or education facilities. Children aged 8 years whose parent(s) or legal guardian(s) resided in the respective areas in 2006 met the case definition for an ASD if their records documented behaviors consistent with the *Diagnostic and Statistical Manual of Mental Disorders, 4th edition,* text revision (DSM-IV-TR) criteria for autistic disorder, pervasive developmental disorder–not otherwise specified (PDD NOS), or Asperger disorder. Presence of an identified ASD was determined through a review of data abstracted from developmental evaluation records by trained clinician reviewers.

Results.—For the 2006 surveillance year, 2,757 (0.9%) of 308,038 children aged 8 years residing in the 11 ADDM sites were identified as having an ASD, indicating an overall average prevalence of 9.0 per 1,000 population (95% confidence interval [CI] = 8.6–9.3). ASD prevalence per 1,000 children aged 8 years ranged from 4.2 in Florida to 12.1 in Arizona and Missouri, with prevalence for the majority of sites ranging between 7.6 and 10.4. For 2006, ASD prevalence was significantly lower in Florida (p<0.001) and Alabama (p<0.05) and higher in Arizona and Missouri (p<0.05) than in all other sites. The ratio of males to females ranged from 3.2:1 in Alabama to 7.6:1 in Florida. ASD prevalence varied by type of ascertainment source, with higher average prevalence in sites with access to health and education records (10.0) compared with sites with health records only (7.5). Although parental or professional concerns regarding development before age 36 months were noted in the evaluation records of the majority of children who were identified as having an ASD, the median age of earliest documented ASD diagnosis was much later (range: 41 months [Florida]—60 months [Colorado]). Of 10 sites that collected data for both the 2002 and 2006 surveillance years, nine observed an increase in ASD prevalence (range: 27%–95% increase; p<0.01), with increases among males in all sites and among females in four of 11 sites, and variation among other subgroups.

Interpretation.—In 2006, on average, approximately 1% or one child in every 110 in the 11 ADDM sites was classified as having an ASD (approximate range: 1:80–1:240 children [males: 1:70; females: 1:315]). The average prevalence of ASDs identified among children aged 8 years increased 57% in 10 sites from the 2002 to the 2006 ADDM surveillance year. Although improved ascertainment accounts for some of the prevalence increases documented in the ADDM sites, a true increase in the risk for children to develop ASD symptoms cannot be ruled out. On average, although delays in identification persisted, ASDs were being diagnosed by community professionals at earlier ages in 2006 than in 2002.

Public Health Actions.—These results indicate an increased prevalence of identified ASDs among U.S. children aged 8 years and underscore the need to regard ASDs as an urgent public health concern. Continued monitoring is needed to document and understand changes over time, including the multiple ascertainment and potential risk factors likely to be contributing. Research is needed to ascertain the factors that put certain persons at risk, and concerted efforts are essential to provide support for persons with ASDs, their families, and communities to improve long-term outcome.

▶ There is continuing need to monitor the prevalence of autism and other pervasive developmental disorders (PDDs). It appears highly likely that going forward, by the way, they will be referred to as the autism spectrum disorders (ASDs). In this report, the Centers for Disease Control's (CDC's) Autism and Developmental Disabilities Monitoring Network provides estimates of the prevalence of ASDs in the United States in 2006. One interesting feature is that the point prevalence is measured for those children aged 8 years. The male dominance seen previously was replicated, and overall the prevalence was estimated at 1 in 110 eight-year olds who had a disorder on the autism spectrum. This represented a 57% increase overall, compared with a similar study performed in 2002. It does represent an urgent problem, both for continued surveillance and for implementation of appropriate health care responses. A limitation is that the diagnoses were made through review of charts and other evaluation records, albeit by trained clinician reviewers. Actually, these rates are not too different from those determined in the United Kingdom. A recent study among school-age children in the United Kingdom reported a prevalence of around 94 to 99 per 10 000 (this study used face-to-face assessments—the Autism Diagnostic Observation Schedule and the Autism Diagnostic Interview, and it allowed for PDD-not otherwise specified/spectrum diagnoses) or roughly 1% to 2% of the school-age population. It is helpful that experts[1] have been able to discern up to 7 different reasons for which there has been the massive increase in prevalence over the past 4 decades—all were based on diagnostic awareness and reduction of stigma rather than on some biological widespread agent. Thus, these 2 English-speaking developed nations displayed similar rates of the ASDs. Both studies bear a positive feature in that the investigators used some added form of diagnostic confirmation beyond institutional statistics.

One additional feature of the CDC study is that the investigators assessed developmental status among participants and found that in the vast majority of cases, deviance from normal development had been identified before age 3 years—this corresponds with current thinking about the natural history of autism, which is often assumed to be silent until age 3 years.

A. H. Mack, MD

Reference

1. Baron-Cohen S, Scott FJ, Allison C, et al. Prevalence of autism-spectrum conditions: UK school-based population study. *Br J Psychiatry.* 2009;194:500-509.

Pediatric Bipolar Disorder Versus Severe Mood Dysregulation: Risk for Manic Episodes on Follow-Up
Stringaris A, Baroni A, Haimm C, et al (Natl Inst of Mental Health, Bethesda, MD)
J Am Acad Child Adolesc Psychiatry 49:397-405, 2010

Objective.—An important question in pediatric bipolar research is whether marked nonepisodic irritability is a manifestation of bipolar disorder in youth. This study tests the hypothesis that youth with severe mood dysregulation (SMD), a category created for the purpose of studying children presenting with severe nonepisodic irritability, will be significantly less likely to develop (hypo-)manic or mixed episodes over time than will youth with bipolar disorder (BD).

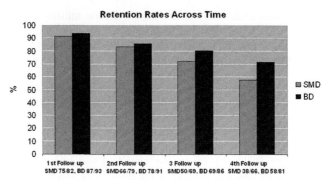

FIGURE 1.—Percentage of patients with severe mood dysregulation (SMD) and bipolar disorder (BD) at each follow-up point is shown in the bars. Note: Underneath each pair of bars are the raw number proportions for each category. (Reprinted from Stringaris A, Baroni A, Haimm C, et al. Pediatric bipolar disorder versus severe mood dysregulation: risk for manic episodes on follow-up. *J Am Acad Child Adolesc Psychiatry.* 2010;49:397-405, with permission from The American Academy of Child & Adolescent Psychiatry.)

Method.—Patients with SMD (N = 84) and narrowly defined BD (N = 93) at baseline were followed up in 6-monthly intervals using the relevant K-SADS modules to ascertain (hypo-)manic or mixed episodes.

Results.—Only one of 84 SMD subjects (1/84 [1.2%]; 95% confidence interval CI = 0.0003 to 0.064) experienced a (hypo-)manic or mixed episode during the study (median follow-up = 28.7 months). The frequency of such episodes was more than 50 times higher in those with narrowly defined BD (58/93 [62.4%]; 95% CI 0.52 to 0.72).

Conclusions.—These data suggest that, over an approximately 2-year follow-up period, youth with SMD are unlikely to develop (hypo-)manic or mixed episodes.

▶ Several lines of information are converging to illuminate different components of the decade-long upsurge in diagnoses of the various types of bipolar disorder. As we have observed in reviews over the past several years, a hard definition separating types of nonspecific irritability or lability from an actual bipolar or mood disorder definition is sorely needed. There also needs to be closure on the assertion that childhood bipolar disorder inherently is different and does not necessarily follow the adult DSM definition. Like others, this report focuses on persons who are actually diagnosed with bipolar disorder and compares them with those who would otherwise be diagnosed with severe mood dysregulation (SMD). Here, of 84 patients diagnosed with SMD, only 1 developed a form of manic, hypomanic, or mixed episodes, as shown in Fig 1. This is important evidence that a background SMD is not sufficient in making a diagnosis of bipolar disorder. As we continue to try to impose standards in the diagnosis of bipolar disorder and irritability, we need descriptive definitions that will withstand the inevitable disuse of SMD—and then maybe we will understand more.

A. H. Mack, MD

Developmental dyslexia in Chinese and English populations: dissociating the effect of dyslexia from language differences

Hu W, Lee HL, Zhang Q, et al (Xuzhou Normal Univ, Jiangsu Province, China; Max-Planck Inst for Biological Cybernetics, Tubingen, Germany; et al)
Brain 133:1694-1706, 2010

Previous neuroimaging studies have suggested that developmental dyslexia has a different neural basis in Chinese and English populations because of known differences in the processing demands of the Chinese and English writing systems. Here, using functional magnetic resonance imaging, we provide the first direct statistically based investigation into how the effect of dyslexia on brain activation is influenced by the Chinese and English writing systems. Brain activation for semantic decisions on written words was compared in English dyslexics, Chinese dyslexics, English normal readers and Chinese normal readers, while controlling for all other experimental parameters. By investigating the effects of dyslexia and language in one study, we show common activation in Chinese and English dyslexics despite different activation in Chinese versus English normal readers. The effect of dyslexia in both languages was observed as less than normal activation in the left angular gyrus and in left middle frontal, posterior temporal and occipitotemporal regions. Differences in Chinese and English normal reading were observed as increased activation for Chinese relative to English in the left inferior frontal sulcus; and increased activation for English relative to Chinese in the left posterior superior temporal sulcus. These cultural differences were not observed in dyslexics who activated both left inferior frontal sulcus and left posterior superior temporal sulcus, consistent with the use of culturally independent strategies when reading is less efficient. By dissociating the effect of dyslexia from differences in Chinese and English normal reading, our results reconcile brain activation results with a substantial body of behavioural studies showing commonalities in the cognitive manifestation of dyslexia in Chinese and English populations. They also demonstrate the influence of cognitive ability and learning environment on a common neural system for reading.

▶ Reading disorder, or developmental dyslexia, is a learning disorder that remains without a clear form of psychopathology. Evidence has pointed to various areas of the central nervous system, particularly following evidence of low activation in the posterior occipital-temporal and/or temporoparietal regions. Furthermore, there has been the assumption that dyslexia is tied to languages that require writing with Arabic letters and numbers. But this study provides information that suggests dyslexia of Chinese written language uses the same pathways. As noted in Fig 2, the same areas of reduced activation occur in the English and English dyslexic population as in their Chinese counterparts. In addition, the study demonstrates that the brain areas previously thought to be specific to the specific language are also affected. As such, there

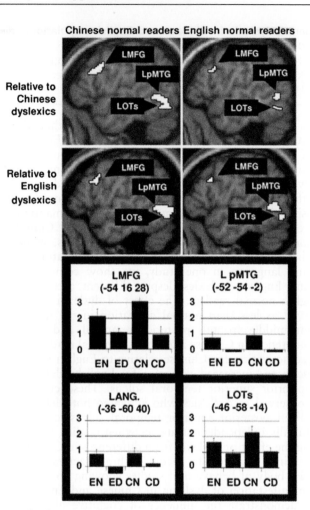

FIGURE 2.—Reduced activation for Chinese and English dyslexics. *Top:* activation (in white) is shown in the left middle frontal gyrus (LMFG), left posterior middle temporal gyrus (LpMTG) and left occipito-temporal sulcus (LOTs) for the comparison of each of the good reader groups to each of the dyslexic groups. Statistical threshold = $P < 0.05$ uncorrected to compare all effects. *Bottom:* parameter estimates for semantic word matching relative to fixation are plotted for each of the regions showing reduced activation for dyslexics compared to normal readers (common to English and Chinese). LANG. = left angular gyrus. See Fig. 3 for details of plots. (Reprinted from Hu W, Lee HL, Zhang Q, et al. Developmental dyslexia in Chinese and English populations: dissociating the effect of dyslexia from language differences. *Brain.* 2010;133:1694-1706. Published by Oxford University Press.)

may be an opportunity for further collaboration. The report provides empirical evidence that may be helpful in the study and treatment of these conditions in the future.

A. H. Mack, MD

Treatment Studies: Pharmacotherapy

A Candidate Gene Analysis of Methylphenidate Response in Attention-Deficit/Hyperactivity Disorder

McGough JJ, McCracken JT, Loo SK, et al (Semel Inst for Neuroscience & Human Behavior and David Geffen School of Medicine at the Univ of California, Los Angeles; Ctr for Neurobehavioral Genetics at the UCLA Semel Inst; et al)
J Am Acad Child Adolesc Psychiatry 48:1155-1164, 2009

Objective.—This study examines the potential role of candidate genes in moderating treatment effects of methylphenidate (MPH) in attention-deficit/hyperactivity disorder (ADHD).

Method.—Eighty-two subjects with ADHD aged 6 to 17 years participated in a prospective, double-blind, placebo-controlled, multiple-dose, crossover titration trial of immediate release MPH three times daily. The subjects were assessed on a variety of parent and clinician ratings and a laboratory math test. Data reduction based on principal components analysis identified statistically derived efficacy and side effect outcomes.

Results.—Attention-deficit/hyperactivity disorder symptom response was predicted by polymorphisms at the serotonin transporter (*SLC6A4*) intron 2 *VNTR* ($p = .01$), with a suggested trend for catechol-O-methyltransferase (*COMT*) ($p = .04$). Gene × dose interactions were noted on math test outcomes for the dopamine D4 receptor (*DRD4*) promoter ($p = .008$), *DRD4* exon 3 *VNTR* ($p = .006$), and *SLC6A4* promoter insertion/deletion polymorphism (*5HTTLPR*) ($p = .02$). Irritability was predicted by *COMT* ($p = .02$). Vegetative symptoms were predicted by *5HTTLPR* ($p = .003$). No significant effects were noted for the dopamine transporter (*SLC6A3*) or synaptosomal-associated protein 25 (*SNAP25*).

Conclusions.—This article confirms and expands previous studies suggesting that genes moderate ADHD treatment response. The ADHD outcomes are not unitary but reflect both behavioral and learning domains that are likely influenced by different genes. Future research should emphasize candidate gene and genome-wide association studies in larger samples, symptom reduction as well as side effects outcomes, and responses over full therapeutic dose ranges to assess differences in both gene and gene × dose interactive effects.

▶ Within the literature on pharmacogenomics, here is some thinking outside of the box. Previous studies had focused on either the dopamine transporter gene or the dopamine receptor. But as a step forward, here is a prospective study that provides evidence as to the effect of gene and dose. Genes are being viewed as potential moderators of efficacy, and it is timely and appropriate to review this study closely as an example of the types of questions that should be addressed now. The authors mention that their findings were not unitary, but they did overall show that genetic variations in a number of specific genes do affect response to methylphenidate. This prospective study is well designed in that their sample size of more than 80 youths was not small; their methods included a crossover design. Overall, the study provided results of great interest, which will need replication and further elucidation and lengthier time periods of study.

A. H. Mack, MD

Adjunctive Divalproex Versus Placebo for Children With ADHD and Aggression Refractory to Stimulant Monotherapy

Blader JC, Schooler NR, Jensen PS, et al (Stony Brook Univ School of Medicine, NY; Zucker Hillside Hosp, Glen Oaks, NY; REACH Inst, NY; et al)
Am J Psychiatry 166:1392-1401, 2009

Objective.—The purpose of the present study was to evaluate the efficacy of divalproex for reducing aggressive behavior among children 6 to 13 years old with attention deficit hyperactivity disorder (ADHD) and a disruptive disorder whose chronic aggression was underresponsive to a prospective psychostimulant trial.

Method.—Children received open stimulant treatment during a lead-in phase that averaged 5 weeks. Agent and dose were assessed weekly and modified to optimize response. Children whose aggressive behavior persisted at the conclusion of the lead-in phase were randomly assigned to receive double-blind, flexibly dosed divalproex or a placebo adjunctive to stimulant for 8 weeks. Families received weekly behavioral therapy throughout the trial. The primary outcome measure was the proportion of children whose aggressive behavior remitted, defined by post-trial ratings of negligible or absent aggression.

Result.—A significantly higher proportion of children randomly assigned to divalproex met remission criteria (eight out of 14 [57%]) than those randomly assigned to placebo (two out of 13 [15%]). Divalproex was generally well tolerated.

Conclusions.—Among children with ADHD whose chronic aggressive behavior is refractory to optimized stimulant treatment, the addition of divalproex increases the likelihood that aggression will remit. A larger trial is necessary to specify with greater precision the magnitude of benefit for adjuvant divalproex.

▶ This study fills a gap in the study of some of the population of youth with attention-deficit/hyperactivity disorder (ADHD) who, in the absence of another axis I disorder, also are aggressive. It is valuable to have an evidence base as to the next step after such youth display aggression, despite a stimulant having been prescribed. If prescribed safely and carefully, might valproate (VPA) be an answer? Both systematic and well controlled, the study also reviewed the safety of VPA in this administration. The mean VPA dose was 571 milligrams per day in a population of N = 13. As is often the case nowadays, the intent to

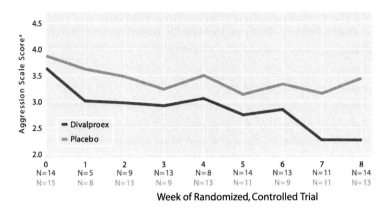

FIGURE 2.—Weekly aggression ratings for children randomly assigned to divalproex or placebo. [a] Logarithmically transformed Retrospective-Modified Overt Aggression Scale score. (Reprinted from Blader JC, Schooler NR, Jensen PS, et al. Adjunctive divalproex versus placebo for children with ADHD and aggression refractory to stimulant monotherapy. *Am J Psychiatry.* 2009;166:1392-1401, with permission from the American Psychiatric Association, Copyright 2010.)

treat model was used. The mean trough concentration for VPA was 68 mg/dL. Note in Fig 2 that the results of the Overt Aggression Scale reduced more in those on VPA than those on placebo. Other groups continue to try to find other ways to reduce the burden of comorbidity or the need for adjunctive treatment in ADHD, as in the study by Thurstone et al,[1] which reviewed the effectiveness of atomoxetine in comorbid ADHD and substance use disorder. Atomoxetine was not statistically significantly better than placebo in the Thurstone study. This study by Blader et al is a systematic and well-controlled trial. A trial of stimulants had begun for all. The regression analysis showed a steeper change each week. Perhaps what is going on is the use of a medication that has an entirely different mode of action. Drawbacks with the study include that there are no girls studied and there is a small N, but it is an example to follow, maybe the best method will be the overlapping use of such different medications. But, to the extent that this is not a suboptimal dose, it provides a manner of a different, evidence-based, or at least studied polypharmacy for aggression.

A. H. Mack, MD

Reference

1. Thurstone C, Riggs PD, Salomonsen-Sautel S, Mikulich-Gilbertson SK. Randomized, controlled trial of atomoxetine for attention-deficit/hyperactivity disorder in adolescents with substance use disorder. *J Am Acad Child Adolesc Psychiatry.* 2010;49:573-582.

Modeled Economic Evaluation of Alternative Strategies to Reduce Sudden Cardiac Death Among Children Treated for Attention Deficit/Hyperactivity Disorder

Denchev P, Kaltman JR, Schoenbaum M, et al (Natl Inst of Mental Health, Bethesda, MD; Natl Heart, Lung, and Blood Inst, Bethesda, MD)
Circulation 121:1329-1337, 2010

Background.—Stimulants are widely used to treat children with attention deficit/hyperactivity disorder and may increase the risk for sudden cardiac death (SCD). We examined the cost-effectiveness of pretreatment screening with ECG for reducing SCD risk in children diagnosed with attention deficit/hyperactivity disorder who are candidates for stimulant medication.

Method and Results.—We constructed a state-transition Markov model with 10 annual cycles spanning 7 to 17 years of age. Taking a societal perspective, we compared the cost-effectiveness of 3 screening strategies: (1) performing a history and physical examination with cardiology referral if abnormal (current standard of care); (2) performing a history and physical examination plus ECG after negative history and physical examination, with cardiology referral if either is abnormal; and (3) performing a history and physical examination plus ECG, with cardiology referral only if ECG is abnormal. Children identified with SCD-associated cardiac abnormalities would be restricted from stimulants and from playing competitive sports. The expected incremental cost-effectiveness over strategy 1 was $39 300 and $27 200 per quality-adjusted life-year for strategies 2 and 3, respectively. Monte Carlo simulation found that the chance of incremental cost-effectiveness was 55% for strategy 2 and 71% for strategy 3 (willingness to pay ≤$50 000 per quality-adjusted life-year). Both strategies 2 and 3 would avert 13 SCDs per 400 000 children seeking stimulant treatment for ADHD, for a cost of $1.6 million per life for strategy 2 and $1.2 million per life for strategy 3.

Conclusions.—Relative to current practice, adding ECG screening to history and physical examination pretreatment screening for children with attention deficit/hyperactivity disorder has borderline cost-effectiveness for preventing SCD. Relative cost-effectiveness may be improved by basing cardiology referral on ECG alone. Benefits of ECG screening arise primarily by restricting children identified with SCD risk from competitive sports.

▶ Here is a helpful analysis by a group of pediatric cardiologists in terms of what makes sense for screening youth who would be beginning stimulant therapy. There is rightfully concern that stimulant medications may cause sudden cardiac death or other cardiac morbidity, and this is based on some data that have demonstrated an association between stimulant exposure and such harm. Although stimulant prescribers may remind us that stimulants have been used with good safety profile since the 1930s, the magnitude of use across the nation could never have been as great as it is today. Across a large number of persons taking stimulants, we will see more cases of cardiac injury. On this scale, it is important that we have good tools for making decisions to do extra evaluations. Of course no life has a price, but we must have information like this to continue making decisions about the prices of health care and the best practice in pediatric psychopharmacology.

A. H. Mack, MD

Comparative Safety of Antidepressant Agents for Children and Adolescents Regarding Suicidal Acts
Schneeweiss S, Patrick AR, Solomon DH, et al (Brigham and Women's Hosp, Boston, MA; et al)
Pediatrics 125:876-888, 2010

Objective.—The objective of this study was to assess the risk of suicide attempts and suicides after initiation of antidepressant medication use by children and adolescents, for individual agents.

Methods.—We conducted a 9-year cohort study by using population-wide data from British Columbia. We identified new users of antidepressants who were 10 to 18 years of age with a recorded diagnosis of depression. Study outcomes were hospitalization attributable to intentional self-harm and suicide death.

Results.—Of 20 906 children who initiated antidepressant therapy, 16 774 (80%) had no previous antidepressant use. During the first year of use, we observed 266 attempted and 3 completed suicides, which yielded an event rate of 27.04 suicidal acts per 1000 person-years (95% confidence interval [CI]: 23.9–30.5 suicidal acts per 1000 person-years). There were no meaningful differences in the rate ratios (RRs) comparing fluoxetine with citalopram (RR: 0.97 [95% CI: 0.54–1.76]), fluvoxamine (RR: 1.05 [95% CI: 0.46–2.43]), paroxetine (RR: 0.80 [95% CI: 0.47–1.37]), and sertraline (RR: 1.02 [95% CI: 0.56–1.84]). Tricyclic agents showed risks similar to those of selective serotonin reuptake inhibitors (RR: 0.92 [95% CI: 0.43–2.00]).

Conclusion.—Our finding of equal event rates among antidepressant agents supports the decision of the Food and Drug Administration to include all antidepressants in the black box warning regarding potentially increased suicidality risk for children and adolescents beginning use of antidepressants.

▶ Here is one more analysis of the risks that might be associated with antidepressant medications demonstrating that the risk of suicidality among adolescents receiving antidepressants may be less than feared. At the least, this report compares the relative safety of the various antidepressants. Of course, because adolescent use of some medications is very rare, the study's authors were correct to use a large cohort, and they succeeded in finding more than 20 000 youth in British Columbia who initiated antidepressants over an 8-year period (1997-2005). Among the various antidepressants used, there was no significant difference in suicide attempts or acts. If nothing else, the study's findings suggest that the Food and Drug Administration was appropriate when it implemented a black box warning on all antidepressants, rather than being selective about them. But criticism of government black box warnings regarding suicidality continues, especially after the implementation of a warning for antiepileptic medications.[1] As many commentators have noted, the best care includes evaluation for depression and suicidality and follow-up treatment and evaluation.

A. H. Mack, MD

Reference

1. Shneker B, Cios JS, Elliott JO. Suicidality, depression screening, and antiepileptic drugs: reaction to the FDA alert. *Neurology.* 2009;72:987-991.

Treatment Studies: Psychotherapies

Impact of Childhood Trauma on Treatment Outcome in the Treatment for Adolescents with Depression Study (TADS)

Lewis CC, Simons AD, Nguyen LJ, et al (Univ of Oregon, Eugene; et al)
J Am Acad Child Adolesc Psychiatry 49:132-140, 2010

Objective.—The impact of childhood trauma was examined in 427 adolescents (54% girls, 74% Caucasian, mean = 14.6, SD = 1.5) with major depressive disorder participating in the Treatment for Adolescents with Depression Study (TADS).

Method.—TADS compared the efficacy of cognitive behavioral therapy (CBT), fluoxetine (FLX), their combination (COMB), and placebo (PBO). Teens were separated into four trauma history groups: (1) no trauma; (2) trauma, no abuse; (3) physical abuse; (4), and sexual abuse. The effects of treatment and trauma history on depression severity across 12 weeks of acute treatment, as measured by the Children's Depression Rating Scale–Revised (CDRS-R), were examined.

Results.—A significant trauma-by-treatment-by-time interaction indicated that trauma history moderated treatment. The Week 12 primary efficacy findings previously reported by TADS were replicated in the no trauma group (n = 201): COMB = FLX > CBT = PBO. No significant differences in treatment arms were observed among the trauma, no abuse, or physical abuse group. Teens with a history of sexual abuse treated with COMB, FLX, and PBO showed significant and equivalent improvement on the CDRS-R (mean <45), whereas the mean CDRS-R for the CBT group tended to remain in the depressed range (mean >45). Baseline suicidality and self-reported depression were significantly related to a history of sexual abuse.

Conclusions.—The study was limited by the level of detail regarding childhood traumatic experiences. Results are discussed in terms of the implications for treating depressed adolescents with traumatic backgrounds.

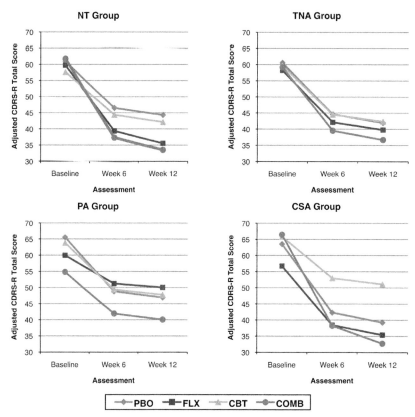

FIGURE 1.—CDRS-R total scores for trauma subgroups across 12 weeks of treatment. 1.1: NT group; 1.2: TNA group; 1.3: PA group; 1.4: CSA group. *Note*: CDRS-R total scores are adjusted for the fixed (treatment, time, treatment-by-time, trauma, trauma-by-time, trauma-by-treatment, trauma-by-treatment-by-time, site) and random effects (patient, patient-by-time) included in the random coefficients regression model. CDRS-R = children's depression rating scale-revised; CSA = childhood sexual abuse or both sexual and physical abuse; NT = no trauma; PA = physical abuse and/or victim of a violent crime; TNA = trauma, no abuse. (Reprinted from Lewis CC, Simons AD, Nguyen LJ, et al. Impact of childhood trauma on treatment outcome in the treatment for adolescents with depression study (TADS). *J Am Acad Child Adolesc Psychiatry*. 2010;49:132-140.)

Clinical Trials Registry Information.—Treatment for Adolescents with Depression Study; *http://www.clinicaltrials.gov*, NCT00006286 (Fig 1).

▶ The Treatment of Adolescents with Depression Study continues to inform the field. Here, the authors have analyzed their cohort of depressed adolescents receiving 1 of their 4 treatment arms, specifically reviewing whether a history of trauma affected treatment outcomes. The findings were that a history of trauma moderated the success of the treatment intervention. Figs 1.1-1.4 display these outcomes in terms of Children's Depression Rating Scale-Revised total scores for trauma subgroups across 12 weeks of treatment. As is seen, the authors specifically reviewed which type of trauma the patient had experienced. This is not an incidental finding: there are now data to support that maltreatment, when ascertained prospectively, is associated with psychopathology in young adults (for example, see study using Composite International Diagnostic Interview).[1] As a result, continued review of the best treatment for this subgroup (or groups) continues to be an important endeavor. It may eventually be found that cognitive behavioral therapy is less appropriate for survivors of trauma than other psychotherapies. In both types of abuse, however, combination treatment had the largest effect, which seems consistent with previous findings in the general group.

A. H. Mack, MD

Reference

1. Scott KM, Smith DR, Ellis PM. Prospectively ascertained child maltreatment and its association with DSM-IV mental disorders in young adults. *Arch Gen Psychiatry.* 2010;67:712-719.

Treatment of Resistant Depression in Adolescents (TORDIA): Week 24 Outcomes
Emslie GJ, Mayes T, Porta G, et al (Univ of Texas Southwestern Med Ctr, Dallas; Univ of Pittsburgh, PA; Kaiser Permanente Ctr for Health Sciences, Portland, OR; et al)
Am J Psychiatry 167:782-791, 2010

Objective.—The purpose of this study was to report on the outcome of participants in the Treatment of Resistant Depression in Adolescents (TORDIA) trial after 24 weeks of treatment, including remission and relapse rates and predictors of treatment outcome.

Method.—Adolescents (ages 12–18 years) with selective serotonin reuptake inhibitor (SSRI)-resistant depression were randomly assigned to either a medication switch alone (alternate SSRI or venlafaxine) or a medication switch plus cognitive-behavioral therapy (CBT). At week 12, responders could continue in their assigned treatment arm and nonresponders received open treatment (medication and/or CBT) for 12 more weeks (24 weeks total). The primary outcomes were remission and relapse, defined by the Adolescent Longitudinal Interval Follow-Up Evaluation as rated by an independent evaluator.

Results.—Of 334 adolescents enrolled in the study, 38.9% achieved remission by 24 weeks, and initial treatment assignment did not affect rates of remission. Likelihood of remission was much higher (61.6% versus 18.3%) and time to remission was much faster among those who had already demonstrated clinical response by week 12. Remission was also higher among those with lower baseline depression, hopelessness, and self-reported anxiety. At week 12, lower depression, hopelessness, anxiety, suicidal ideation, family conflict, and absence of comorbid dysthymia, anxiety, and drug/alcohol use and impairment also predicted remission. Of those who responded by week 12, 19.6% had a relapse of depression by week 24.

Conclusions.—Continued treatment for depression among treatment-resistant adolescents results in remission in approximately one-third of patients, similar to adults. Eventual remission is evident within the first 6 weeks in many, suggesting that earlier intervention among non-responders could be important.

▶ The field continues to benefit from this well-designed longitudinal study of more than 300 children who had treatment-resistant depression. As can be seen in Fig 3 in the original article, the impact of the intervention of adding cognitive behavioral therapy (CBT) to a regimen of a selective serotonin reuptake inhibitor (SSRI) has significant effects; the impact that this report shows continues to grow up to 24 weeks into the intervention. Looking backward, however, it is interesting to see that it is around week 6 that the largest change had occurred on the Children's Depression Rating Scale-Revised scores and that divergence was clear between those who were remitting and those who were not. The message of the Treatment of Resistant Depression in Adolescents (TORDIA) study is that among nonresponders to SSRIs, around 40% will subsequently remit with a change to another SSRI or to venlafaxine. But this study and others continue to not demonstrate tremendous benefit from CBT—at least not as first-line treatment or in the case of greater severity—this will need to be investigated further to determine why this has been found. Of note, 1 benefit of the TORDIA study has been the accumulation of other data, such as the neurobiological status of those who have suicidal events: a study of the TORDIA data[1] shows that the *FKBP5* genotypes of the glucocorticoid receptor were associated with suicidal events in this cohort, which provides ideas about further genomic investigation.

A. H. Mack, MD

Reference

1. Brent D, Melhem N, Ferrell R, et al. Association of FKBP5 polymorphisms with suicidal events in the Treatment of Resistant Depression in Adolescents (TORDIA) study. *Am J Psychiatry.* 2010;167:190-197.

Services and Outcomes

Psychiatric Symptoms Among Juveniles Incarcerated in Adult Prison

Murrie DC, Henderson CE, Vincent GM, et al (Univ of Virginia School of Medicine, Charlottesville; Sam Houston State Univ, Huntsville, TX; Univ of Massachusetts Med School, Worcester)
Psychiatr Serv 60:1092-1097, 2009

Objective.—Although studies reveal substantial mental health treatment needs among youths in the juvenile justice system, far less is known about young offenders transferred to adult criminal court. This statewide study examined the mental health needs of young offenders who committed serious crimes and were transferred to adult court and subsequently incarcerated in a prison for adults.

Methods.—Sixty-four boys aged 16 and 17 years who were incarcerated in the Texas adult correctional system completed the Massachusetts Youth Screening Instrument-Version 2 (MAYSI-2), a mental health screening measure widely used in the juvenile justice system. Scores from the youths in adult prison were compared with those of a matched sample of youths in juvenile correctional facilities, drawn from the MAYSI-2 normative data.

Results.—Youths in adult prison reported substantial symptoms of mental health problems. Most youths surveyed (51%) scored above the highest clinical cutoff (the "warning" range) on at least one MAYSI-2 subscale. For every clinical subscale except suicide ideation, the majority of youths (54% to 70%, depending on the subscale) scored above the "caution" range. Juveniles in adult prison reported higher rates of symptoms than did those in juvenile correctional facilities (effect sizes ranged from d=.18 to d=.65, depending on the subscale).

Conclusions.—Although the mental health needs of youths in the juvenile justice system are well documented, this study reveals that mental health treatment needs appear to be even more pronounced in the small subgroup of youths transferred to the adult criminal justice system and incarcerated in adult prison.

▶ It is important to draw a distinction between juveniles who are in the juvenile justice system versus those in the adult criminal justice system, although those in either system usually carry risk factors for mental disorders. Over the past decade, the child psychiatry literature has included several studies on the rates of disorder among those in the juvenile justice system, but few have assessed, as this study does, those who enter the adult criminal justice system, a system intended to mete out punishment (as opposed to the therapeutic jurisprudence of the juvenile system). This study compares 64 males in the adult system versus juveniles in the juvenile system who were matched—the comparison being measured was the Massachusetts Youth Screening Instrument, a screening instrument widely used in juvenile facilities. The findings demonstrated that those in adult facilities had greater symptomatology. What can be taken from this endeavor? The juvenile justice facilities may be less stressful than adult facilities, that juvenile offenders (those in the adult system) have as many, if not more, risks for mental illness and disabling conditions, and that further efforts to find these cases are needed. The age of those entering the adult criminal justice system continues to drop,[1] and our efforts need to be more and more vigilant as we try to catch up with these trends affecting our nation's youth.

A. H. Mack, MD

Reference

1. Deitch M, Barstow A, Lukens L, Reyna R. *From Time Out to Hard Time: Young Children in the Adult Criminal Justice System.* Austin, TX: The University of Texas at Austin, LBJ School of Public Affairs; 2009.

Adolescent Prescription ADHD Medication Abuse Is Rising Along With Prescriptions for These Medications

Setlik J, Bond GR, Ho M (Univ of Cincinnati, OH)

Pediatrics 124:875-880, 2009

Objective.—We sought to better understand the trend for prescription attention-deficit/hyperactivity disorder (ADHD) medication abuse by teenagers.

Methods.—We queried the American Association of Poison Control Center's National Poison Data System for the years of 1998–2005 for all cases involving people aged 13 to 19 years, for which the reason was intentional abuse or intentional misuse and the substance was a prescription medication used for ADHD treatment. For trend comparison, we sought data on the total number of exposures. In addition, we used teen and preteen ADHD medication sales data from IMS Health's National Disease and Therapeutic Index database to compare poison center call trends with likely availability.

Results.—Calls related to teenaged victims of prescription ADHD medication abuse rose 76%, which is faster than calls for victims of substance abuse generally and teen substance abuse. The annual rate of total and teen exposures was unchanged. Over the 8 years, estimated prescriptions for teenagers and preteenagers increased 133% for amphetamine products, 52% for methylphenidate products, and 80% for both together. Reports of exposure to methylphenidate fell from 78% to 30%, whereas methylphenidate as a percentage of ADHD prescriptions decreased from 66% to 56%. Substance-related abuse calls per million adolescent prescriptions rose 140%.

Conclusions.—The sharp increase, out of proportion to other poison center calls, suggests a rising problem with teen ADHD stimulant medication abuse. Case severity increased over time. Sales data of ADHD medications suggest that the use and call-volume increase reflects availability, but the increase disproportionately involves amphetamines.

▶ All clinicians who are asked to provide stimulant medications are aware of the individual and the public health risks and the liability, which can come from the prescription of these controlled agents. On one hand, there is an intention to provide proper diagnosis and treatment for those with the condition, but the availability of these medications in the wrong hands can lead to dangerous consequences. Studies such as this one demonstrate those risks, as they use collected information from 2 different emergency/poison control databases.

Clearly, the frequency of problems related to stimulants is rising. But it is important to try to learn more about why. Are all of these cases of patients, or are these reports made by nonpatients who have obtained stimulants in inappropriate ways? Moreover, one might ask about a next step—how could the health community answer such questions? For now, the best information is to be aware of this trend and for individual practitioners to exercise care and caution in the prescription of stimulants—the most effective pharmacotherapy for attention-deficit/hyperactivity disorder.

A. H. Mack, MD

Adolescent Outcomes of Childhood Attention-Deficit/Hyperactivity Disorder in a Diverse Community Sample
Bussing R, Mason DM, Bell L, et al (Division of Child and Adolescent Psychiatry at the Univ of Florida in Gainesville; et al)
J Am Acad Child Adolesc Psychiatry 49:595-605, 2010

Objective.—To describe adolescent outcomes of childhood attention-deficit/hyperactivity disorder (ADHD) in a diverse community sample.

Method.—ADHD screening of a school district sample of 1,615 students aged 5 to 11 years was followed by a case-control study 8 years later. High-risk youths meeting full (n = 94) and subthreshold (n = 75) DSM-IV ADHD criteria were matched with demographically similar low-risk peers (n = 163). Outcomes domains included symptom, functional impairment, quality of life, substance use, educational outcomes, and juvenile justice involvement.

Results.—In all, 44% of youths with childhood ADHD had not experienced remission. Compared with unaffected peers, adolescents with childhood ADHD were more likely to display oppositional defiant disorder (odds ratio [OR] = 12.9, 95% confidence interval [CI] 5.6-30.0), anxiety/depression (OR = 10.3, 95% CI 2.7-39.3), significant functional impairment (OR = 3.4, 95% CI 1.7-6.9), reduced quality of life (OR = 2.5, 95% CI 1.3-4.7), and involvement with the juvenile justice system (OR = 3.1, 95% CI 1.0-9.1). Subthreshold ADHD, but not full ADHD, increased the risk of grade retention, whereas both conditions increased the risk of graduation failure. Oppositional defiant disorder (ODD), but not childhood ADHD, increased the risk of cannabis and alcohol use. None of the adolescent outcomes of childhood ADHD were moderated by gender, race or poverty.

Conclusions.—ADHD heralds persistence of ADHD and comorbid symptoms into adolescence, as well as significant risks for functional impairment and juvenile justice involvement. Subthreshold ADHD symptoms typically do not qualify affected students for special educational interventions, yet increase the risk for adverse educational outcomes. Findings stress the importance of early ADHD recognition, especially its comorbid presentation with ODD, for prevention and intervention strategies.

▶ Consistent with the most recent assessments of the data from the Multimodal Treatment Study of Children with ADHD (MTA), this group reviews the persistence of attention-deficit/hyperactivity disorder (ADHD) and associated psychological and social deficits that accompany it throughout adolescence. Like the MTA study before it, the authors demonstrate the significant biological, psychological, and social morbidities that persist with an earlier ADHD diagnosis. This is an excellently designed study: the authors not only utilize 1 school district but also go into various areas, such as juvenile justice facilities. This is important because we need to prepare our patients appropriately and we need to assist our adult colleagues (or our adult practices) when interacting with adults claiming to have ADHD. This review assessed adolescent outcomes, in terms of psychopathology, risk behaviors, substance use, juvenile justice, and quality of life. In this cohort, 44% of those had not remitted in terms of ADHD. This study demonstrates the persistence of these symptoms into adolescence, and it would be helpful to see studies that were as crisp in the adult ADHD period.

A. H. Mack, MD

Brief, Personality-Targeted Coping Skills Interventions and Survival as a Non–Drug User Over a 2-Year Period During Adolescence
Conrod PJ, Castellanos-Ryan N, Strang J (King's College London and South London and Maudsley NHS Foundation Trust, UK)
Arch Gen Psychiatry 67:85-93, 2010

Context.—Selective interventions targeting personality risk are showing promise in the prevention of problematic drinking behavior, but their effect on illicit drug use has yet to be evaluated.

Objective.—To investigate the efficacy of targeted coping skills interventions on illicit drug use in adolescents with personality risk factors for substance misuse.

Design.—Randomized controlled trial.

Setting.—Secondary schools in London, United Kingdom.

Participants.—A total of 5302 students were screened to identify 2028 students aged 13 to 16 years with elevated scores on self-report measures of hopelessness, anxiety sensitivity, impulsivity, and sensation seeking. Seven hundred thirty-two students provided parental consent to participate in this trial.

Intervention.—Participants were randomly assigned to a control no-intervention condition or a 2-session group coping skills intervention targeting 1 of 4 personality profiles.

Main Outcome Measures.—The trial was designed and powered to primarily evaluate the effect of the intervention on the onset, prevalence, and frequency of illicit drug use over a 2-year period.

Results.—Intent-to-treat repeated-measures analyses on continuous measures of drug use revealed time × intervention effects on the number of drugs used ($P < .01$) and drug use frequency ($P < .05$), whereby the control group showed significant growth in the number of drugs used as well as more frequent drug use over the 2-year period relative to the intervention group. Survival analysis using logistic regression revealed that the intervention was associated with reduced odds of taking up the use of marijuana ($\beta = -0.3$; robust SE = 0.2; $P = .09$; odds ratio = 0.7; 95% confidence interval, 0.5-1.0), cocaine ($\beta = -1.4$; robust SE = 0.4; $P < .001$; odds ratio = 0.2; 95% confidence interval, 0.1-0.5), and other drugs ($\beta = -0.7$; robust SE = 0.3; $P = .03$; odds ratio = 0.5; 95% confidence interval, 0.3-0.9) over the 24-month period.

Conclusion.—This study extends the evidence that brief, personality-targeted interventions can prevent the onset and escalation of substance misuse in high-risk adolescents.

Trial Registration.—clinicaltrials.gov Identifier: NCT00344474.

▶ Prevention of substance use among adolescents could not be more of a public health urgency. Unfortunately, too few methods have been shown to be successful. The effects of this intervention are well documented as seen in Fig 2 in the original article, in which use among those who underwent this intervention was less than those who did not. So what is special about this method? First, that the interventions were intensive as they included group interventions targeted at those at risk. Second, that the interventions focused not on resistance to peer pressure but rather became operationalized in terms of the psychological experiences that lead to use. That correlates with the study's stated intention to focus on coping skills during ongoing abstinence. This was a powerful study in that the patient population was greater than 5000. Its generalizability to US populations will be an important next research area. It is an intervention with great potential.

A. H. Mack, MD

Serious Emotional Disturbance Among Youths Exposed to Hurricane Katrina 2 Years Postdisaster

McLaughlin KA, Fairbank JA, Gruber MJ, et al (Harvard Med School, Boston, MA; Duke Univ Med Ctr, Durham, NC; et al)
J Am Acad Child Adolesc Psychiatry 48:1069-1078, 2009

Objective.—To estimate the prevalence of serious emotional disturbance (SED) among children and adolescents exposed to Hurricane Katrina along with the associations of SED with hurricane-related stressors, sociodemographics, and family factors 18 to 27 months after the hurricane.

Method.—A probability sample of prehurricane residents of areas affected by Hurricane Katrina was administered by a telephone survey. Respondents provided information on up to two of their children ($n = 797$) aged 4 to 17 years. The survey assessed hurricane-related stressors and lifetime history of psychopathology in respondents, screened for 12-month SED in respondents' children using the Strengths and Difficulties Questionnaire, and determined whether children's emotional and behavioral problems were attributable to Hurricane Katrina.

Results.—The estimated prevalence of SED was 14.9%, and 9.3% of the youths were estimated to have SED that is directly attributable to Hurricane Katrina. Stress exposure was associated strongly with SED, and 20.3% of the youths with high stress exposure had hurricane-attributable SED. Death of a loved one had the strongest association with SED among prehurricane residents of New Orleans, whereas exposure to physical adversity had the strongest association in the remainder of the sample. Among children with stress exposure, parental psychopathology and poverty were associated with SED.

Conclusions.—The prevalence of SED among youths exposed to Hurricane Katrina remains high 18 to 27 months after the storm, suggesting a substantial need for mental health treatment resources in the hurricane-affected areas. The youths who were exposed to hurricane-related stressors, have a family history of psychopathology, and have lower family incomes are at greatest risk for long-term psychiatric impairment.

▶ Hurricane Katrina and its aftermath continues to be present in our collective perception as natural and man-made disasters with the potential for having

---

TABLE 2.—Distribution of Exposure to Hurricane-Related Stressors (Weighted $N = 797$)

| | New Orleans Metro | | Remainder of Hurricane Area | | Total | |
	%	SE	%	SE	%	SE
Property loss[a]	60.4	2.4	48.1	2.8	52.4	2.0
Physical adversity	36.1	2.4	41.3	2.7	39.5	2.0
Housing adversity[a]	46.6	2.5	31.2	2.5	36.5	1.9
Psychological adversity	24.3	2.2	23.9	2.4	24.1	1.7
Income loss	21.5	2.0	19.7	2.2	20.3	1.6
Loved one victimized	17.7	1.9	13.8	1.9	15.2	1.4
Death of a loved one[a]	18.3	2.0	12.6	2.0	14.6	1.5
Physical illness or injury	11.0	1.6	14.0	1.9	13.0	1.4
Victimization	10.5	1.6	7.9	1.6	8.8	1.2
Life-threatening experience	4.2	1.1	2.0	0.8	2.8	0.6
No. of stressors						
1–2	42.2	2.4	46.3	2.8	44.9	2.0
3–4	29.1	2.2	23.0	2.3	25.1	1.7
5+	15.5	1.9	11.6	1.7	13.0	1.3
Any[a]	86.8	1.6	80.9	2.2	83.0	1.6

Note: Metro = metropolitan area.
[a]Significant difference at the .05 level, two-sided test in the prevalence of exposure between prehurricane respondents of the New Orleans metro and the remainder of the hurricane area.

stimulated cases of posttraumatic stress disorder (PTSD). But it is important to think beyond PTSD—not only in terms of the effects of the original events but also in terms of the lasting damage that has beset New Orleans and the nearby communities (see Table 2 for 1 enumeration among those in this sample). What is measured is not a diagnosis but a concept measured as serious emotional disturbance, and McLaughlin et al describe its prevalence and attempt to relate it to other variables, which is a highly sophisticated approach. This report considers the psychopathology of children as well as families and finds vast and widespread psychiatric morbidity, which calls for equally widespread treatment access and care. Its attention to the type of traumatic or stressful event or to demographics may help in focusing treatment.

A. H. Mack, MD

Association of Hospitalization for Infection in Childhood With Diagnosis of Autism Spectrum Disorders: A Danish Cohort Study
Atladóttir HÓ, Thorsen P, Schendel DE, et al (Univ of Århus, Denmark; Natl Ctr on Birth Defects and Developmental Disabilities, Atlanta, GA; et al)
Arch Pediatr Adolesc Med 164:470-477, 2010

Objective.—To investigate the association between hospitalization for infection in the perinatal/neonatal period or childhood and the diagnosis of autism spectrum disorders (ASDs).

Design.—A population-based cohort study.

Setting.—Denmark.

Participants.—All children born in Denmark from January 1, 1980, through December 31, 2002, comprising a total of 1 418 152 children.

Exposure.—Infection requiring hospitalization.

Main Outcome Measure.—The adjusted hazard ratio (HR) for ASDs among children hospitalized for infection compared with other children.

Results.—A total of 7379 children were diagnosed as having ASDs. Children admitted to the hospital for any infectious disease displayed an increased rate of ASD diagnoses (HR, 1.38 [95% confidence interval, 1.31-1.45]). This association was found to be similar for infectious diseases of bacterial and viral origin. Furthermore, children admitted to the hospital for noninfectious disease also displayed an increased rate of ASD diagnoses (HR, 1.76 [95% confidence interval, 1.68-1.86]), and admissions for infection increased the rate of mental retardation (2.18 [2.06-2.31]).

Conclusions.—The association between hospitalization for infection and ASDs observed in this study does not suggest causality because a general association is observed across different infection groups. Also, the association is not specific for infection or for ASDs. We discuss a number of noncausal explanatory models.

▶ Perhaps more significant than any publication over the past year was the formal rejection of the work that had been the basis of the paranoia over vaccinations as potential causes of autism. There have been continued bona fide investigations into the possibility that some infections may cause autism or the pervasive developmental disorders. However, the authors are able to demonstrate that such a relationship does not account for autism either. In particular, this review of all children born in Denmark from 1980-2002 provides a huge cohort; the finding that a history of hospitalization for infection is important, but not causal, because the infections were of a variety of classes. Perhaps the hospitalization experience itself is causative, or perhaps those with autism are at greater risk for this type of medical experience. Further study may provide explanation, without leading us down another inappropriate cul-de-sac.

A. H. Mack, MD

Prenatal and Infant Exposure to Thimerosal From Vaccines and Immunoglobulins and Risk of Autism
Price CS, Thompson WW, Goodson B, et al (Abt Associates Inc, Cambridge, MA; Ctrs for Disease Control and Prevention, Atlanta, GA; et al)
Pediatrics 126:656-664, 2010

Objective.—Exposure to thimerosal, a mercury-containing preservative that is used in vaccines and immunoglobulin preparations, has been hypothesized to be associated with increased risk of autism spectrum disorder (ASD). This study was designed to examine relationships between prenatal and infant ethylmercury exposure from thimerosal-containing vaccines and/or immunoglobulin preparations and ASD and 2 ASD subcategories: autistic disorder (AD) and ASD with regression.

Methods.—A case-control study was conducted in 3 managed care organizations (MCOs) of 256 children with ASD and 752 controls matched by birth year, gender, and MCO. ASD diagnoses were validated through standardized in-person evaluations. Exposure to thimerosal in vaccines and immunoglobulin preparations was determined from electronic immunization registries, medical charts, and parent interviews. Information on potential confounding factors was obtained from the interviews and medical charts. We used conditional logistic regression to assess associations between ASD, AD, and ASD with regression and exposure to ethylmercury during prenatal, birth-to-1 month, birth-to-7-month, and birth-to-20-month periods.

Results.—There were no findings of increased risk for any of the 3 ASD outcomes. The adjusted odds ratios (95% confidence intervals) for ASD associated with a 2-SD increase in ethylmercury exposure were 1.12 (0.83–1.51) for prenatal exposure, 0.88 (0.62–1.26) for exposure from birth to 1 month, 0.60 (0.36–0.99) for exposure from birth to 7 months, and 0.60 (0.32–0.97) for exposure from birth to 20 months.

Conclusions.—In our study of MCO members, prenatal and early-life exposure to ethylmercury from thimerosal-containing vaccines and immunoglobulin preparations was not related to increased risk of ASDs.

▶ The continued scientific push back to unfounded concerns about the cause of the serious pervasive developmental disorders (PDDs) includes several new approaches to determine the risk that vaccines or preservatives may have caused these conditions. This study is one such novel approach as it first uses a managed care organization population and second that it uses a case control method. Here the risk of thimerosal is specifically studied. The choice of population is important because it uses a group in which compliance with vaccinations may have been greater than in the general population. A benefit of the case control method is that by matching subjects there is greater strength of the controls. Further benefits of this design are that it breaks down diagnosis by type of PDD and prenatal exposure to the substance. It is interesting to consider that in screening controls, the study used the Social Communication Questionnaire to exclude those with an undiagnosed PDD, and some were excluded because of high scores on the questionnaire. This report is the most helpful addition to the fears over thimerosal and vaccines and hopefully will provide information that clinicians may use to improve declines in vaccination rates throughout the United States.

A. H. Mack, MD

Miscellaneous

Effects of Catechol-*O*-Methyltransferase on Normal Variation in the Cognitive Function of Children

Barnett JH, Heron J, Goldman D, et al (Univ of Cambridge, UK; Cambridge Cognition Ltd, UK; Univ of Bristol, UK; et al)
Am J Psychiatry 166:909-916, 2009

Objective.—Genetic variants that contribute to the risk of psychiatric disorders may also affect normal variation in psychological function. Indeed, the behavioral effects of many genetic variants may be better understood as process-specific rather than disease-specific. A functional valine-to-methionine (Val[158]Met) polymorphism in the catechol-O-methyltransferase (COMT) gene has been associated with cognitive function and brain metabolic activity accompanying such tasks. Not all studies are consistent, and less is known about the effect of this polymorphism during development. The authors tested the hypothesis that a more informative COMT haplotype predicts normal cognitive development in a large population-based cohort of children enrolled in the Avon Longitudinal Study of Parents and Children.

Method.—Effects on verbal and performance IQ as well as verbal inhibition were assessed at age 8, and effects on working memory were assessed at age 10. From the five COMT single nucleotide polymorphisms (SNPs) genotyped, the effect of a functional three-SNP haplotype consisting of Val^{158}Met and two synonymous SNPs (rs6269 and rs4818), which together exert a major influence on the level of COMT expression and enzyme activity, was evaluated.

Results.—This three-SNP haplotype predicted both verbal inhibition and working memory, and there was a genotype-by-sex interaction on verbal IQ. The effect of COMT genotype (diplotype) on cognition was curvilinear, which is consistent with the "inverted U" model of dopamine effect on frontal cortical efficiency. In addition, the SNP rs2075507 (previously rs2097603) was independently associated with verbal inhibition, while rs165599 showed no main cognitive effects. However, rs165599 showed a genotype-by-sex interaction with working memory.

Conclusions.—Genetic variation at several loci in the COMT gene affects normal cognitive function in children.

▶ We usually focus on the effects of genetic variation upon illness, but this report provides information about normal variation in cognitive functioning. Two of the study's figures help to portray its findings. Fig 2 in the original article refers to variances in verbal intelligence quotient (IQ) assessment according to catechol-*O*-methyltransferase diplotype for 8-year-old boys but perhaps not for girls; there is a trend among this group of increased verbal IQ. Fig 3 in the original article demonstrates that different types of the rs165599 genotype may be associated with alterations in working memory span among girls aged 10 years, and perhaps the opposite effects may be seen in boys of the same age. It is important for all of us to continue to generate further literacy and comprehension of genetics, as the understanding of mental health is more and more entwined with genetic bases.

A. H. Mack, MD

Practice Parameter for the Assessment and Treatment of Children and Adolescents With Posttraumatic Stress Disorder
Cohen JA, AACAP Work Group On Quality Issues (AACAP Communications Dept, WA)
J Am Acad Child Adolesc Psychiatry 49:414-430, 2010

This Practice Parameter reviews the evidence from research and clinical experience and highlights significant advances in the assessment and treatment of posttraumatic stress disorder since the previous Parameter was published in 1998. It highlights the importance of early identification of posttraumatic stress disorder, the importance of gathering information from parents and children, and the assessment and treatment of comorbid disorders. It presents evidence to support trauma-focused psychotherapy, medications, and a combination of interventions in a multimodal approach.

▶ Pediatricians are impressive because they can attend to the needs of humans ranging from 1-day old to young adults. Child psychiatrists too must master this range and beyond, and the content of this practice parameter includes the stuff that demands the full capacities of the child psychiatrist. The evaluation and treatment of posttraumatic stress disorder (PTSD) in children can range from exposures to violence, witnessing accidents, and many other situations over which children may have little control. Furthermore, the presentation of the condition, when it occurs, may be vastly different among those in this age range, and the ability to assess symptoms or even the fact of a traumatic event requires special skills. And so this practice parameter was sorely needed and is a welcome development as it addresses so many of the problems that arise in this situation. And, as in other recent American Academy of Child and Adolescent Psychiatry practice parameters, the publication is centered around a limited number of recommendations, which cover knowledge, skills, and attitudes. The first recommendation, of the need to screen all patients for traumatic experiences or PTSD symptoms, is something that applies to all clinicians. It provides an excellent review of psychotherapies for children and adolescents with PTSD. All child and adolescent clinicians should read this document closely.

A. H. Mack, MD

2 Psychotherapy

Introduction

In reviewing the titles of this year's collection of studies pertaining to psychotherapy, I am struck by the breadth of treatments, mental health disorders, physical health disorders, target populations, and perspectives that are represented. A number of the studies describe randomized clinical trials (RCTs), the "gold standard" in tests of the efficacy or effectiveness of a given intervention. Yet, even among the RCTs, there are rigorous trials of psychodynamic psychotherapy, behavior therapy, cognitive behavioral analysis system (CBAS), family therapy, cognitive behavior therapy, and cognitive therapy. Further, there is an RCT exploring outcomes with online therapy, a growing area of treatment development and assessment.

In addition to addressing a range of psychiatric disorders (eg, anxiety disorders, depression, bipolar disorder, eating disorders, and Tourette syndrome), some studies explore interventions associated with patients who suffer from diabetes, HIV, and cancer. Among the target populations that were studied are children, adolescents, the elderly, and soldiers, with attention paid to ethnic minorities and health disparities.

Finally, in addition to outcome studies, some of the articles that were reviewed address psychotherapy process variables, an important contribution to a field that is demanding to know more about the mechanisms of change in psychosocial interventions. Overall, this breadth and variety suggest that psychotherapy research is alive and well, branching out to explore a range of topics that are salient to enhancing the evidence base with regard to psychosocial intervention.

Janice L. Krupnick, PhD

Outcome Studies

Attachment-Based Family Therapy for Adolescents with Suicidal Ideation: A Randomized Controlled Trial

Diamond GS, Wintersteen MB, Brown GK, et al (Univ of Pennsylvania School of Medicine, Philadelphia; Thomas Jefferson Univ, Philadelphia, PA; et al)
J Am Acad Child Adolesc Psychiatry 49:122-131, 2010

Objective.—To evaluate whether Attachment-Based Family Therapy (ABFT) is more effective than Enhanced Usual Care (EUC) for reducing suicidal ideation and depressive symptoms in adolescents.

Method.—This was a randomized controlled trial of suicidal adolescents between the ages of 12 and 17, identified in primary care and emergency departments. Of 341 adolescents screened, 66 (70% African American) entered the study for 3 months of treatment. Assessment occurred at baseline, 6 weeks, 12 weeks, and 24 weeks. ABFT consisted of individual and family meetings, and EUC consisted of a facilitated referral to other providers. All participants received weekly monitoring and access to a 24-hour crisis phone. Trajectory of change and clinical recovery were measured for suicidal ideation and depressive symptoms.

Results.—Using intent to treat, patients in ABFT demonstrated significantly greater rates of change on self-reported suicidal ideation at post-treatment evaluation, and benefits were maintained at follow-up, with a strong overall effect size (ES = 0.97). Between-group differences were similar on clinician ratings. Significantly more patients in ABFT met criteria for clinical recovery on suicidal ideation post-treatment (87%; 95% confidence interval [CI] = 74.6–99.6) than patients in EUC (51.7%; 95% CI = 32.4–54.32). Benefits were maintained at follow-up (ABFT, 70%; 95% CI = 52.6–87.4; EUC 34.6%; 95% CI = 15.6–54.2; odds ratio = 4.41). Patterns of depressive symptoms over time were similar, as were results for a subsample of adolescents with diagnosed depression. Retention in ABFT was higher than in EUC (mean = 9.7 versus 2.9).

Conclusions.—ABFT is more efficacious than EUC in reducing suicidal ideation and depressive symptoms in adolescents. Additional research is warranted to confirm treatment efficacy and to test the proposed mechanism of change (the Family Safety Net Study).

Clinical Trial Registry Information.—Preventing Youth Suicide in Primary Care: A Family Model, URL: http://www.clinicaltrials.gov, unique identifier: NCT00604097.

▶ This article addresses an important problem concerning depression and suicidal ideation/attempts in adolescents. It was actually surprising to read in the introduction that so little treatment research has been done with this population, and the study's results with cognitive behavioral therapy and/or antidepressant medication have not been that effective for severely depressed and suicidal adolescents. The authors make a persuasive case for developing and assessing an alternative approach. The model they describe is quite interesting. This manualized family therapy approach is theory based (relying on interpersonal theories), integrative (incorporating behavioral, cognitive, and psychoeducational interventions within a treatment that is primarily process oriented and emotion focused), and focused, with 5 specific tasks that are accomplished with the adolescent alone, parents alone, and parents and adolescent together. It nicely addresses the developmental tasks of an adolescent to separate and become autonomous while aiming to enhance his/her support from parents. There are many things to like about this study. It includes the elements of a gold standard RCT, for example, randomization to treatment, assessments of treatment fidelity, etc. It also addresses a tough to recruit sample of low-income, minority adolescents. It is not surprising that these researchers were not able to recruit the original sample size for which they had hoped. Nevertheless, they did quite well with regard to participant retention. They rightly point out in their section on study limitations that it is not clear whether the significantly better outcomes achieved in the family therapy were due to treatment dose rather than the treatment type. Since retention was so much better in their treatment than in the treatment provided by the community, those in ABFT received a good deal of treatment. Nevertheless, this seems to be an intervention model with a good deal of promise.

J. L. Krupnick, PhD

Clinical Effectiveness of Individual Cognitive Behavioral Therapy for Depressed Older People in Primary Care: A Randomized Controlled Trial

Serfaty MA, Haworth D, Blanchard M, et al (Univ College London; et al)
Arch Gen Psychiatry 66:1332-1340, 2009

Context.—In older people, depressive symptoms are common, psychological adjustment to aging is complex, and associated chronic physical illness limits the use of antidepressants. Despite this, older people are rarely offered psychological interventions, and only 3 randomized controlled trials of individual cognitive behavioral therapy (CBT) in a primary care setting have been published.

Objective.—To determine the clinical effectiveness of CBT delivered in primary care for older people with depression.

Design.—A single-blind, randomized, controlled trial with 4- and 10-month follow-up visits.

Patients.—A total of 204 people aged 65 years or older (mean [SD] age, 74.1 [7.0] years; 79.4% female; 20.6% male) with a Geriatric Mental State diagnosis of depression were recruited from primary care.

Interventions.—Treatment as usual (TAU), TAU plus a talking control (TC), or TAU plus CBT. The TC and CBT were offered over 4 months.

Outcome Measures.—Beck Depression Inventory-II (BDI-II) scores collected at baseline, end of therapy (4 months), and 10 months after the baseline visit. Subsidiary measures were the Beck Anxiety Inventory, Social Functioning Questionnaire, and Euroqol. Intent to treat using

Generalized Estimating Equation and Compliance Average Causal Effect analyses were used.

Results.—Eighty percent of participants were followed up. The mean number of sessions of TC or CBT was just greater than 7. Intent-to-treat analysis found improvements of -3.07 (95% confidence interval [CI], -5.73 to -0.42) and -3.65 (95% CI, -6.18 to -1.12) in BDI-II scores in favor of CBT vs TAU and TC, respectively. Compliance Average Causal Effect analysis compared CBT with TC. A significant benefit of CBT of 0.4 points (95% CI, 0.01 to 0.72) on the BDI-II per therapy session was observed. The cognitive therapy scale showed no difference for nonspecific, but significant differences for specific factors in therapy. Ratings for CBT were high (mean [SD], 54.2 [4.1]).

Conclusion.—Cognitive behavioral therapy is an effective treatment for older people with depressive disorder and appears to be associated with its specific effects.

Trial Registration.—isrctn.org Identifier: ISRCTN18271323.

▶ Depression is a common disorder among the elderly and one that is frequently mistaken for dementia. This makes it particularly important that depressed older people are identified and provided with appropriate and effective treatment. Screening is essential, particularly because numerous studies have shown that depression is often missed. Recruitment in a primary care setting is an excellent idea, given that many depressed older people are unlikely to seek out specialty mental heath care, but primary care physicians frequently fail to ask about or note depression in their patients. This study is an important one in terms of its design and its findings. There is a good sample size, and longer than usual follow-up—10 months rather than the usual 3 months or 6 months. In addition, the researchers were effective in following up 80% of their research participants. An important part of the design was the inclusion of a "talking control" arm that was used to assess the effects of attention. This enabled the researchers to determine that it was not only having someone to talk to, but rather the specific techniques of the mental health intervention that led to positive changes. The adaptations in the cognitive behavioral therapy (CBT) approach that were made for an older sample were interesting, for example , increased structure of the sessions and techniques to facilitate recall. It was not clear, however, what was meant by the modifications "to reflect an English perspective." The quality of life measure that was used, the Euroqol, is not typically used in studies conducted in the United States and might also reflect this English perspective. Since interpersonal therapy has been adapted for use with depressed older people, it is good to have research evidence that a CBT approach works as well, providing different treatment strategies that can be selected based on patient preferences or specific characteristics of the patient.

J. L. Krupnick, PhD

Changes in Self-Schema Structure in Cognitive Therapy for Major Depressive Disorder: A Randomized Clinical Trial

Dozois DJA, Bieling PJ, Patelis-Siotis I, et al (Univ of Western Ontario, London, Canada; St. Joseph's Healthcare McMaster Univ, Hamilton, Canada)
J Consult Clin Psychol 77:1078-1088, 2009

Negative cognitive structure (particularly for interpersonal content) has been shown in some research to persist past a current episode of depression and potentially to be a stable marker of vulnerability for depression. Given that cognitive therapy (CT) is highly effective for treating the acute phase of a depressive episode and that this treatment also reduces the risk of relapse and recurrence, it is possible that CT may alter these stable cognitive structures. In the current study, patients were randomly assigned to CT + pharmacotherapy ($n = 21$) or to pharmacotherapy alone ($n = 21$). Both groups evidenced significant and similar reductions in level of depression (as measured with the Beck Depression Inventory–II and the Hamilton Rating Scale for Depression), as well as automatic thoughts and dysfunctional attitudes. However, group differences were found on cognitive organization in favor of individuals who received the combination of CT + pharmacotherapy. The implications of these results for understanding mechanisms of change in therapy and the prophylactic nature of CT are discussed.

▶ As the authors of this article point out, this study responded to the call for research that further elucidates the deeper structures involved in cognitive change. One could go further in noting that understanding of the deeper structures is important because it appears to be associated with prevention of relapse in depressive disorder. There is a great deal of evidence pointing to a considerable degree of relapse with this disorder and determining ways to reduce vulnerability to relapse is an important public health issue. Confirming that cognitive therapy can alter some of the deeper underlying cognitive structures that give rise to depression and helping to identify possible mechanisms associated with the reduced risk of depressive relapse provides important information for researchers, clinicians, and patients. There were some study weaknesses that should also be noted, however. For example, the sample was quite small (only 21 research participants in each group). Further investigation with a larger sample is needed before these findings have real credibility. Also, the authors emphasize the real worldness of the setting and sample, ie, patients were treated in a tertiary care setting. Yet, the exclusion criteria were quite similar to those seen in efficacy trials. Further, the sample was almost exclusively white (90%), predominantly female (74%), and highly educated, thereby limiting the generalizability of the findings.

J. L. Krupnick, PhD

Mindfulness-Based Cognitive Therapy for Individuals Whose Lives Have Been Affected by Cancer: A Randomized Controlled Trial

Foley E, Baillie A, Huxter M, et al (Macquarie Univ, Sydney, New South Wales, Australia; Lismore Community Mental Health, New South Wales, Australia; et al)

J Consult Clin Psychol 78:72-79, 2010

Objective.—This study evaluated the effectiveness of mindfulness-based cognitive therapy (MBCT) for individuals with a diagnosis of cancer.

Method.—Participants ($N = 115$) diagnosed with cancer, across site and stage, were randomly allocated to either the treatment or the wait-list condition. Treatment was conducted at 1 site, by a single therapist, and involved participation in 8 weekly 2-hr sessions that focused on mindfulness. Participants meditated for up to 1 hr daily and attended an additional full-day session during the course. Participants were assessed before treatment and 10 weeks later; this second assessment occurred immediately after completion of the program for the treatment condition. The treatment condition was also assessed at 3 months postintervention. All postinitial assessments were completed by assessors who were blind to treatment allocation.

Results.—There were large and significant improvements in mindfulness (effect size [ES] $= 0.55$), depression (ES $= 0.83$), anxiety (ES $= 0.59$), and distress (ES $= 0.53$) as well as a trend for quality of life (ES $= 0.30$) for MBCT participants compared to those who had not received the training. The wait-list group was assessed before and after receiving the intervention and demonstrated similar change.

Conclusions.—These improvements represent clinically meaningful change and provide evidence for the provision of MBCT within oncology settings.

▶ Mindfulness-based treatments have become very popular in recent years, especially in terms of mindfulness-based cognitive therapy to prevent depression relapse. Thus, it is not surprising to see this type of intervention adapted for cancer patients who are experiencing anxiety and depression because these types of symptoms are common among these patients. In addition, the fact that there is evidence for the efficacy of Kabat-Zinn's mindfulness-based stress reduction intervention with cancer patients makes it not too much of a stretch to think that the current adaptation might be helpful for cancer patients with depression and anxiety. The focus on cognitive processes, such as reactive and ruminative states of mind, makes a lot of sense for this population because cancer patients are likely to suffer from rumination about their illness. Despite the fact that this article was published in one of the premier psychotherapy outcome journals, there are some aspects of the study that are potentially problematic. For example, there is generally concern about the use of a wait-list these days as the control or comparison group. Perhaps a more active treatment might have been used for comparison purposes. Another problem is the use of only a single therapist; it is generally a good idea to have at least 2 therapists to reduce the likelihood that positive effects are not due possibly to the charismatic personality of a single therapist. In addition, in one page of the article, the authors describe the average baseline levels of the sample as being in the "mild anxiety range for both conditions"; yet, in the Discussion section of the article, the authors write that the sample had "high levels of anxiety." Thus, it is not clear how distressed the sample really was at the baseline. As the authors themselves point out, there are questions about the generalizability of the findings because there was considerable self-selection for the study, and the level of motivation in the sample may as well have increased the effect size of the intervention. Nevertheless, as the authors write, the study does provide support for the use of mindfulness training within oncology settings. The types of adaptations that the authors made to mindfulness-based stress reduction therapy for this sample seem appropriate and useful, and this low-intensity form of intervention does indeed seem "likely to reduce distress and build resilience."

J. L. Krupnick, PhD

Behavior Therapy for Children With Tourette Disorder: A Randomized Controlled Trial

Piacentini J, Woods DW, Scahill L, et al (Univ of California at Los Angeles; Univ of Wisconsin–Milwaukee; Yale Child Study Ctr, New Haven, CT; et al)
JAMA 303:1929-1937, 2010

Context.—Tourette disorder is a chronic and typically impairing childhood-onset neurologic condition. Antipsychotic medications, the first-line treatments for moderate to severe tics, are often associated with adverse effects. Behavioral interventions, although promising, have not been evaluated in large-scale controlled trials.

Objective.—To determine the efficacy of a comprehensive behavioral intervention for reducing tic severity in children and adolescents.

Design, Setting, and Participants.—Randomized, observer-blind, controlled trial of 126 children recruited from December 2004 through May 2007 and aged 9 through 17 years, with impairing Tourette or chronic tic disorder as a primary diagnosis, randomly assigned to 8 sessions during 10 weeks of behavior therapy (n = 61) or a control treatment consisting of supportive therapy and education (n = 65). Responders received 3 monthly booster treatment sessions and were reassessed at 3 and 6 months following treatment.

Intervention.—Comprehensive behavioral intervention.

Main Outcome Measures.—Yale Global Tic Severity Scale (range 0-50, score > 15 indicating clinically significant tics) and Clinical Global Impressions–Improvement Scale (range 1 [very much improved] to 8 [very much worse]).

Results.—Behavioral intervention led to a significantly greater decrease on the Yale Global Tic Severity Scale (24.7 [95% confidence interval {CI}, 23.1-26.3] to 17.1 [95% CI, 15.1-19.1]) from baseline to end point compared with the control treatment (24.6 [95% CI, 23.2-26.0] to 21.1

[95% CI, 19.2-23.0]) (*P* < .001; difference between groups, 4.1; 95% CI, 2.0-6.2) (effect size = 0.68). Significantly more children receiving behavioral intervention compared with those in the control group were rated as being very much improved or much improved on the Clinical Global Impressions–Improvement scale (52.5% vs 18.5%, respectively; *P* < .001; number needed to treat = 3). Attrition was low (12/126, or 9.5%); tic worsening was reported by 4% of children (5/126). Treatment gains were durable, with 87% of available responders to behavior therapy exhibiting continued benefit 6 months following treatment.

Conclusion.—A comprehensive behavioral intervention, compared with supportive therapy and education, resulted in greater improvement in symptom severity among children with Tourette and chronic tic disorder.

Trial Registration.—clinicaltrials.gov Identifier: NCT00218777.

▶ This article describes an excellent study. It is excellent both because it provides compelling evidence of the efficacy of a psychosocial intervention for children with Tourette disorder and also because it meets the gold standard in every respect for a randomized controlled trial. Given that the first-line treatments for moderate to severe tics are antipsychotic medications, it is important to find a less dangerous way of treating this disorder in children and adolescents. As the authors note, Tourette disorder can be associated with considerable impairment and social isolation in school-aged children. However, antipsychotics are associated with tardive dyskinesia, weight gain, and cognitive dulling. Thus, the disorder can be a crippling one for children, but the existing treatment carries the risk of troubling side effects. The habit reversal training that was developed to counter severe tics seems easy to implement and achieves nearly as good effects as medications (see Table 2 in the original article regarding key outcome measures). One can have confidence in the study results because the methodology of the study was very sound. The control treatment controlled for time and attention, research participants were randomized, and several methods were used to maintain the treatment blind. It is likely that the results achieved by clinicians in the community will not be as sturdy as those achieved in the tightly controlled, carefully monitored university setting. This is typically the case as a treatment moves from the university to the community. However, the behavioral intervention it describes provides a promising and useful way to treat a disorder that can wreak havoc on a child or adolescent's life.

J. L. Krupnick, PhD

Short-Term Psychodynamic Psychotherapy and Cognitive-Behavioral Therapy in Generalized Anxiety Disorder: A Randomized, Controlled Trial
Leichsenring F, Salzer S, Jaeger U, et al (Justus-Liebig-Univ Giessen, Germany; Georg-August-Univ Goettingen, Germany; the Asklepios Clinic, Tiefenbrunn, Germany; et al)
Am J Psychiatry 166:875-881, 2009

Objective.—While several studies have shown that cognitive-behavioral therapy (CBT) is an efficacious treatment for generalized anxiety disorder, few studies have addressed the outcome of shortterm psychodynamic psychotherapy, even though this treatment is widely used. The aim of this study was to compare short-term psychodynamic psychotherapy and CBT with regard to treatment outcome in generalized anxiety disorder.

Method.—Patients with generalized anxiety disorder according to DSM-IV were randomly assigned to receive either CBT (N = 29) or short-term psychodynamic psychotherapy (N = 28). Treatments were carried out according to treatment manuals and included up to 30 weekly sessions. The primary outcome measure was the Hamilton Anxiety Rating Scale, which was applied by trained raters blind to the treatment conditions. Assessments were carried out at the completion of treatment and 6 months afterward.

Results.—Both CBT and short-term psychodynamic psychotherapy yielded significant, large, and stable improvements with regard to symptoms of anxiety and depression. No significant differences in outcome were found between treatments in regard to the primary outcome measure. These results were corroborated by two self-report measures of anxiety. In measures of trait anxiety, worry, and depression, however, CBT was found to be superior.

Conclusions.—The results suggest that CBT and short-term psychodynamic psychotherapy are beneficial for patients with generalized anxiety disorder. In future research, large-scale multicenter studies should examine more subtle differences between treatments, including differences in the patients who benefit most from each form of therapy.

▶ Given that the evidence base for the treatment of anxiety disorders has disproportionately favored cognitive-behavioral therapy (CBT) in recent years, one might almost forget that psychodynamic psychotherapy is still often used by practitioners for these conditions. Thus, it is good to see a study that compares CBT with psychodynamic treatment in a randomized controlled trial. The finding that both approaches yield significant, large, and stable improvements, with no significant differences with regard to the primary outcome allows practitioners from different theoretical perspectives to feel comfortable in using whichever modality better suits them and their patients.

It is interesting that this study was conducted in Germany, rather than the United States. In most United States studies, the duration of treatment would likely have been 10 or 12 sessions rather than 30, as it was in this study. This is probably more a function of the different systems of research funding and insurance coverage than a conclusion that a certain number of sessions are needed to address the problem under investigation.

It is also interesting that the study found that CBT was superior in terms of measures of trait anxiety, worry, and depression. Perhaps these findings could be used to further adapt psychodynamic approaches to the treatment of generalized anxiety that focus on cognitive issues in this disorder. These findings could be useful in terms of making both types of treatments even more effective in addressing some of the core problems in this type of disorder.

J. L. Krupnick, PhD

Clinical effectiveness of online computerised cognitive–behavioural therapy without support for depression in primary care: randomised trial
de Graaf LE, Gerhards SAH, Arntz A, et al (Maastricht Univ, The Netherlands; et al)
Br J Psychiatry 195:73-80, 2009

Background.—Computerised cognitive–behavioural therapy (CCBT) might offer a solution to the current undertreatment of depression.

Aims.—To determine the clinical effectiveness of online, unsupported CCBT for depression in primary care.

Method.—Three hundred and three people with depression were randomly allocated to one of three groups: Colour Your Life; treatment as usual (TAU) by a general practitioner; or Colour Your Life and TAU combined. Colour Your Life is an online, multimedia, interactive CCBT programme. No assistance was offered. We had a 6-month follow-up period.

Results.—No significant differences in outcome between the three interventions were found in the intention-to-treat and per protocol analyses.

Conclusions.—Online, unsupported CCBT did not outperform usual care, and the combination of both did not have additional effects. Decrease in depressive symptoms in people with moderate to severe depression was moderate in all three interventions. Online CCBT without support is not beneficial for all individuals with depression.

▶ This study started out with good intentions, but I fear that it ultimately was not terribly well conceptualized. There is considerable literature indicating high rates of depression in primary care and a terrible history of its identification there. Thus, the idea that an effort was being made to identify patients with depression and a comparative effectiveness trial for its treatment was being initiated seemed to be a good idea. Also, the use of an online method of delivering cognitive-behavioral therapy (CBT) seemed to also provide a way to provide at least a minimum dose of an evidence-based treatment, which sounded very reasonable. The major problem with the way this study was conceived, however, is that there was no ongoing contact for research participants who were randomized to the online CBT only. It seems likely that depressed individuals, even with an interactive program, are unlikely to complete the program or to derive as much benefit as they might if there were another person checking in on them. It seems that the lack of assistance may have been a key problem in boosting the effectiveness of this program.

It should be noted that other online CBT programs, eg, one for individuals with substance abuse and another for veterans with posttraumatic stress disorder, seem to be achieving positive results. However, these programs are used as adjunctive treatments, allowing for regular contact with a therapist.

Curiously, the combination of general practitioner provided treatment plus the online program did not provide any benefits over and beyond usual care. Perhaps the usual care component did not address any of the issues that were targeted in the CBT program?

This study does seem to shed more light on the importance of the therapy relationship. If the techniques of CBT have proven effectiveness in the treatment of depression, but there is no assistance in determining whether the patients are using the program or interpreting it correctly, maybe its effectiveness is diminished. If the treatment as usual is not modified to address the issues being raised in the online intervention, maybe it does not reinforce the techniques/concepts being introduced online.

J. L . Krupnick, PhD

Childhood Sexual Abuse Differentially Predicts Outcome of Cognitive-Behavioral Therapy for Deliberate Self-Harm

Spinhoven P, Slee N, Garnefski N, et al (Leiden Univ, The Netherlands; et al)
J Nerv Ment Dis 197:455-457, 2009

This study examined the association of childhood abuse with deliberate self-harm and related psychopathology and the impact of childhood abuse on treatment outcome as assessed in a randomized controlled trial of cognitive-behavioral therapy for 90 young people who recently engaged in Deliberate Self-Harm (DSH). Participants with a history of childhood sexual abuse manifested more Axis I disorders and reported higher levels of DSH, depression, suicidal cognitions, anxiety, and dissociation. After statistically controlling for baseline differences in DSH and related psychopathology, participants with a reported history of childhood sexual abuse showed a significantly lower risk of repeated DSH in the Cognitive-Behavioral Therapy condition compared with those receiving treatment-as-usual (TAU). Our results suggest that a structured treatment format and focus on adequate emotion regulation skills may be essential elements in the treatment of persons with DSH and a history of childhood sexual abuse.

▶ This brief report focused on the treatment outcomes of 90 patients, almost all women, who received cognitive-behavioral treatment in addition to treatment as usual for deliberate self-harm (DSH). It reports some important findings, particularly that the addition of 10 or 12 cognitive-behavioral therapy (CBT) sessions focused specifically on the prevention of DSH significantly reduced the likelihood of later self-harm. Because this is a particularly problematic behavior among many patients with borderline personality, this is a valuable contribution to the treatment literature.

Although there is ample literature to confirm the serious negative impact of sexual abuse, this article provides additional data that confirm this event(s) as one that is associated with multiple psychological and psychiatric problems. It clearly is more disorganizing and disruptive to healthy emotional development than physical abuse alone. Surprisingly, the CBT intervention was more effective for individuals with a childhood sexual abuse history than for those without this history. This is counterintuitive because most previous studies suggest that patients with more initial impairment have less successful therapy outcomes.

It is not clear how this intervention differs from dialectical behavior therapy (DBT), which was developed initially on the same population, ie, those who demonstrated deliberate self-harming behaviors. Both treatments focus on emotional awareness, distress tolerance, and problem-solving skills. The authors suggest the merit of CBT in this study is that it's being individualized and tailored to the specific presenting problem. Does that differ from DBT as typically practiced? It would be useful to know whether the additional problem dimensions addressed in this approach offers anything different from DBT in its focus or approach.

J. L. Krupnick, PhD

What Are the Components of CBT for Psychosis? A Delphi Study
Morrison AP, Barratt S (Univ of Manchester, UK; Greater Manchester West, UK)
Schizophr Bull 36:136-142, 2010

There is strong evidence supporting the implementation of cognitive behavior therapy (CBT) for people with psychosis. However, there are a variety of approaches to the delivery and conceptual underpinnings within different research groups, and the degree of consensus or disagreement regarding what are the intrinsic components has not been explored. This study uses the Delphi method to try to establish what a group of experts in CBT for psychosis view as important. Experts were invited to participate in 3 rounds of producing and rating statements that addressed areas such as principles, assessment, models, formulation, change strategies, homework, and therapists' assumptions in order to consolidate consensus of opinion. Seventy-seven items were endorsed as important or essential for CBT for psychosis by >80% of the panel. These recommendations should ensure greater fidelity in clinical practice, allow greater evaluation of adherence within clinical trials, facilitate the development of competency frameworks, and be of value in relation to training and dissemination of CBT for psychosis.

▶ The authors of this study make some interesting and valid points. In particular, is their assertion that, even though cognitive behaviour therapy (CBT) is a manualized treatment, there is considerable variation in how it is implemented. This is probably true of all manualized treatments, not to mention those that are not manualized. Aiming to identify and codify the aspects of the treatment that experts in the field deem to be essential is a worthwhile endeavor, although it should be noted that it is not really possible to know which techniques account for change without an actual dismantling study in which specific components are isolated and tested in terms of treatment outcome. This study reflects an early, but important, way to identify those components that might be more rigorously assessed in such a study, however. A significant problem with the results they obtained is that so many of the "recommended elements of CBT for psychosis" seem so generic. For example, in terms of "engagement" with the client, the recommended elements include items that would seem relevant for any type of treatment. For example, they include items, such as, "Interventions should be informed by client feedback," and "The client should be allowed and encouraged to express positive and negative reactions regarding therapy." These could most likely be included as elements of client engagement that would be recommended in any form of psychotherapy; they do not seem specific to CBT and these types of nonspecific statements appear throughout their "recommended elements" list.

J. L. Krupnick, PhD

Patient Personality and Outcome in Short-Term Psychodynamic Psychotherapy
Cromer TD, Hilsenroth MJ (The City Univ of New York; Adelphi Univ, Garden City, NY)
J Nerv Ment Dis 198:59-66, 2010

The current study examines pretherapy patient personality characteristics that may be related to outcome in Short-Term Psychodynamic Psychotherapy. The prognostic ability of the Capacity for Dynamic Process Scale (CDPS; Thackrey et al., *A Collection of Psychological Scales*. 1993:57–63) was examined in a sample of 71 outpatient adults seeking treatment at a university-based community clinic. The relationship of CDPS to various outcome variables, including both patient and clinician perspectives, were investigated. A Principal Components Factor Analysis of the items comprising the CDPS was used to identify salient item clusters representing the insight, affective, or relational capacities of patients. Results indicated that the CDPS Total score was positively correlated to several of the outcome measures, but not at a level of significance. Certain CDPS items, and to a greater extent items composing the Insight subscale, demonstrated significant positive relationships to a number of patient and clinician rated outcome measures. Results from the study will be discussed in regard to their applied clinical implications.

▶ Several short-term psychodynamic psychotherapists have provided guidelines for which patients they believe can benefit most from this type of treatment. For example, Sifneos, in his book *Short-Term Anxiety-Provoking Psychotherapy: A Treatment Manual,* identified such characteristics as motivation for change, above-average intelligence, and history of at least one meaningful relationship as pretreatment characteristics that are likely to be associated with positive therapy outcomes. The contribution that this article makes is the application of validated measures to assess pretreatment capacities and then linking them to outcome, identifying with greater specificity and empirical support which patient capacities are most likely to lead to good outcomes. The results of their factor analysis do not yield any great surprises. Patient characteristics, such as the capacity for insight, verbal fluency, and introspectiveness would, on the face of it, seem to bode well for individuals engaging in a type of treatment that focuses on these abilities. It should be noted that there were aspects of the study design that run counter to the way a psychotherapy study is typically conducted. For example, it is unusual for the person who conducts assessments to be the same person who conducts the actual psychotherapy. With the same person filling these dual roles, there is generally too much potential for bias in the ratings. For this particular type of study, this may not have posed as great a problem as it would for an outcome study, however.

J. L. Krupnick, PhD

Disparity in Use of Psychotherapy Offered in Primary Care Between Older African-American and White Adults: Results from a Practice-Based Depression Intervention Trial
Joo JH, Morales KH, de Vries HF, et al (Univ of Pennsylvania, Philadelphia)
J Am Geriatr Soc 58:154-160, 2010

The purpose of this study was to assess ethnic differences in use of psychotherapy (having met at least once with a psychotherapist) for late-life depression in primary care. Participants were identified through a two-stage, age-stratified (60–74, ≥75) depression screening of randomly sampled patients from 20 practices in New York City, Philadelphia, and Pittsburgh in a practice-randomized trial. Practices were randomly assigned to usual care or to an intervention with a depression care manager who worked with primary care physicians to provide algorithm-based care. Depression status based on clinical interview and any use of psychotherapy within the 2-year follow-up interval were the primary dependent variables under study. The focus was on 582 persons with complete data. Participants were sorted into major depression (n = 385, 112 African American and 273 white) and clinically significant minor depression (n = 197, 51 African American and 146 white) based on clinical diagnostic assessment. Persons who selfidentified as African American were less likely than whites to use interpersonal therapy (IPT) if they had minor depression, even after adjusting for potentially influential variables including age, cognitive functioning, and whether the dose of antidepressant was adequate (adjusted odds ratio (AOR) = 0.22, 95%

confidence interval (CI) = 0.06–0.80). Ethnicity was not significantly associated with IPT use in persons with major depression (AOR = 0.71, 95% CI = 0.37–1.37). Older African Americans with minor depression were less likely than whites to use psychotherapy. Targeted strategies are needed to mitigate the disparity in use of psychotherapy.

▶ This is a nicely conducted study that provides further research data about racial disparities in the use of psychotherapy for depression. It is indeed curious that ethnicity was not found to be significantly associated with psychotherapy use with major depression, but there were significant differences with minor depression. Since minor depression may be associated with significant impairment, however, this is still a matter that needs attention. There has been considerable attention paid in recent years to health disparities between whites and minorities, with minorities frequently receiving less adequate treatment. There are also multiple reports of minorities failing to receive psychotherapy or dropping out of treatment prematurely. There are various reasons for this, including mistrust of the mental health system and failures to engage with providers. It was particularly interesting to read in this article that the majority of older adults indicate a preference for psychotherapy over antidepressants, yet only 1% of those interviewed 3 months after an interview about this had reported 4 or more sessions of counseling. Clearly, there are problems in getting psychotherapy to depressed older adults in general. This problem is significantly worse in older African Americans with minor depression. The authors' conclusion that "targeted strategies are needed to mitigate the disparity in the use of psychotherapy" for this population is well taken.

J. L. Krupnick, PhD

Cognitive Behavioral Analysis System of Psychotherapy and Brief Supportive Psychotherapy for Augmentation of Antidepressant Nonresponse in Chronic Depression: The REVAMP Trial
Kocsis JH, Gelenberg AJ, Rothbaum BO, et al (Weill Cornell Med College, New York; Univ of Wisconsin, and Healthcare Technology Systems, Inc, Madison; Emory Univ School of Medicine, Atlanta, GA; et al)
Arch Gen Psychiatry 66:1178-1188, 2009

Context.—Previous studies have found that few chronically depressed patients remit with antidepressant medications alone.

Objective.—To determine the role of adjunctive psychotherapy in the treatment of chronically depressed patients with less than complete response to an initial medication trial.

Design.—This trial compared 12 weeks of (1) continued pharmacotherapy and augmentation with cognitive behavioral analysis system of psychotherapy (CBASP), (2) continued pharmacotherapy and augmentation with brief supportive psychotherapy (BSP), and (3) continued optimized pharmacotherapy (MEDS) alone. We hypothesized that adding

CBASP would produce higher rates of response and remission than adding BSP or continuing MEDS alone.

Setting.—Eight academic sites.

Participants.—Chronically depressed patients with a current *DSM-IV*–defined major depressive episode and persistent depressive symptoms for more than 2 years.

Interventions.—Phase 1 consisted of open-label, algorithm-guided treatment for 12 weeks based on a history of antidepressant response. Patients not achieving remission received next-step pharmacotherapy options with or without adjunctive psychotherapy (phase 2). Individuals undergoing psychotherapy were randomized to receive either CBASP or BSP stratified by phase 1 response, ie, as nonresponders (NRs) or partial responders (PRs).

Main Outcome Measures.—Proportions of remitters, PRs, and NRs and change on Hamilton Scale for Depression (HAM-D) scores.

Results.—In all, 808 participants entered phase 1, of which 491 were classified as NRs or PRs and entered phase 2 (200 received CBASP and MEDS, 195 received BSP and MEDS, and 96 received MEDS only). Mean HAM-D scores dropped from 25.9 to 17.7 in NRs and from 15.2 to 9.9 in PRs. No statistically significant differences emerged among the 3 treatment groups in the proportions of phase 2 remission (15.0%), partial response (22.5%), and nonresponse (62.5%) or in changes on HAM-D scores.

Conclusions.—Although 37.5% of the participants experienced partial response or remitted in phase 2, neither form of adjunctive psychotherapy significantly improved outcomes over that of a flexible, individualized pharmacotherapy regimen alone. A longitudinal assessment of later-emerging benefits is ongoing.

▶ This is a major and important study, although clearly one that yielded unanticipated and probably undesired results. When there are 8 participating academic sites and 491 research participants, a lot of time, energy, and resources went into the conduct of this investigation. The study followed the gold standard in terms of the features of a treatment outcome study. Further, it addressed an important population, ie, chronically depressed patients whose depressive symptoms persisted for more than 2 years.

It is discouraging that only 37.5% of research participants who were randomized into phase 2 of the study, ie, those who did not achieve a complete response to an initial medication trial, achieved remission or a partial response. Thus, more than half of those who were entered into the second phase of the study continued to suffer from depression. The investigators had been optimistic, based on the earlier study of cognitive behavioral analysis system of psychotherapy (CBASP), that they had a method for helping patients with chronic depression. Yet, this study showed that this intervention proved to not be all that they had hoped. This is disappointing news.

Some of their ideas, eg, that with this population a 12-session therapy is not of sufficient duration, make a lot of sense. The same can be said of the suggestion that it might be a good idea to explore particular subsamples, eg, pregnant or nursing women, those with histories of early adversity (by which I imagine they mean child abuse, for example), and those who are motivated for psychotherapy, to see if they have disproportionately better outcomes with CBASP than the participants in this study.

It was particularly striking to read that one-third (32%) of this sample was unemployed at study entry. Perhaps more emphasis on social role functioning might be advisable in treating this population because they clearly have significant impairment in functioning.

J. L. Krupnick, PhD

Women With Bulimic Eating Disorders: When Do They Receive Treatment for an Eating Problem?

Mond JM, Hay PJ, Darby A, et al (LaTrobe Univ, Bundoora, Australia; Univ of Western Sydney, Campbelltown, Australia; James Cook Univ, Townsville, Australia; et al)
J Consult Clin Psychol 77:835-844, 2009

Variables associated with the use of health services were examined in a prospective, community-based study of women with bulimic-type eating disorders who did ($n = 33$) or did not ($n = 58$) receive treatment for an eating problem during a 12-month follow-up period. Participants who received treatment for an eating problem differed from those who did not in several respects, including higher body weight, higher levels of eating disorder psychopathology, general psychological distress, and impairment in role functioning, deficits in specific aspects of coping style, greater awareness of an eating problem, and greater likelihood of prior treatment for a problem with weight. However, the variables most strongly associated with treatment seeking were greater perceived impairment in role functioning specifically associated with an eating problem and greater perceived inability to suppress emotional difficulties. These were the only variables that were significantly associated with treatment seeking in multivariable analysis. The findings suggest that individuals' recognition of the adverse effects of eating-disordered behavior on quality of life may need to be addressed in prevention and early intervention programs for eating disorders.

▶ This is an interesting article and well worth reading for at least 2 reasons. One is the study design. It is a prospective study that uses a community sample. These are design issues that provide access to the larger group of individuals who are suffering from eating disorders, rather than only those who have sought out mental health treatment, and it provides, as well, the ability to follow them and their choices over time. It also provides an intriguing look at the different ways that individuals may perceive and categorize their problems, thereby driving the types of practitioners they seek in dealing with their problems. Unfortunately, the vast majority of individuals who need mental health care do not receive it at all, and many who do seek care obtain it from sources that are not likely to be terribly effective. That certainly proved to be the case in this sample of women with bulimic eating disorders. It does make sense that those who seemed to be struggling more with their emotions and those who perceived greater impairment in their role functioning were more likely than those who felt more able to function in their social roles and who could more effectively manage their emotions, even if that meant suppressing them rather than dealing with them, to seek professional help. In other words, those who were more distressed were more likely to seek help. More interesting is the observation that people may conceptualize their problems differently and seek help accordingly. For example, if someone sees weight as a medical problem, she is more likely to seek help from a primary care provider. Or, others might seek help for a comorbid mental health issues, such as depression. If this is the case, they are unlikely to receive specific treatments aimed at individuals with eating disorders, which have greater evidence for efficacy. As the authors point out, early intervention and education might play a role in pointing people in the direction in which they might receive the most effective treatment for their disorder.

J. L. Krupnick, PhD

Psychological Treatments of Binge Eating Disorder

Wilson GT, Wilfley DE, Agras WS, et al (The State Univ of New Jersey, Piscataway; Washington Univ School of Medicine in St Louis, MO; Stanford Univ School of Medicine, CA)

Arch Gen Psychiatry 67:94-101, 2010

Context.—Interpersonal psychotherapy (IPT) is an effective specialty treatment for binge eating disorder (BED). Behavioral weight loss treatment (BWL) and guided self-help based on cognitive behavior therapy (CBTgsh) have both resulted in short-term reductions in binge eating in obese patients with BED.

Objective.—To test whether patients with BED require specialty therapy beyond BWL and whether IPT is more effective than either BWL or CBTgsh in patients with a high negative affect during a 2-year follow-up.

Design.—Randomized, active control efficacy trial.

Setting.—University outpatient clinics.

Participants.—Two hundred five women and men with a body mass index between 27 and 45 who met *DSM-IV* criteria for BED.

Intervention.—Twenty sessions of IPT or BWL or 10 sessions of CBTgsh during 6 months.

Main Outcome Measures.—Binge eating assessed by the Eating Disorder Examination.

Results.—At 2-year follow-up, both IPT and CBTgsh resulted in greater remission from binge eating than BWL ($P < .05$; odds ratios: BWL vs CBTgsh, 2.3; BWL vs IPT, 2.6; and CBTgsh vs IPT, 1.2). Self-esteem ($P < .05$) and global Eating Disorder Examination ($P < .05$) scores were moderators of treatment outcome. The odds ratios for low and high global Eating Disorder Examination scores were 2.8 for BWL, 2.9 for CBTgsh, and 0.73 for IPT; for self-esteem, they were 2.4 for BWL, 1.9 for CBTgsh, and 0.9 for IPT.

Conclusions.—Interpersonal psychotherapy and CBTgsh are significantly more effective than BWL in eliminating binge eating after 2 years. Guided self-help based on cognitive behavior therapy is a first-line treatment option for most patients with BED, with IPT (or full cognitive behavior therapy) used for patients with low self-esteem and high eating disorder psychopathology.

Trial Registration.—clinicaltrials.gov Identifier: NCT00060762.

▶ One of the major health concerns about Americans at this time is overweight and obesity, making effective treatment of this condition a vital issue in United States health care. A whole industry has grown up to help individuals lose weight—which they often do—but typically people regain all the weight they have lost plus a few extra pounds. This makes the assessment of interventions for binge eating disorder (BED), a condition frequently associated with excessive weight, important. Previous studies have shown that both interpersonal psychotherapy (IPT) and cognitive behavior therapy (CBT), adapted for eating disorders, are effective treatments, but there may not be many clinicians who are trained to provide these interventions. This makes the finding that a guided self-help method can be the first line of attack both efficient and cost-effective. The idea of a stepped care approach seems to be gaining ground in many studies, suggesting that the most expensive and sometimes least available treatments, such as specialized mental health care be recommended only for those with the greatest need. Two aspects of this study make it particularly useful: that it had a long follow-up (2 years) and that it identified those for whom specialty therapy (IPT or CBT) is indicated. Particularly in the case of conditions that are likely to relapse, such as BED, it is important to have long-term follow-up. Many interventions, including diets, may work in the short-term, but those with greater "staying power" yield better results. The authors point to a problem that should get more attention. As they note, only 18% of the sample were minority group members and they had a significantly higher attrition rate. Given the high levels of obesity among African Americans and Latinos, as well as some other minority groups, this study provides further evidence that more attention needs to be paid to the issue of recruitment and retention of minorities for studies such as these.

J. L. Krupnick, PhD

A Community-Based Treatment for Native American Historical Trauma: Prospects for Evidence-Based Practice

Gone JP (Univ of Michigan, Ann Arbor)
J Consult Clin Psychol 77:751-762, 2009

Nineteen staff and clients in a Native American healing lodge were interviewed regarding the therapeutic approach used to address the legacy of Native American historical trauma. On the basis of thematic content analysis of interviews, 4 components of healing discourse emerged. First, clients were understood by their counselors to carry pain, leading to adult dysfunction, including substance abuse. Second, counselors believed that such pain must be confessed in order to purge its deleterious influence. Third, the cathartic expression of such pain was said by counselors to inaugurate lifelong habits of introspection and self-improvement. Finally, this healing journey entailed a reclamation of indigenous heritage, identity, and spirituality that program staff thought would neutralize the pathogenic effects of colonization. Consideration of this healing discourse suggests that one important way for psychologists to bridge evidence-based and culturally sensitive treatment paradigms is to partner with indigenous programs in the exploration of locally determined therapeutic outcomes for existing culturally sensitive interventions that are maximally responsive to community needs and interests.

▶ This is a fascinating article about treatment development and outcome assessment for Native Americans. It describes the origins of a community-based treatment that was developed by conducting interviews with administrators, counselors, and clients of a program that offers psychological help to Aboriginal people. The author takes issue with the usual point of departure in trying to address the needs of minority patients, suggesting that adapting existing evidence-based therapies is not the most useful way to make intervention most relevant for non-Europeans. He suggests that a treatment that originates from the community it aims to serve can be more therapeutic than modifying an existing therapy that was derived from western sources.

At the heart of this treatment model is the notion of the soul-destroying consequences of historical trauma, ie, the colonization of Native peoples and the robbing of their culture and language. There is a heavy emphasis on the consequences of the sexual and physical abuse that many Native Americans experienced in the context of the residential schools to which they were sent.

The main point of this article is that mainstream psychological services, even if they are modified in some minor ways to address some of the cultural sensitivities of those receiving these services, are doomed to fail because they are based upon European and European American culture. In the case of the Native Americans, it is not helpful to think of someone as having a substance disorder. Rather, the focus should be on the trauma, whether it is physical, sexual, and/or historical, that led to the emotional pain that led to the desire to numb the pain.

Interestingly, many of the themes that emerged from the community-based treatment are not that dissimilar from western-oriented psychotherapy. For example, western therapies incorporate the idea that individuals carry pain from their childhoods that can lead to adult dysfunction. Western therapies also include the idea that expression of one's emotional pain is part of the healing process. The emphasis on spiritual practices as a means of healing is also incorporated into some types of treatment. What the author convincingly conveys, however, is the importance of truly understanding the nature of the pain that a particular group has undergone, not only as individuals but also as a group or culture. The need to bring an understanding of the group's culture in determining appropriate assessment of the intervention is also addressed.

J. L. Krupnick, PhD

Racial and Ethnic Disparities in Use of Psychotherapy: Evidence From U.S. National Survey Data
Chen J, Rizzo J (City Univ of New York, Staten Island; Stony Brook Univ, NY)
Psychiatr Serv 61:364-372, 2010

Objective.—This study investigated racial and ethnic disparities in psychotherapy use and expenditures in the United States and identified important factors associated with these disparities.

Methods.—Using the Medical Expenditure Panel Survey from 1996 to 2006, the investigators performed bivariate and multivariable analyses to estimate racial and ethnic disparities in the probability of receiving any psychotherapy, total psychotherapy expenditures, and out-of-pocket-payment share for 7,376 patients with depressive or anxiety disorders. Blinder-Oaxaca decomposition techniques were used to identify the most important factors associated with these disparities.

Results.—Caucasians were more likely to use psychotherapy than Latinos (57% versus 52%, p<.001), but there was no significant difference between Caucasians and African Americans in the probability of receiving any psychotherapy. Caucasians self-paid 29% of the total cost for each visit, significantly higher than the shares paid by Latinos (19%) and African Americans (14%). Racial-ethnic differences in the propensity to utilize psychotherapy vanished in multivariable regression, but Caucasians still paid a significantly higher out-of-pocket share than others. English proficiency was the most important factor associated with racial-ethnic disparities in psychotherapy use. The extensive Medicaid coverage among Latinos and African Americans was the main reason for their lower out-of-pocket payment for psychotherapy compared with Caucasians.

Conclusions.—This study found little evidence of racial and ethnic disparities in access to psychotherapy services. Health care reforms affecting mental health coverage under Medicaid would significantly affect psychotherapy expenditure and use among Latinos and African Americans.

▶ This article is of particular interest because of its conclusion that there was little evidence of racial and ethnic disparities in access to psychotherapy services. This finding flies in the face of previous studies, including the 1999 US Surgeon General's report that indicated that ethnic minority groups are significantly undertreated and have less access to psychotherapy services. Of particular note is the use of a nationally representative data set from 1996 to 2006, indicating that this study used a large, relatively recent, representative set of figures on which to base their conclusions. The study points to issues other than socioeconomic status in drawing conclusions. While African Americans and Latinos were more likely than whites to have public health insurance, this did not seem to be the determining factor in whether different groups sought psychosocial intervention. Rather, there were differences that were more based on cultural factors, such as language barriers and possibly citizenship status, that made more of a difference in seeking help than financial barriers. These findings emphasize the need to further adapt treatments to better fit racial-ethnic interpretations of emotional symptoms as well as dealing with the stigma that certain racial-ethnic groups might attach to mental health treatment seeking. This is of particular importance, given the repeated finding that Latinos and African Americans are more likely than whites to suffer from worse mental health status.

J. L. Krupnick, PhD

Changing Network Support for Drinking: Network Support Project 2-Year Follow-Up
Litt MD, Kadden RM, Kabela-Cormier E, et al (Univ of Connecticut Health Ctr, Farmington)
J Consult Clin Psychol 77:229-242, 2009

The Network Support Project was designed to determine whether a treatment could lead patients to change their social network from one that supports drinking to one that supports sobriety. This study reports 2-year posttreatment outcomes. Alcohol-dependent men and women ($N = 210$) were randomly assigned to 1 of 3 outpatient treatment conditions: network support (NS), network support + contingency management (NS + CM), or case management (CaseM, a control condition). Analysis of drinking rates indicated that the NS condition yielded up to 20% more days abstinent than the other conditions at 2 years posttreatment. NS treatment also resulted in greater increases at 15 months in social network support for abstinence, as well as in AA attendance and AA involvement than did the other conditions. Latent growth modeling suggested that social network changes were accompanied by increases in self-efficacy and coping that were strongly predictive of long-term drinking outcomes.

The findings indicate that a network support treatment can effect long-term adaptive changes in drinkers' social networks and that these changes contribute to improved drinking outcomes in the long term.

▶ This is an important study, not only because it is well conducted in terms of its methodological sophistication, but also because of its relatively long-term follow-up of treatment for a disorder with a high rate of relapse. As the authors indicate in the introduction, one-third of individuals who are treated for alcohol problems relapse in the first 3 months after treatment is completed while 65% of patients continue to drink 1 year after alcoholism treatment. Therefore, following patients for 2 years posttreatment is important in determining the long-term efficacy of the intervention.

The role of social networks in understanding many health problems has been reported quite a bit in recent years. Some groundbreaking research has been conducted that show the centrality of social networks in disorders/behaviors/conditions as disparate as obesity, smoking, and substance abuse. This article identifies the importance of increasing the number of abstinent friends as a crucial piece of alcoholism treatment.

Another important component of the study is the emphasis not only on the outcome of a network support intervention relative to 2 other treatments, but also its elucidation of 2 proposed mechanisms of change, ie, self-efficacy and coping. The former is identified as an area of emphasis in motivational interviewing as well as in network support intervention, so this may turn out to be a crucial part of any effective intervention for problem drinking.

It is interesting that the network intervention alone was more effective than this intervention plus contingency management. One might think that getting 2 interventions believed to be effective might be at least as effective as just the one, and this was not the case. It is always fascinating when research results are counterintuitive. Maybe, it also lends credence to the idea that parents should not pay their children for good grades. The intrinsic satisfaction of achieving one's goals outweighs the external reinforcement. The success of network support in encouraging and reinforcing participation in Alcoholics Anonymous (AA) is also impressive.

J. L. Krupnick, PhD

Partner Violence Before and After Couples-Based Alcoholism Treatment for Female Alcoholic Patients
Schumm JA, O'Farrell TJ, Murphy CM, et al (Harvard Med School, Boston, MA; VA Boston Healthcare System, West Roxbury, MA; Univ of Maryland, Baltimore County)
J Consult Clin Psychol 77:1136-1146, 2009

This study examined partner violence before and in the 1st and 2nd year after behavioral couples therapy (BCT) for 103 married or cohabiting women seeking alcohol dependence treatment and their male partners; it used a demographically matched nonalcoholic comparison sample. The treatment sample received $M = 16.7$ BCT sessions over 5–6 months. Follow-up rates for the treatment sample at Years 1 and 2 were 88% and 83%, respectively. In the year before BCT, 68% of female alcoholic patients had been violent toward their male partner, nearly 5 times the comparison sample rate of 15%. In the year after BCT, violence prevalence decreased significantly to 31% of the treatment sample. Women were classified as remitted after treatment if they demonstrated abstinence or minimal substance use and no serious consequences related to substance use. In Year 1 following BCT, 45% were classified as remitted, and 49% were classified as remitted in Year 2. Among remitted patients in the year after BCT, violence prevalence of 22% did not differ from the comparison sample and was significantly lower than the rate among relapsed patients (38%). Results for male-perpetrated violence and for the 2nd year after BCT were similar to the 1st year. Results supported predictions that partner violence would decrease after BCT and that clinically significant violence reductions to the level of a nonalcoholic comparison sample would occur for patients whose alcoholism was remitted after BCT. These findings replicate previous research among men with alcoholism.

▶ This is a well-conducted study that includes most of the gold standard elements of a strong efficacy study, for example, a manualized treatment, commonly used psychometrically valid instruments, measurement of adherence and competence, etc. Predoctoral psychology interns are typically not considered to be sufficiently experienced to serve as therapists in many efficacy studies, but it seems that they had extensive training and supervision. What is most interesting about this study is its focus on female alcoholic patients and partner violence. One typically thinks of partner violence as associated with men as the perpetrators. There is ample evidence that alcohol is frequently involved in partner violence when the perpetrator of the violence is a man, but less information when the alcoholic member of the dyad is a woman. Here it seems that the substance abuse makes the alcoholic woman vulnerable to receipt of violence or to perpertrate violence. The strength of this study is the 2-year follow-up because the rates of relapse in substance abuse treatment are high. It would have been more helpful, however, for the authors to break down their results in terms of verbal aggression and physical aggression since the latter is of much greater concern. Nevertheless, the couples approach seems to be an effective one in reducing partner violence among women who remitted following the treatment of alcoholism.

J. L. Krupnick, PhD

Outcomes of an integrated cognitive behaviour therapy (CBT) treatment program for co-occurring depression and substance misuse in young people

Hides L, Carroll S, Catania L, et al (Univ of Melbourne, Victoria, Australia; et al)

J Affective Disord 121:169-174, 2010

Background.—There are high rates of co-occurring depression among young people with substance use disorders. While there is preliminary evidence for the effectiveness of integrated cognitive behaviour therapy (CBT) in combination with antidepressants among alcohol and substance dependent adolescents and adults with co-existing depression, no studies have examined the effectiveness of integrated CBT interventions in the absence of pharmacotherapy. The aim of the current study was to determine the outcomes of an integrated CBT intervention for co-occurring depression and substance misuse in young people presenting to a mental health setting.

Methods.—Sixty young people (aged 15 to 25), with a DSM-IV diagnosis of Major Depressive Disorder and concurrent substance misuse (at least weekly use in the past month) or disorder were recruited from a public youth mental health service in Melbourne, Australia. Participants received 10 sessions of individual integrated CBT treatment delivered with case management over a 20-week period.

Results.—The intervention was associated with significant improvements in depression, anxiety, substance use, coping skills, depressive and substance use cognitions and functioning at mid- (10 weeks) and post- (20 weeks) treatment. These changes were maintained at 6 months follow-up (44 weeks).

Conclusions.—These results provide preliminary evidence for the effectiveness of the integrated CBT intervention in young people with co-occurring depression and substance misuse. Further studies using randomised controlled designs are required to determine its efficacy.

▶ This article describes a pilot study that is hardly definitive , but it does provide some useful and promising data. The added value of this study over at least a few that preceded it using the same treatment approach is that it offered the psychosocial treatment without concurrent antidepressant medication. Since there has been a good deal of concern about the use of antidepressants with adolescents (despite suicide rates among adolescents falling while such medication was widely prescribed), there is understandably greater interest in finding treatments that might be effective without the use of medication. What is not particularly clear is whether this study added components that were not present in the earlier studies of integrated cognitive behavior therapy for co-occurring depression and substance misuse in young people. This study included both case management and mindfulness skills, whereas the others may not have. It would be interesting to know a bit more about what the weekly 1-hour case management appointments consisted of, which mindfulness skills were taught, and what the authors concluded about the addition of these components. It was also interesting to note that more than half of the research participants were unemployed, and 41.5% had met criteria for childhood conduct disorder. This seems relevant in terms of potential prevention efforts. Since such a substantial proportion of young people with comorbid depression and substance misuse disorders also had conduct disorders during childhood, one could think about targeting this population when they are younger to try to stave off the later difficulties.

J. L. Krupnick, PhD

Design of a family-based lifestyle intervention for youth with type 2 diabetes: the TODAY study
The TODAY Study Group (Washington Univ School of Medicine, St Louis, MO)
Int J Obes 34:217-226, 2010

Type 2 diabetes is associated with obesity and is increasing at an alarming rate in youth. Although weight loss through lifestyle change is one of the primary treatment recommendations for adults with type 2 diabetes, the efficacy of this approach has not been tested with youth. This paper provides a summary of the reviews and meta-analyses of pediatric weight-loss interventions that informed the design and implementation of an intensive, family-based lifestyle weight management program for adolescents with type 2 diabetes and their families developed for the Treatment Options for type 2 Diabetes in Adolescents and Youth (TODAY) study. A total of 1092 youth have been screened, and 704 families have been randomized for inclusion in this 15-center clinical trial sponsored by the National Institutes of Health. The TODAY study is designed to test three approaches (metformin, metformin plus rosiglitazone and metformin plus an intensive lifestyle intervention) to the treatment of a diverse cohort of youth, 10–17 years of age, within 2 years of their diagnosis. The principal goal of the TODAY Lifestyle Program (TLP) is to decrease baseline weight of youth by 7–10% (or the equivalent for children who are growing in height) through changes in eating and physical activity habits, and to sustain these changes through ongoing treatment contact. The TLP is implemented by interventionists called Personal Activity and Nutrition Leaders (PALs) and delivered to youth with type 2 diabetes, and at least one family support person. The TLP provides a model for taking a comprehensive, continuous care approach to the treatment of severe overweight in youth with comorbid medical conditions such as type 2 diabetes.

▶ While this report does not address a psychotherapy study per se, it does describe the design of a behavioral intervention that is aimed at weight reduction and lifestyle changes in severely overweight youths with comorbid type 2 diabetes. What is most impressive about this study is its size and scope, including 15 centers and 704 participating families. The design is based on theory and previous empirical studies, and it includes 3 phases—an acute phase, a maintenance phase, and a continued contact phase. This approach makes a lot of sense because it is well known that behavioral change involving weight reduction and maintenance is a long-term process. Interestingly, the lead author of this article, describing the study and rationale for the approach, has done considerable psychotherapy research, investigating interpersonal and behavioral approaches for the treatment of binge eating disorder. Thus she and, undoubtedly, her many colleagues in this endeavor are experienced researchers in the treatment of eating disorders and behavioral treatments. Of particular note is that the study sample is almost three-fourths minority, with a similar number of Hispanic and black research participants. Since these are the populations that suffer disproportionately from obesity and type 2 diabetes, it is great that the researchers were able to recruit and retain these families. The adaptations that the researchers made to retain their families are also the strength of the approach. For example, they agreed to meet people in the community if it was too difficult for research participants to go to the clinic. They also included funds for a toolbox, allowing them to purchase goods, such as a calculator to add up calories. In this way, they were able to individualize a standardized treatment, making it relevant and useful for the specific individuals and families who participated. The provisions made to anticipate relapse are also assets to enhance the likely success of the intervention. It is increasingly being recognized that behavioral interventions are an important component in the treatment of many medical conditions. This study looks like a carefully thought-through way to make a difference in the national epidemic of obesity.

J. L. Krupnick, PhD

Multisystemic Therapy for Adolescents With Poorly Controlled Type 1 Diabetes: Reduced diabetic ketoacidosis admissions and related costs over 24 months

Ellis D, Naar-King S, Templin T, et al (Wayne State Univ, Detroit, MI; et al)
Diabetes Care 31:1746-1747, 2008

Objective.—The study aim was to determine if multisystemic therapy (MST), an intensive home-based psychotherapy, could reduce hospital admissions for diabetic ketoacidosis (DKA) in youth with poorly controlled type 1 diabetes over 24 months. Potential cost savings from reductions in admissions were also evaluated.

Research Design and Methods.—A total of 127youth were randomly assigned to MST or control groups and also received standard medical care.

Results.—Youth who received MST had significantly fewer hospital admissions than control subjects ($\chi^2 = 11.77$, 4 d.f., $n = 127$; $P = 0.019$). MST-treated youth had significantly fewer admissions versus their baseline rate at 6-month ($P = 0.004$), 12-month ($P = 0.021$), 18-month ($P = 0.046$), and 24-month follow-up ($P = 0.034$). Cost to provide MST was 6, 934 USD per youth; however, substantial cost offsets occurred from reductions in DKA admissions.

Conclusions.—The study demonstrates the value of intensive behavioral interventions for high-risk youth with diabetes for reducing one of the most serious consequences of medication noncompliance.

▶ This report focuses on a specific aspect of a larger study on the efficacy of an intensive home-based family therapy for youth with chronically poor metabolic control in type 1 diabetes. Earlier reports on this sample indicated that research participants receiving this treatment, relative to a control group that received standard medical care, had fewer hospital admissions due to serious nonadherence to treatment, both at termination of treatment and also 6 months later. This report looked at hospital admissions at the conclusion of the trial, ie, at 24-month follow-up and comparative costs for each of the groups. The results showed that the multisystemic therapy (MST) group had significantly fewer hospital admissions at each assessment point and, not surprisingly, this led to substantial cost savings because of fewer hospital admissions.

This study is particularly interesting at a time when the issue of health care reform and the rising costs of health care are center stage in discussions of public policy. The results of the study point the way to a psychosocial approach that is both effective and cost saving.

There are considerable data that suggest metabolic control of diabetes is particularly difficult among adolescents who may resist taking their insulin because they do not want to be different from others their age and who may feel ashamed of their differences. They may also want to eat the same way that their friends are eating, leading to difficulties in maintaining glucose levels. What is particularly interesting in this study is the demonstration of the role that the family and the larger community has to play in helping these adolescents maintain their health regimens. Rather than relying on the emotional resources of the adolescent him/herself, this approach focused on the individual's support system, ie, family, school, and health care system, as well, obviously to good effect. It is also notable that the treatment was home based, making the intervention one that adapted to the needs of the patients/families and increasing the likelihood of the intervention actually being received.

Two issues are of particular salience here. One is the use of adapting methods to increase the likelihood of their receipt. The other is the importance of assessing costs. Demonstrating methods to improve health in a cost-effective manner is of great importance. Also, demonstrating the ways that psychosocial interventions play a role in the management of physical illness is another important contribution.

J. L. Krupnick, PhD

Group-Based Randomized Trial of Contingencies for Health and Abstinence in HIV Patients
Petry NM, Weinstock J, Alessi SM, et al (Univ of Connecticut Health Ctr, Farmington, CT; et al)
J Consult Clin Psychol 78:89-97, 2010

Objective.—Contingency management (CM) treatments are usually applied individually for drug abstinence, but CM can also be targeted toward health behaviors and implemented in groups. This study evaluated effects of a group-based CM intervention that focused on reinforcing health behaviors.

Method.—HIV-positive patients with cocaine or opioid use disorders ($n = 170$) were randomized to weekly CM or 12-step (TS) groups for 24 weeks (mean attendance was 10.8 ± 8.1 sessions for CM participants and 9.0 ± 6.9 session for TS participants). During the treatment period, both groups received compensation for attendance ($10 per session) and submission of urine samples (about $2 per sample). In addition, participants received $25 for submitting samples and completing evaluations at Months 1, 3, 6, 9, and 12; 65–75 of the 81 participants assigned to TS and 71–80 of the 89 participants assigned to CM completed these evaluations. During the treatment period, patients in the CM group received chances to win prizes contingent upon completing health activities and submitting substance-free specimens ($M = \$260$, $SD = \$267$).

Results.—Mean attendance was 10.8 ± 8.1 sessions for CM participants and 9.0 ± 6.9 sessions for TS participants. CM participants submitted a significantly greater number of consecutive drug-free specimens than did TS participants (5.2 ± 6.0 vs. 3.7 ± 5.6), but proportions of negative samples did not differ between groups during treatment or at follow-up evaluations. From pre- to posttreatment, CM participants showed greater reductions in viral loads and HIV-risk behaviors than did TS participants, but these effects were not maintained throughout the follow-up period.

Conclusions.—These data suggest the efficacy of group-based CM for HIV-positive substance abusers, but more research is needed to extend the long-term benefits.

▶ This study addressed a very difficult population, that is, patients with substance abuse/dependence disorders and HIV infection. Since contingency management treatments have support for the treatment of drug abusers, it is not surprising that the authors sought to test its efficacy for drug abusers with HIV infection. Their finding that this type of treatment was more effective than a 12-step intervention in terms of reducing sexual risk behavior and patients' viral load suggests that this is a type of treatment that is worth pursuing. There were aspects of the study that are quite problematic. As the authors themselves indicate, there is a real question of generalizability when research participants are paid to attend sessions. This may be what is needed to get people to sessions, but one must question how many sessions would be attended if these rewards were not provided. If the sessions were not attended as regularly as they were, would participants have made the gains that they achieved? There is also the question of what gains are being retained, if behavior reverts back once the reinforcement is withdrawn. In contrast to other types of interventions, it is not clear what skills or insights are being internalized, or do participants comply only when reinforcement is actively dispensed? Since HIV infection is now a chronic illness, with the need for strong adherence to a medication regimen, ongoing compliance is essential. It would have been valuable for the authors to discuss the benefits and drawbacks of using contingency management as a group-based treatment, rather than individual treatment.

J. L. Krupnick, PhD

Testing the Efficacy of Theoretically Derived Improvements in the Treatment of Social Phobia
Rapee RM, Gaston JE, Abbott MJ (Macquarie Univ, Sydney, Australia; Univ of Sydney, Australia)
J Consult Clin Psychol 77:317-327, 2009

Recent theoretical models of social phobia suggest that targeting several specific cognitive factors in treatment should enhance treatment efficacy over that of more traditional skills-based treatment programs. In the current study, 195 people with social phobia were randomly allocated to 1 of 3 treatments: standard cognitive restructuring plus in vivo exposure, an "enhanced" treatment that augmented the standard program with several additional treatment techniques (e.g., performance feedback, attention retraining), and a nonspecific (stress management) treatment. The enhanced treatment demonstrated significantly greater effects on diagnoses, diagnostic severity, and anxiety during a speech. The specific treatments failed to differ significantly on self-report measures of social anxiety symptoms and life interference, although they were both significantly better than the nonspecific treatment. The enhanced treatment also showed significantly greater effects than standard treatment on 2 putative process measures: cost of negative evaluation and negative views of one's skills and appearance. Changes on these process variables mediated differences between the treatments on changes in diagnostic severity.

▶ An important lesson that can be gleaned from this study is that, even if one already has a treatment with demonstrated efficacy, there is always room for improvement. The authors write that existing cognitive-behavioral therapy (CBT) treatments for social phobia, comprising exposure and cognitive restructuring, have produced changes of approximately 0.9 standard deviations at the end of treatment, and these changes have been maintained for up to 12 months. The goal of this study was to determine whether a new and improved enhanced treatment that targeted several specific cognitive factors could improve upon the traditional treatment. Because cognitive restructuring has long been considered key in this approach for this disorder, recent findings about specific cognitive distortions were incorporated into the enhanced treatment. In terms of theory building and basing treatments on theoretical underpinnings, it makes sense to integrate new findings.

A puzzling aspect of the authors' approach is their use of group rather than individual therapy. They note that the group format may have limited variance among the treatments that were used while also indicating that there is some evidence that group treatment of social phobia may not produce as large effects as individual delivery. Given this, it is not clear why they chose to use a group modality.

Overall, this was a well-conducted study, using therapists who were well versed in the treatment method, appropriate measures, and the standard intention-to-treat analyses. They included assessments of treatment integrity to ascertain that the treatments provided were consistent with the techniques of that method. There was a large N. The study makes an important contribution to the literature in indicating specific process variables that made a difference to treatment outcome.

J. L. Krupnick, PhD

Expressive Writing for Gay-Related Stress: Psychosocial Benefits and Mechanisms Underlying Improvement
Pachankis JE, Goldfried MR (Yeshiva Univ, Bronx, NY; Stony Brook Univ, Bronx, NY)
J Consult Clin Psychol 78:98-110, 2010

Objective.—This study tested the effectiveness of an expressive writing intervention for gay men on outcomes related to psychosocial functioning.

Method.—Seventy-seven gay male college students (mean age = 20.19 years, $SD = 1.99$) were randomly assigned to write for 20 min a day for 3 consecutive days about either (a) the most stressful or traumatic gay-related event in their lives or (b) a neutral topic. We tested an exposure-based hypothesis of written emotional expression by asking half of the participants who were assigned to write about gay-related stress to read their previous day's narrative before writing, whereas the other half did not. Posttest and 3-month follow-up outcomes were assessed with common measures of overall psychological distress, depression, physical health symptoms, and positive and negative affect. Gay-specific social functioning was assessed with measures of gay-related rejection sensitivity, gay-specific self-esteem, and items regarding openness and comfort with one's sexual orientation.

Results.—Participants who wrote about gay-related stress, regardless of whether they read their previous day's writing, reported significantly greater openness with their sexual orientation 3 months following writing than participants who wrote about a neutral topic, $F(1, 74) = 6.66$, $p < .05$, $\eta^2 = .08$. Additional analyses examined the impact of emotional engagement in the writing, severity of the expressed topic, previous disclosure of writing topic, tendency to conceal, and level of perceived social support on mental health outcomes.

Conclusions.—The findings suggest that an expressive writing task targeting gay-related stress can improve gay men's psychosocial functioning, especially openness with sexual orientation. The intervention seems to be particularly beneficial for those men who write about more severe topics and for those with lower levels of social support. The findings suggest future tests of expressive writing tasks for different aspects of stigma-related stress.

▶ This study adds to the already extensive literature on the usefulness of expressive writing about stress and trauma that was initiated by Pennebaker and colleagues in the 1980s. It extends this type of intervention to deal with stresses related to being a gay man in today's society, an identity that may be accompanied by discrimination, job loss, and even physical violence. Of particular usefulness in this study was the exploration of various process variables to try to understand how and why this intervention works. It was interesting that the component of exposure, operationalized as reading the writing before proceeding with the next day's writing, did not turn out to be essential in promoting change. It is also notable that high engagement with the writing without a corrective third party, in terms of helping the research participant revise erroneous schemas or attitudes was not useful. This suggests that a writing intervention with more therapist involvement, perhaps commenting on the writing as it is progressing, might be more effective than just having people write as a way of coming to terms with their shame and other negative emotions about their sexual orientation or any other stress. This is a nonstigmatizing low-cost method of reaching individuals that could be particularly effective with people who are reluctant to seek out specialty care mental health services.

J. L. Krupnick, PhD

Specific Personality Traits Evoke Different Countertransference Reactions: An Empirical Study
Rossberg JI, Karterud S, Pedersen G, et al (Ullevaal Univ Hosp, Oslo, Norway; The Norwegian Network of Psychotherapeutic Day Hosps, Oslo; et al)
J Nerv Ment Dis 196:702-708, 2008

The main aim of this study was to examine the relationship between patients' self-reported personality characteristics, treatment outcome and therapists' countertransference reactions. Eleven therapists filled in the Feeling Word Checklist 58 (FWC-58) for each patient admitted to a day treatment program. The patients completed the Circumplex of Interpersonal Problems (CIP) at admission and discharge. Outcome measures were assessed at the end of treatment. At the start of treatment, therapists reported fewer feelings of rejection and being on guard in response to patients who reported high avoidant, exploitable, overly nurturing and intrusive CIP subscale traits. At the end of the treatment, the CIP subscales of being domineering, vindictive and cold correlated with fewer positive and more negative countertransference feelings. The study revealed a strong relationship between improvement and countertransference feelings. This study confirms clinical narratives on relationships between the therapists' countertransference reactions and patients' reported interpersonal problems and outcome.

▶ This is a relatively slight study looking at the relationship between patients' self-reported personality characteristics, therapists' reactions to certain types of patients, and overall treatment outcome. Not surprisingly, certain patient characteristics correlated with more negative feelings on the therapists' part. Unfortunately, because this was a correlational study, one does not learn the point at which the therapists' negative feelings emerged. Thus, it is not possible to understand the process by which certain patient characteristics became problematic for the therapist. Did certain patients just wear their therapists down over time because they were domineering, cold, and vindictive or did the therapists have negative feelings because they felt unable to help these patients? Perhaps the patients with those characteristics were sicker patients who were more difficult to engage. It seems likely that patients who reported a high level of conscientiousness, a trait associated with fewer feelings of rejection in the therapists, worked harder in therapy, making the therapists feel that they were getting somewhere.

The authors note that therapists could use their countertransference feelings of being rejected and inadequate as a warning signal that the treatment is likely to have a less positive outcome. It would have been helpful if they had some advice about how to use reactions to help the patient. It seems likely that therapists would know when a treatment is not going well. The challenge is figuring out a way to turn that around. It is far easier to treat patients who are likable and capable of engaging in a therapeutic relationship. Finding a way to empathize with individuals who make one feel inadequate and rejected is far more difficult. The fact that the authors took an empirical approach to this problem is a positive step because research will not necessarily confirm clinical assumptions. The testing of methods for enhancing the therapeutic alliance with difficult to treat patients would be a useful next step.

J. L. Krupnick, PhD

Cost-effectiveness of psychotherapy for cluster B personality disorders
Soeteman DI, Verheul R, Delimon J, et al (Erasmus Med Ctr, Rotterdam, The Netherlands; Univ of Amsterdam, The Netherlands; VISPD, Halsteren, The Netherlands)
Br J Psychiatry 196:396-403, 2010

Background.—Recommendations on current clinical guidelines are informed by limited economic evidence.

Aims.—A formal economic evaluation of three modalities of psychotherapy for patients with cluster B personality disorders.

Method.—A probabilistic decision-analytic model to assess the cost-effectiveness of out-patient, day hospital and in-patient psychotherapy over 5 years in terms of cost per recovered patient-year and cost per quality-adjusted life-year (QALY). Analyses were conducted from both societal and payer perspectives.

Results.—From the societal perspective, the most cost-effective choice switched from out-patient to day hospital psychotherapy at a threshold of €12 274 per recovered patient-year; and from day hospital to in-patient psychotherapy at €113 298. In terms of cost per QALY, the optimal strategy changed at €56 325 and €286 493 per QALY respectively. From the payer perspective, the switch points were at €9895 and €155 797 per recovered patient-year, and €43 427 and €561 188 per QALY.

Conclusions.—Out-patient psychotherapy and day hospital psychotherapy are the optimal treatments for patients with cluster B personality disorders in terms of cost per recovered patient-year and cost per QALY.

▶ Given the current concerns about health care expenditures and, particularly, concerns about the use and potential abuse of mental health care services, studies on the cost-effectiveness of psychotherapy are always welcome. It is unfortunate that there are no more studies of this type that are conducted. It is of particular interest that the authors turned their attention to psychotherapy for personality disorders because treatments of this sort are typically of longer duration and greater expense. At the same time, patients with personality disorders, such as borderline personality disorder and antisocial personality disorder, are also extremely costly to society in terms of the services they use. It was surprising to me that the authors addressed cluster B personality disorders as a group, especially because the literature has typically suggested that antisocial personality disorder is not effectively treated in psychotherapy. The authors make a case for there being a "partially common nature to these disorders," noting that "several treatments with demonstrated efficacy for borderline personality disorder are being adapted and tested for antisocial personality disorder." One gets the sense from this article that the focus is more on these 2 disorders than the other disorders in the B cluster (ie, histrionic and narcissistic personality disorders). There are many strengths to this study, including the focus on both payer and societal perspectives, the longer term look (ie, over 5 years) at outcomes, and state-of-the-art economic methods. At the same time, I was not sure about the division of treatment into outpatient, day hospital, and inpatient status, as the treatment groups provide a lot of clarity when studying the cluster B population. In the case of patients with borderline personality disorder, it would seem that at some points, based on the patient's clinical status, any one of these approaches would have validity. For example, a patient with borderline personality disorder might need to be hospitalized if he/she made a suicide attempt or might need a day hospital for a period of time posthospitalization, even if these options were more costly than the outpatient treatment. Except for court-mandated treatment, it's not clear how frequently patients with antisocial personality disorder wind up in any kind of psychotherapy. It would seem that patients with histrionic or narcissistic personality disorders would be less likely to need day hospital or inpatient treatment. In short, I am all in favor of cost-effectiveness analyses, but I'm less enthusiastic about grouping and analyzing all cluster B personality disorders for such examination.

J. L. Krupnick, PhD

Cognitive–Behavioral Therapy Versus Usual Clinical Care for Youth Depression: An Initial Test of Transportability to Community Clinics and Clinicians
Weisz JR, Southam-Gerow MA, Gordis EB, et al (Harvard Univ and Judge Baker Children's Ctr, MA; Virginia Commonwealth Univ; State Univ of New York; et al)
J Consult Clin Psychol 77:383-396, 2009

Community clinic therapists were randomized to (a) brief training and supervision in cognitive-behavioral therapy (CBT) for youth depression or (b) usual care (UC). The therapists treated 57 youths (56% girls), ages 8–15, of whom 33% were Caucasian, 26% were African American, and 26% were Latino/Latina. Most youths were from low-income families and all had *Diagnostic and Statistical Manual of Mental Disorders* (4th ed.; American Psychiatric Association, 1994) depressive disorders (plus multiple comorbidities). All youths were randomized to CBT or UC and treated until normal termination. Session coding showed more use of CBT by CBT therapists and more psychodynamic and family approaches by UC therapists. At posttreatment, depression symptom measures were at subclinical levels, and 75% of youths had no remaining depressive disorder, but CBT and UC groups did not differ on these outcomes. However, compared with UC, CBT was (a) briefer (24 vs. 39 weeks), (b) superior in parent-rated therapeutic alliance, (c) less likely to require additional services (including all psychotropics combined and depression medication in particular), and (d) less costly. The findings showed advantages for CBT in parent engagement, reduced use of medication and other services, overall cost, and possibly speed of improvement—a hypothesis that warrants testing in future research.

▶ This is a nicely conducted study that addresses an important topic, ie, transporting evidence-based psychological treatments to sites outside of university-based clinics. It has frequently been found that outcomes in university-based efficacy trials are much better than those in effectiveness trials where there is far less control over patient selection and extensive training and supervision of therapists. Further, those methods that have the greatest evidence base are often not practiced out in the "real world." This study attempted to bridge that gap by providing brief training and supervision of cognitive-behavioral therapy (CBT), a treatment with a substantial evidence base, but less frequent application at community clinics, and comparing outcomes with usual care.

The outcomes of the 2 groups, ie, CBT versus usual care, were not significantly different, but the authors point out the advantages of the CBT method in that it was briefer, less costly, and required fewer additional services. All of these differences would suggest that CBT offered important advantages over the other approaches used. What the authors do not emphasize though is the fact that the CBT group was getting regular supervision and oversight of their work, making it possible that even though the CBT was a relatively new treatment for the therapists who used it, the deck may have been "stacked" in the CBT direction because of the supervision of experts in this method. For this reason, it would be useful to do a follow-up study to see if the therapists who were trained in CBT continued to use the method and whether further down the line, when the CBT therapists were no longer having supervision or as much attention paid to their work, the results are comparable.

What is particularly striking about this study is its thoughtfulness. The authors provided good empirical reasons for every study design choice they made. In addition, they took care to try to be even-handed about their approach. For example, they did not select only the best therapists to provide CBT, even though they had hypothesized that CBT would be the superior treatment for youths with depression. They made a point of addressing all 3 major effectiveness trial dimensions (as described in the article), allowing the reader to have great confidence in their results. Of greatest note is their conclusion that evidence-based treatments can be taught to clinicians in practice with relatively little time and cost.

J. L. Krupnick, PhD

Battlemind Debriefing and Battlemind Training as Early Interventions With Soldiers Returning From Iraq: Randomization by Platoon
Adler AB, Bliese PD, McGurk D, et al (Walter Reed Army Inst of Res, Heidelberg, Germany; Walter Reed Army Inst of Res, Silver Spring, MD)
J Consult Clin Psychol 77:928-940, 2009

Researchers have found that there is an increase in mental heath problems as a result of military-related traumatic events, and such problems increase in the months following return from combat. Nevertheless, researchers have not assessed the impact of early intervention efforts with this at-risk population. In the present study, the authors compared different early interventions with 2,297 U.S. soldiers following a year-long deployment to Iraq. Platoons were randomly assigned to standard postdeployment stress education, Battlemind debriefing, and small and large group Battlemind training. Results from a 4-month follow-up with 1,060 participants showed those with high levels of combat exposure who received Battlemind debriefing reported fewer posttraumatic stress symptoms, depression symptoms, and sleep problems than those in stress education. Small group Battlemind training participants with high combat exposure reported fewer posttraumatic stress symptoms and sleep problems than stress education participants. Compared to stress education participants, large group Battlemind training participants with high combat exposure reported fewer posttraumatic stress symptoms and lower levels of stigma and, regardless of combat exposure, reported fewer depression symptoms. Findings demonstrate that brief early interventions have the potential to be effective with at-risk occupational groups.

▶ Arguably, some of the most interesting treatment development and comparative treatment effectiveness research going on at the moment, particularly with regard to posttraumatic stress disorder (PTSD), pertains to interventions for military personnel. The armed forces are, understandably, very concerned about the high rates of personnel returning from deployments in Iraq and Afghanistan with PTSD and comorbid conditions. A particular emphasis has been on the development of interventions that might prevent or diminish the effects of combat stress, known to be a major precipitant for PTSD. This study compared the efficacy of different types of interventions adapted for military personnel who had experienced combat deployment, using standard stress education as a treatment as usual condition. One of the comparison groups was a kind of debriefing they called Battlemind debriefing. Given recent studies that indicate that debriefing as a stress-related intervention might be unhelpful or even harmful, the authors make a point of differentiating their debriefing method with some other debriefings. As they indicate in this article, the military is a good occupational context in which to examine psychological debriefing efficacy and group debriefing is consistent with military tradition. Their hypotheses in this domain proved to be true, given the finding that this type of intervention was more effective than standard stress education. Something that was particularly striking was the size of the groups that were studied. Typically, group sizes in psychotherapy studies include approximately 6 to 8 members, but with the military, small groups ranged from 18 to 45 individuals, and large groups had 126 to 225 members. Stress education was conducted in groups of 51 to 257. One really has to shift gears in thinking about groups when considering these interventions. It is unfortunate that the follow-up rate was so low (approximately half the sample was lost to follow-up). However, this was a function of deployment rather than lack of interest in the study, and there is probably not much that could be done under the circumstances to increase retention rates. Overall, the adaptations that were made to make the interventions specific to the population were creative and clearly paid off in terms of the improved responses to the Battlemind interventions relative to stress education.

J. L. Krupnick, PhD

The Impact of Narcissism on Drop-Out From Cognitive–Behavioral Therapy for the Eating Disorders: A Pilot Study

Campbell MA, Waller G, Pistrang N (Univ College London, UK; King's College London, UK)
J Nerv Ment Dis 197:278-281, 2009

This study examined the relationship between narcissism and drop-out from the early stage of cognitive behavioral therapy (CBT) for the eating disorders. Narcissism was defined in terms of both its core elements and the narcissistic defense styles. The participants were 41 patients presenting for CBT at a specialist eating disorders service. Each completed measures of narcissism and eating disorder psychopathology. Attendance at sessions was also recorded. The presence of the narcissistically abused personality defense style was associated with a higher likelihood of dropping out of outpatient CBT. This "martyred" form of narcissism appears to have a significant role in the adherence to treatment for the eating disorders. The limitations and the clinical implications of this preliminary research are discussed, and future directions for research are suggested.

▶ This is a relatively small study ($N = 41$ patients), and only a pilot study, but it makes some interesting points regarding successful treatment for cognitive-behavioral therapy (CBT) for eating disorders. It addresses the issue of treatment retention for patients with this type of problem and, of course, patients are more likely to derive success from treatment if they complete a full course of sessions than if they terminate prematurely. The focus in this study was looking at the role of personality pathology in predicting treatment retention.

The finding that patients who have a certain type of narcissistic vulnerability are more likely than patients who do not have this vulnerability to discontinue treatment is intriguing. The view that others are hostile and over-demanding, making the patient feel martyred, has obvious implications for the development of the therapeutic alliance. These are issues that typically are not focused on in CBT treatments, but perhaps should be.

J. L. Krupnick, PhD

Unique and Common Mechanisms of Change Across Cognitive and Dynamic Psychotherapies

Gibbons MBC, Crits-Christoph P, Barber JP, et al (Univ of Pennsylvania)
J Consult Clin Psychol 77:801-813, 2009

The goal of this article was to examine theoretically important mechanisms of change in psychotherapy outcome across different types of treatment. Specifically, the role of gains in self-understanding, acquisition of compensatory skills, and improvements in views of the self were examined. A pooled study database collected at the University of Pennsylvania Center for Psychotherapy Research, which includes studies conducted from 1995 to 2002 evaluating the efficacy of cognitive and psychodynamic therapies for a variety of disorders, was used. Patient samples included major depressive disorder, generalized anxiety disorder, panic disorder, borderline personality disorder, and adolescent anxiety disorders. A common assessment battery of mechanism and outcome measures was given at treatment intake, termination, and 6-month follow-up for all 184 patients. Improvements in self-understanding, compensatory skills, and views of the self were all associated with symptom change across the diverse psychotherapies. Changes in self-understanding and compensatory skills across treatment were predictive of follow-up symptom course. Changes in self-understanding demonstrated specificity of change to dynamic psychotherapy.

▶ The study of change mechanisms in psychotherapy has assumed a great deal of interest and investigation in recent years. Researchers are interested in identifying the techniques and therapeutic behaviors that are linked to outcome as both a way of scientifically understanding what takes place in the so-called black box of treatment and as a means to improve existing interventions. The assumption is that by disentangling the specific therapist behaviors that lead to therapeutic change, clinicians can be encouraged to use those techniques and treatments that can incorporate more of those types of interventions. Since the theoretical bases of different types of therapeutic approaches differ, it has been assumed that the active ingredients in different types of therapy would be different. For example, psychoanalytic theory posits that interpretation of the transference is the key mechanism in psychodynamic psychotherapy, whereas focus on interpersonal relationships has been found to be related to positive outcome in interpersonal psychotherapy. Cognitive therapy focuses on the central role of changing maladaptive thoughts and attitudes while exposure therapy posits that it is essential to activate the fear structure to eliminate conditioned anxiety. What makes this study particularly interesting is its exploration of theoretically relevant mechanism variables across different types of treatment. One of the findings, that self-understanding changed more in dynamic psychotherapies than in cognitive therapies, was expected, given that the encouragement of insight is a major focus in this type of treatment. The finding that changes in compensatory skills were common across the dynamic and cognitive therapies was more of a surprise because the focus on skills is more commonly associated with the cognitive approaches. This article makes an important contribution to our understanding of the issues and foci that lead to change in psychotherapy.

J. L. Krupnick, PhD

Expressed Emotion Moderates the Effects of Family-Focused Treatment for Bipolar Adolescents
Miklowitz DJ, Axelson DA, George EL, et al (Univ of Colorado, Boulder; Univ of Pittsburgh School of Medicine, PA; et al)
J Am Acad Child Adolesc Psychiatry 48:643-651, 2009

Objective.—Family interventions have been found to be effective in pediatric bipolar disorder (BD). This study examined the moderating effects of parental expressed emotion (EE) on the 2-year symptomatic outcomes of adolescent BD patients assigned to family-focused therapy for adolescents (FFT-A) or a brief psychoeducational treatment (enhanced care [EC]).

Method.—A referred sample of 58 adolescents (mean age 14.5 ± 1.6 years, range 13–17 years) with BD I, II, or not otherwise specified was randomly allocated after a mood episode to FFT-A or EC, both with protocol pharmacotherapy. Levels of EE (criticism, hostility, or emotional overinvolvement) in parents were assessed through structured interviews. Adolescents and parents in FFT-A underwent 21 sessions in 9 months of psychoeducation, communication training, and problem-solving skills training, whereas adolescents and parents in EC underwent 3 psychoeducation sessions. Independent "blind" evaluators assessed adolescents' depressive and manic symptoms every 3 to 6 months for 2 years.

Results.—Parents rated high in EE described their families as lower in cohesion and adaptability than parents rated low in EE. Adolescents in high-EE families showed greater reductions in depressive and manic symptoms in FFT-A than in EC. Differential effects of FFT-A were not found among adolescents in low-EE families. The results could not be attributed to differences in medication regimens.

Conclusions.—Parental EE moderates the impact of family intervention on the symptomatic trajectory of adolescent BD. Assessing EE before family interventions may help determine which patients are most likely to benefit from treatment.

▶ This article describes a well-conducted study that extends findings about family-focused therapy for adults with bipolar illness to adolescents. There is a good deal of evidence for the efficacy of the family-focused approach for patients with bipolar disorder, so it is an advance to learn a bit more about the subgroups for whom this approach is effective and the factors that might contribute to its efficacy. As the article notes, there has been considerable focus in psychotherapy research in the past couple of years on trying to identify the mechanisms of change in psychosocial treatments that have been found effective in outcome studies. This study addressed just that issue, finding that family-focused therapy was more effective in reducing depressive and manic symptoms in patients with bipolar illness whose families have high expressed emotion (EE). This makes sense because it is these families that have the more dysfunctional communication patterns. This is a factor that has previously been studied quite a bit in families of patients with schizophrenia, so it is not unexpected that it would be explored in another diagnostic group. It also seems that measuring this family characteristic could be quite useful in determining the type of psychosocial intervention that would be of greatest use for a given family in which a member has bipolar illness.

J. L. Krupnick, PhD

Mediators of Psychotherapy Outcome

Personality, Stressful Life Events, and Treatment Response in Major Depression
Bulmash E, Harkness KL, Stewart JG, et al (Queen's Univ, Kingston, Ontario, Canada)
J Consult Clin Psychol 77:1067-1077, 2009

The current study examined whether the personality traits of self-criticism or dependency moderated the effect of stressful life events on treatment response. Depressed outpatients ($N = 113$) were randomized to 16 weeks of cognitive–behavioral therapy, interpersonal psychotherapy, or antidepressant medication (ADM). Stressful life events were assessed with the Bedford College Life Events and Difficulties Schedule. Severe events reported during or immediately prior to treatment predicted poor response in the ADM condition but not in the psychotherapy conditions. In contrast, nonsevere life events experienced prior to onset predicted superior response to treatment. Further, self-criticism moderated the relation of severe life events to outcome across conditions, such that in the presence of severe stress those high in self-criticism were less likely to respond to treatment than were those low in self-criticism.

▶ The links among personality, stressful life events, and vulnerability to depression have been studied for more than 3 decades, but the associations among personality, stressful life events, and treatment response are less explored. The potential for identifying ways to help depressed patients who do not benefit from evidence-based interventions makes this a fruitful area for investigation. This is a well-conducted study, using randomization to manualized treatments, and commonly used measures to assess depression as well as commonly accepted definitions for treatment response and remission. A major advance in the assessment of life events is the use of the Life Events and Difficulties Schedule (LEDS), an interviewer-rated measure, rather than the use of self-report instruments. Most of the inclusion/exclusion criteria were the same as in treatment studies of depression, although it is not clear why potential research participants with borderline personality (individuals who frequently suffer from depression) were excluded. One might argue that their sample was skewed in the direction of greater treatment responsiveness because of all the comorbidities that were excluded. The confirmation that individuals who are high in self-criticism are less likely to have good outcomes in the face of severe stress is an important finding, with implications for the way such individuals may be helped. This is potentially very useful information given the high number of individuals who do not receive adequate help from even standardized treatments as typically administered. The identification of pretreatment factors that promote or hinder treatment response, as well as potential ways to enhance treatment efficacy, provide important contributions to the literature.

J. L. Krupnick, PhD

3 Alcohol and Substance Abuse

Introduction

The passage in the United States Congress of a major overhaul of health care, leading to increased benefits for the uninsured and parity for mental health including addictions is likely in the next 5 years to widen access to care for patients with substance-related disorders. The government is trying to get primary care doctors and the health care system to diagnose greater numbers of patients with substance abuse problems earlier in order to prevent the costly complications of chronic use that ultimately add to both increased suffering and increased health care costs. The need for research on the most effective targeted treatments for addictive disorders has never been greater, and the need for new pharmaceutical drugs and possibly vaccines that could help is also great.

This year, proposals for a new nomenclature for substance-related disorders in preparation for DSM-V have been brought forth, with severity criteria replacing "abuse," and the term "addiction" reintroduced after years of being removed because of negative stereotypes. In the DSM-II, "addiction" was linked with personality disorders, and in the 1960s it was felt necessary to drop the term because it stigmatized this population. The return of the term may indicate that destigmatization efforts and the surgeon general's use of the term "addiction" have led to an evolving acceptance of it. Controversy over whether these and other changes in nomenclature are needed has been considerable.

Richard J. Frances, MD

Neuroscience Advances

Nicotine Dependence Is Characterized by Disordered Reward Processing in a Network Driving Motivation

Bühler M, Vollstädt-Klein S, Kobiella A, et al (Univ of Heidelberg, Germany; et al)

Biol Psychiatry 67:745-752, 2010

Background.—Drug addiction is characterized by an unhealthy priority for drug consumption with a compulsive, uncontrolled drug-intake pattern due to a disordered motivational system. However, only some individuals become addicted, whereas others maintain regular but controlled drug use. Whether the transition occurs might depend on how individuals process drug relative to nondrug reward.

Methods.—We applied functional magnetic resonance imaging to measure mesocorticolimbic activity to stimuli predicting monetary or

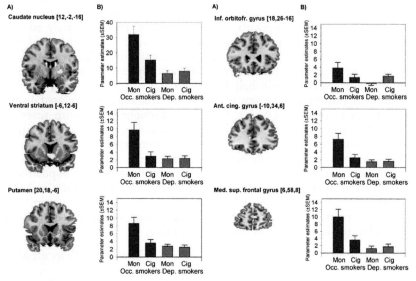

FIGURE 4.—Anticipatory brain activity to monetary and cigarette reward predicting stimuli in dependent compared with occasional smokers in the motivation task. (A) Statistical parametric maps and (B) blood oxygen level–dependent response data of single peak voxels (mean ± SEM) showing that occasional smokers activated significantly more in response to stimuli predicting increasing monetary reward compared with cigarette reward with no significant differences in anticipatory brain activity in the group of dependent smokers (significant interaction between dependence [occasional smokers, dependent smokers] and reward category [money, cigarettes]). The statistical parametric maps were overlaid on a template T1-weighted magnetic resonance image at $p \leq .001$ uncorrected. Slices correspond to local maxima illustrated in Table 1. Ant, anterior; Cig, cigarettes; cing, cingulate; dep., dependent; Inf., inferior; Med sup, medial superior; Mon, Money; Occ., occasional; orbitofr., orbitofrontal. (Reprinted from Bühler M, Vollstädt-Klein S, Kobiella A, et al. Nicotine dependence is characterized by disordered reward processing in a network driving motivation. *Biol Psychiatry.* 2010;67:745-752, with permission from the Society of Biological Psychiatry.)

cigarette reward, together with behavioral assessment of subsequent motivation to obtain the respective reward on a trial-by-trial basis, in 21 nicotine-dependent and 21 nondependent, occasional smokers.

Results.—Occasional smokers showed increased reactivity of the mesocorticolimbic system to stimuli predicting monetary reward relative to cigarette reward and subsequently spent more effort to obtain money. In the group of dependent smokers, we found equivalent anticipatory activity and subsequent instrumental response rates for both reward types. Additionally, anticipatory mesocorticolimbic activation predicted subsequent motivation to obtain reward.

Conclusions.—This imbalance in the incentive salience of drug relative to nondrug reward-predicting cues, in a network that drives motivation to obtain reward, could represent a central mechanism of drug addiction.

▶ Motivation is a key factor in all dependent behavior, and how it is affected by drugs is indeed a very important subject. Motivation to use or stop use of tobacco products is an area that is fertile for research. This article finds support for addiction to tobacco being affected by hijacking of the brain's reward systems by nicotine in the case of tobacco dependence (Fig 4). I might also infer that study is on motivational approaches to treatment as well as studies of how psychotherapy using the transtheoretical model and motivational interviewing treatments leads to effects on reversing brain changes also are needed. The issue of how an individual gains back free will and control over impulses in recovery is the key to understand the process of rehabilitation.

R. J. Frances, MD

Auditory P300 Event-Related Potentials and Neurocognitive Functions in Opioid Dependent Men and Their Brothers

Singh SM, Basu D, Kohli A, et al (Postgraduate Inst of Med Education & Res (PGIMER), Chandigarh, India)
Am J Addict 18:198-205, 2009

Event-related-potentials (especially P300) and cognitive functioning as potential endophenotypes have not been studied in opioid dependence. We compared auditory P300 and cognitive functions in opioid-dependent men, their brothers and normal controls in an exploratory study with a view to find shared genetic factors in the development of opioid dependence. Twenty abstinent opioid-dependent males, their brothers and twenty matched controls were administered Wisconsin card sorting test (WCST), digit span test, trail making test-B, and auditory event-related potentials (P300) from an oddball task were recorded. The opioid dependent group performed the worst, the brothers group was intermediate, and the control group performed the best on tests of WCST, digit span and trail making test-B. The opioid dependent group had the smallest amplitudes and longest latencies of P300, and was followed by the brothers group who had an intermediate position and the control group who had the largest amplitudes and the shortest latencies. P300 and executive neuro-cognitive functions can be considered endophenotypes for the genetic study of vulnerability to opioid dependence. These are reflective of executive dysfunction and disrupted behavioral inhibition and the intermediate position of brothers suggests a common genetic substrate as a component of the etiology.

▶ The P300 event-related evoked potential has long been studied as a biological marker for alcoholism. The search for biological markers for addiction is now worldwide, and this Indian study extends the earlier findings to opioid-dependent men. The most interesting finding is that the P300 evoked potentials, an indication of executive neurocognitive functions, were intermediary in the brothers of opioid-dependent individuals, compared with controls and their dependent brothers. This indicates that the P300 changes are not only just the result of addiction, but also lay the basis to a genetic predisposition, with P300 as a biological marker, perhaps even with the potential for etiologic significance. The fact that a high percentage of opioid addicts also may be prone to alcoholism could be a factor in this finding, and the whole question of the biologic underpinnings and the genetics of choice of a "king drug" in those prone to addiction needs further study.

R. J. Frances, MD

Risk Factors

A Developmental Twin Study of Church Attendance and Alcohol and Nicotine Consumption: A Model for Analyzing the Changing Impact of Genes and Environment
Kendler KS, Myers J (Virginia Commonwealth Univ School of Medicine, Richmond)
Am J Psychiatry 166:1150-1155, 2009

Objective.—Church attendance is one of the most consistent predictors of alcohol and nicotine consumption. The authors sought to clarify changes in the role of genetic and environmental factors in influencing church attendance and the interrelationship between church attendance and alcohol and nicotine use from early adolescence into adulthood.

Method.—The authors used data from two interview waves 6 years apart of 1,796 male twins from a population-based register, in which respondents were asked about current and past church attendance and psychoactive drug use. Structural twin models were fitted and tested using the Mx software program.

Results.—As twins developed from childhood through adulthood, the influence of shared environmental factors on church attendance declined dramatically while genetic factors increased. In early and late adolescence, the negative correlations between church attendance and alcohol and nicotine consumption resulted largely from shared environmental factors. In

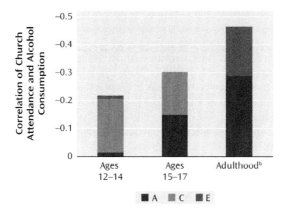

FIGURE 2.—Magnitude and Sources of the Correlation Between Church Attendance and Level of Alcohol Consumption Among 1,796 Male Twins, by Age[a]. [a] The sources of the correlation are additive genetic effects (A), shared or common environmental effects (C), and individual-specific environmental effects (E). These estimates were taken from the best-fitting model, as depicted in Table 1. [b] Mean age in adulthood, 40.3 years (SD=9.0). (Reprinted from Kendler KS, Myers J. A developmental twin study of church attendance and alcohol and nicotine consumption: a model for analyzing the changing impact of genes and environment. *Am J Psychiatry.* 2009;166:1150-1155, with permission of the American Psychiatric Association, Copyright 2009.)

adulthood, the inverse relationship between church attendance and substance use became stronger and arose largely from genetic factors.

Conclusions.—As individuals mature, they increasingly shape their own social environment in large part as a result of their genetically influenced temperament. When individuals are younger and living at home, frequent church attendance reflects a range of familial and social-environmental influences that reduce levels of substance use. In adulthood, by contrast, high levels of church attendance largely index genetically influenced temperamental factors that are protective against substance use. Using genetically informative designs such as twin studies, it is possible to show that the causes of the relationship between social risk factors and substance use can change dramatically over development.

▶ This fascinating twin study uses church attendance as a model for analyzing the changing impact of genes and environment through the life cycle on alcohol and nicotine consumption, and it finds a greater impact for environment, including positive protective factors of church attendance in this largely protestant Virginia set of twins, in childhood and adolescence (Fig 2). In adults and with increasing age, genetics come to play a greater contributing role. The role of spirituality in recovery has long been emphasized in 12 step programs, and in prevention, throughout the history of religion. In recent times, the field has come to recognize more the battle between motivation to avoid risk, or to seek recovery and the pull of temptations, habit patterns, and genetic vulnerability to addiction. Recognizing the complex biopsychosocial interaction of factors that lead to both addiction and recovery is needed to come up with effective approaches to prevention and recovery. This study may be culturally bound to some extent; however, the same mixture of factors are likely to be present across cultures, and the question of how to instill values that may protect against addiction needs further study. Religion may not be the only way to instill these protective values. What factors can help people better control self-harming behaviors and improve self esteem and self care? Pharmacologic treatments for comorbid anxiety, depression, and attention-deficit/hyperactivity disorder (ADHD), cognitive psychotherapies, spiritual approaches—including 12-step approaches—all need to be considered when crafting public policy and treatment plans.

R. J. Frances, MD

Are Women at Greater Risk? An Examination of Alcohol-Related Consequences and Gender
Sugarman DE, Demartini KS, Carey KB (Syracuse Univ, NY)
Am J Addict 18:194-197, 2009

Men typically drink more than women; however, women achieve higher BACs (blood alcohol concentration) than men at equivalent consumption levels. This study investigated the unique effect of gender on individual alcohol problems by controlling both consumption and intoxication in a sample of 1,331 undergraduate drinkers. Gender independently influenced the risk of experiencing seven of nine negative consequences: (a) being female increased risk for tolerance, blacking out, passing out, drinking after promising not to, and getting injured; (b) being male increased risk for damaging property and going to school drunk. Gender patterns should be explored in a wider set of alcohol-related problems.

▶ It is good to see that the last 15 years has led to a major increase in literature on alcohol problems and addiction in women. This study finds that while antisocial and violent behavior results from male excessive consumption of alcohol, women tend to be at risk for tolerance, blackouts, drinking out of control, self-deception, and of getting injured. Also, there are risks to binge drinking—women who try to match men in drinking similar amounts and who are not heeding warnings that equivalent doses have a bigger impact on women than men because of differences in first pass metabolism and fat distribution. Greater awareness on college campuses of recommendations for 1 drink per day for women is important. College-aged women who binge are also more likely to subject fetuses to fetal alcohol problems and are more likely to have unwanted pregnancies and be at risk for sexually transmitted diseases. College programs for prevention of binge drinking need to have a special focus on helping women for all of these reasons.

R. J. Frances, MD

Dual Diagnosis

Impact of Substance Use Disorders on Recovery From Episodes of Depression in Bipolar Disorder Patients: Prospective Data From the Systematic Treatment Enhancement Program for Bipolar Disorder (STEP-BD)

Ostacher MJ, for STEP-BD Investigators (Harvard Med School, Boston, MA; et al)
Am J Psychiatry 167:289-297, 2010

Objective.—Bipolar disorder is highly comorbid with substance use disorders, and this comorbidity may be associated with a more severe course of illness, but the impact of comorbid substance abuse on recovery from major depressive episodes in these patients has not been adequately examined. The authors hypothesized that comorbid drug and alcohol use disorders would be associated with longer time to recovery in patients with bipolar disorder.

Method.—Subjects (N = 3,750) with bipolar I or bipolar II disorder enrolled in the Systematic Treatment Enhancement Program for Bipolar Disorder (STEP-BD) were followed prospectively for up to 2 years. Prospectively observed depressive episodes were identified for this analysis. Subjects with a past or current drug or alcohol use disorder were compared with those with no history of drug or alcohol use disorders on time to recovery from depression and time until switch to a manic, hypomanic, or mixed episode.

Results.—During follow up, 2,154 subjects developed a new-onset major depressive episode; of these, 457 subjects switched to a manic, hypomanic, or mixed episode prior to recovery. Past or current substance use disorder did not predict time to recovery from a depressive episode relative to no substance use comorbidity. However, those with current or past substance use disorder were more likely to experience switch from depression directly to a manic, hypomanic, or mixed state.

Conclusions.—Current or past substance use disorders were not associated with longer time to recovery from depression but may contribute to greater risk of switch into manic, mixed, or hypomanic states. The mechanism conferring this increased risk merits further study.

▶ This study surprisingly did not find that a comorbid substance problem increased time to recovery from depression, although it did increase flipping from depression to mania. This conflicts with the generally held view that the substance use increases treatment resistance in a variety of ways, including, but not limited to, medication compliance. Therefore, the study's findings need to be confirmed by additional study. One important clinical implication is that those treating depression and bipolar depression need to encourage those with dual diagnosis to continue their medications even if they are using or relapsing to substance use. Also, clinicians need to be alert to the increased risk of dually diagnosed patients flipping into mania.

R. J. Frances, MD

Current alcohol use and risk for hypomania in male students: generally more or more binging?

Meyer TD, Wolkenstein L (Newcastle Univ, UK; Univ of Tübingen, Germany)
Compr Psychiatry 51:171-176, 2010

Background.—Alcohol use disorders and bipolar disorder are highly comorbid. Some studies suggest that alcohol abuse or misuse might even precede the onset of bipolar disorder, but few studies have looked at the daily drinking pattern beyond diagnostic categories. We therefore examined if risk for hypomania is associated with a specific drinking pattern when using a calendar-based interview.

Method.—A total of 120 students who completed the Hypomanic Personality Scale were independently interviewed with the FORM 90 to assess daily drinking and the Composite Diagnostic Interview to derive *Diagnostic and Statistical Manual of Mental Disorders, Fourth Edition,* diagnoses.

Results.—Conducting regression analyses, we found that an alcohol-related disorder was related to the amount and frequency of drinking, as expected. Risk for hypomania was specifically related to an unstable drinking pattern and binge drinking, but not generally higher consumption.

Conclusion.—Risk for hypomania was associated with unstable alcohol consumption and binge drinking, even after controlling for alcohol-related disorders. This supports the idea that instability in different areas of behavior is characteristic of vulnerability to hypomania.

▶ This article confirms that unstable and binge drinking are associated with vulnerability to hypomania even after controlling for alcohol-related disorders, an interesting finding. Screening for hypomania, especially in college-age students, should include looking for binge patterns of alcohol and likely also other substance abuse. The issue of causation is not resolved with this association. It may be that the binging is a symptom or prodrome of the mania, self-medication for a vulnerability to affective disorder, or active intoxication may bring out the vulnerability that might be avoided if alcohol and substance abuse were avoided in the first place, or some combination of the above. Longitudinal studies may help answer this difficult question. Which is worse: the wrath of grapes or the grapes of wrath? Those who advocate a self-medication hypothesis sometimes overvalue the cause of drinking being the underlying "other" psychiatric disorder, while others may overvalue the role of addiction as primary and causing all other problems. The clinical evidence is that the interaction is likely to be complex, and sorting out factors for each individual may be difficult. Watching for bipolar disorder when screening for alcohol abuse and watching for alcohol abuse when screening for mood disorders is clearly useful.

R. J. Frances, MD

Acute Negative Affect Relief from Smoking Depends on the Affect Situation and Measure but Not on Nicotine

Perkins KA, Karelitz JL, Conklin CA, et al (Univ of Pittsburgh, PA)
Biol Psychiatry 67:707-714, 2010

Background.—Smoking acutely relieves negative affect (NA) due to smoking abstinence but may not relieve NA from other sources, such as stressors.

Methods.—Dependent smokers ($n = 104$) randomly assigned to one of three smoking conditions (nicotine or denicotinized cigarettes, or no smoking) completed four negative mood induction procedures (one per session): 1) overnight smoking abstinence, 2) challenging computer task, 3) public speech preparation, and 4) watching negative mood slides. A fifth session involved a neutral mood control. The two smoking groups took four puffs on their assigned cigarette and then smoked those same cigarettes ad libitum during continued mood induction. All subjects rated their level of NA and positive affect on several measures (Mood Form, Positive and Negative Affect Scale, Stress-Arousal Checklist, and State-Trait Anxiety Inventory-state). They also rated craving and withdrawal.

Results.—Negative affect relief from smoking depended on the NA source (i.e., mood induction procedure) and the affect measure. Smoking robustly relieved NA due to abstinence on all four measures but only modestly relieved NA due to the other sources and typically on only some measures. Smoking's effects on positive affect and withdrawal were similar to effects on NA, but relief of craving depended less on NA source. Smoking reinforcement only partly matched the pattern of NA relief. Few responses differed between the nicotine and denicotinized smoking groups.

Conclusions.—Acute NA relief from smoking depends on the situation and the affect measure used but may not depend on nicotine intake. These results challenge the common assumption that smoking, and nicotine in particular, broadly alleviates NA (Fig 3).

▶ This article presents novel data indicating that the negative affect relief from smoking is situation-specific and not solely based on nicotine withdrawal relief, as has been often thought to be the case in the past (Fig 3). There are complex psychosocial and biological reasons people smoke and why people may get very situation-specific desired affects, whether it appears to be relief of negative affects or reinforcement of positive affects. Unconditioned stimuli and the complexity of behavioral pharmacological effects clearly play an important role that has not been fully taken into account in earlier studies, and this study points in the direction of tools that can help future studies of this area, not only for tobacco use but also for other substance abuse as well, where withdrawal alone may not be the sole cause of increase in negative affect. Situation-specific stressors could be taken into account when developing specific behavioral

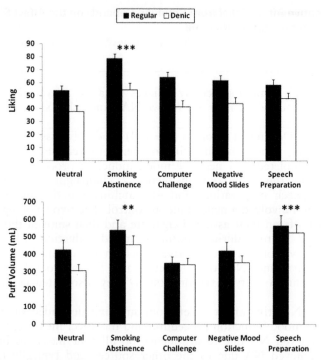

FIGURE 3.—Smoking reward (top) and puff volume during the ad libitum smoking period (bottom) as functions of mood induction procedure and nicotine versus denicotinized smoking group. The main effect of nicotine was significant for reward but not for puff volume. $**p < .01$; $***p < .001$ for the difference from neutral mood control procedure. Denic, denicotinized. (Reprinted from Perkins KA, Karelitz JL, Conklin CA, et al. Acute negative affect relief from smoking depends on the affect situation and measure but not on nicotine. *Biol Psychiatry*. 2010;67:707-714, with permission from the Society of Biological Psychiatry.)

treatment approaches to address the emergence of negative affect and to prevent relapse.

R. J. Frances, MD

Acute cannabis use causes increased psychotomimetic experiences in individuals prone to psychosis

Mason O, Morgan CJA, Dhiman SK, et al (Univ College London, UK)

Psychol Med 39:951-956, 2009

Background.—Epidemiological evidence suggests a link between cannabis use and psychosis. A variety of factors have been proposed to mediate an individual's vulnerability to the harmful effects of the drug, one of which is their psychosis proneness. We hypothesized that highly psychosis-prone individuals would report more marked psychotic experiences under the acute influence of cannabis.

Method.—A group of cannabis users ($n = 140$) completed the Psychotomimetic States Inventory (PSI) once while acutely intoxicated and again when free of cannabis. A control group ($n = 144$) completed the PSI on two parallel test days. All participants also completed a drug history and the Schizotypal Personality Questionnaire (SPQ). Highly psychosis-prone individuals from both groups were then compared with individuals scoring low on psychosis proneness by taking those in each group scoring above and below the upper and lower quartiles using norms for the SPQ.

Results.—Smoking cannabis in a naturalistic setting reliably induced marked increases in psychotomimetic symptoms. Consistent with predictions, highly psychosis-prone individuals experienced enhanced psychotomimetic states following acute cannabis use.

Conclusions.—These findings suggest that an individual's response to acute cannabis and their psychosis-proneness scores are related and both may be markers of vulnerability to the harmful effects of this drug.

▶ Awareness of the dangers of marijuana use among youth waxes and wanes, and young people and often their families still generally don't take the risks of use seriously, and in many schools recreational use of marijuana is almost taken for granted. While "Reefer Madness" has practically become a cult film, and some California doctors inappropriately prescribe medical marijuana for psychiatric problems, there is clearly a need to disseminate findings such as from this study. This British group joins a chorus of studies indicating that those at risk for psychiatric problems are likely to exacerbate or bring out vulnerabilities such as psychosis proneness. The finding that those individuals who respond to intoxication with marijuana with enhanced psychomimetic symptoms are especially at risk provides an important clue to interviewing users and screening for proneness to psychosis (Table 2). Also, the higher prevalence of schizotypal proneness in the marijuana-using group compared with the control group

TABLE 2.—Means (Standard Deviations) for the Subfactors of the PSI Across Day and Group

Subfactor of the PSI	Day 0 Control	Cannabis	F, p	Days 3–5 Control	Cannabis	F, p
Thought disorder	1.90 (2.32)	3.84 (4.43)	21.2, <0.001	1.26 (2.29)	1.8 (2.60)	3.38, 0.067
Perceptual distortion	1.19 (2.45)	5.04 (4.73)	74.26, <0.001	0.83 (2.14)	0.66 (1.64)	0.56, N.S.
Cognitive disorganization	4.42 (3.54)	11.56 (6.91)	120.93, <0.001	3.50 (4.01)	3.67 (3.36)	0.14, N.S.
Anhedonia	4.11 (2.54)	5.17 (3.32)	9.17, 0.003	4.03 (2.72)	4.26 (2.35)	0.54, N.S.
Manic experience	3.88 (2.50)	4.97 (3.01)	11.01, 0.001	3.28 (2.18)	3.58 (2.26)	1.3, N.S.
Paranoia/ suspiciousness	1.47 (2.31)	2.71 (4.22)	9.50, 0.002	0.99 (2.27)	0.96 (1.88)	0.021, N.S.

PSI, Psychotomimetic States Inventory.

confirms findings of other studies. Early screening for proness to both substance abuse and mental illness, with preventive treatment, should be a major public health goal and part of public policy.

R. J. Frances, MD

Correlates of Self-Medication for Anxiety Disorders: Results From the National Epidemiolgic Survey on Alcohol and Related Conditions
Robinson JA, Sareen J, Cox BJ, et al (Univ of Manitoba, Winnipeg, Canada)
J Nerv Ment Dis 197:873-878, 2009

Self-medication is a common behavior among individuals with anxiety disorders, yet few studies have examined the correlates of this behavior. The current study addresses this issue by exploring the pattern of mental health service use and quality of life among people who self-medicate for anxiety. Data came from the National Epidemiologic Survey on Alcohol and Related Conditions and was limited to the subsample of individuals meeting criteria for an anxiety disorder in the past 12 months ($n = 4880$). Multiple regression analyses compared 3 groups–(1) no self-medication, (2) self-medication with alcohol, and (3) self-medication with drugs, on mental health service use and quality of life. After adjusting for potentially confounding covariates, individuals who engaged in self-medication had significantly higher service use compared with people with anxiety disorders who did not self-medicate (adjusted odds ratio = 1.41, 95% CI = 1.06–1.89). Self-medication was also associated with a lower mental health-related quality of life compared with those who did not self-medicate. Clinicians should recognize and respond to the unique needs of this particular subpopulation of individuals with anxiety disorders.

▶ Self-medication for anxiety and anxiety disorders with alcohol and drugs is very common, and this article helps demonstrate how ineffective and harmful it is to do so (Table 3 in the original article). Addiction can cause anxiety problems and dependence that leads to withdrawal anxiety as well. The negative effects of substances on coping skills and increased marital, health, and job problems also add to stress and anxiety. Reportedly, Hippocrates said that wine drives away terror and fear; however, more often the wrath of grapes is worse than the grapes of wrath. It is often difficult to convince patients of this, as they get immediate relief from substance misuse and may not trust the doctors' medications. However, studies such as this one, with its emphasis on quality of life, can be helpful in giving therapists the confidence in trying to motivate patients to forgo self-medication for better self-care. Learning coping skills, building self-efficacy, and finding appropriate psychopharmacologic treatments are helpful in treating these dual-diagnosis patients.

R. J. Frances, MD

Comorbidity

Alcohol Abstinence and Orthotopic Liver Transplantation in Alcoholic Liver Cirrhosis
Immordino G, Gelli M, Ferrante R, et al (Gremaq Universite de Toulouse, France)
Transplant Proc 41:1253-1255, 2009

Patients diagnosed with acute alcoholic hepatitis (AAH) are routinely managed medically and not considered suitable for orthotopic liver transplantation (OLT). The eligibility for OLT in these patients has been questioned due to the social stigma associated with alcohol abuse, based on the fact that AAH is "self-induced" with an unacceptably high recidivism rate. Many centers in Europe and the United States require abstinence periods between 6 and 12 months before OLT listing. AAH outcomes in the literature are poor, in particular due to patient noncompliance during the immediate 3 months preceeding OLT. Between January 1997 and December 2007, 246 patients were evaluated in our center for alcoholic liver disease: 133 (54%) were listed for OLT (I-OLT), including 110 (83%) who underwent transplantation and 8 (6%) still listed as well as 15 (11%) removed from consideration. One hundred thirteen (46%) patients had no indication for OLT (NO I-OLT), including 18 (16%) who died, 81 (71%) still monitored, and 14 (12%) lost to follow-up. Patient survival rates post-OLT were 79%, 74%, 68%, and 64% at 1, 3, 5, and 10 years, respectively. Explant (native liver) pathologic examination revealed AAH in 8 (7.2%) patients who underwent OLT. In this group, patient survival and the post-OLT recidivism rate were statistically identical to the overall group of transplant recipients.

▶ This large liver transplant team in France found no worse prognosis in patients with acute alcoholic hepatitis who received liver transplants, compared with other transplant recipients (Table 1). Stigma for patients with alcoholism has resulted in barriers to treatment in a variety of ways, and in this instance the prejudice can lead to unnecessary deaths. The findings suggest that

TABLE 1.—Characteristics of the Patients (n = 246)

	I-OLT Group (n = 110)	NO I-OLT Group (n = 113)	*P*
Age, mean ± SD (range)	53.2 ± 8.3 (30–68)	49.9 ± 9.9 (33–64)	NS
Gender, M/F, n (%)	95/15 (86/14)	64/26 (56/44)	NS
Child score, n ± SD (range)	10 ± 1.8 (6–13)	6.5 ± 2.2 (5–13)	<.001
MELD score, n ± SD (range)	14.0 ± 4.0 (4–35)	11.5 ± 5.3 (6–40)	.019
Etiology AA/MC, n (%)	67/43 (61/39)	77/36 (68/32)	NS
Presence of HCC, n (%)	35 (26.4)	13 (15.2)	NS
Previous IVDA, n (%)	27 (27.9)	—	—

Abbreviations: M, male; F, female; MELD, model for end-stage liver disease; AA, alcoholism alone; MC, miscellaneous causes; HCC, hepatocellular carcinoma; IVDA, intravenous drug abuse; NS, not significant.

case-by-case decisions regarding risk for recidivism would prevent some deaths of individuals who have to wait too long and don't survive as a result. While there are moral aspects to whether patients will cooperate with treatment recommendations, it is important that physicians remember that addiction has genetic and biological causes, as well as psychosocial ones, and is considered a disease. In addition, alcohol rehabilitation is often more successful when patients have been faced with the reality of a life-threatening disease, which generally heightens their motivation.

R. J. Frances, MD

Pharmacologic Treatment

Nicotinic Acetylcholine Receptor β2 Subunit (*CHRNB2*) Gene and Short-Term Ability to Quit Smoking in Response to Nicotine Patch

Perkins KA, Lerman C, Mercincavage M, et al (Univ of Pittsburgh, PA; Univ of Pennsylvania, Philadelphia)
Cancer Epidemiol Biomarkers Prev 18:2608-2612, 2009

Genes coding for nicotinic acetylcholine receptors may influence response to nicotine replacement therapy for smoking cessation. We examined the association of a $3'$ untranslated region polymorphism (rs2072661) in the nicotinic acetylcholine receptor β2 subunit (*CHRNB2*) gene with quitting success in response to nicotine versus placebo patch during a short-term test of patch effects. In a within-subjects cross-over design, smokers of European descent ($n = 156$) received 21 mg nicotine and placebo patch in counter-balanced order, during two separate 5-day simulated quit attempts, each preceded by a week of *ad libitum* smoking. Abstinence was assessed daily by $CO < 5$ ppm. Smokers with the *CHRNB2* GG genotype had more days of abstinence during the nicotine versus placebo patch week compared with those with the AG or AA genotypes ($P < 0.01$). Moreover, nicotine patch increased the probability of quitting on the target quit day, quitting anytime during the patch week, and avoiding relapse among those with the GG genotype but not the AA/AG genotypes, although the nicotine × genotype interaction was significant only for quitting on the target quit day ($P < 0.05$). Regardless of patch condition, quitting on the target quit day was more likely in those with the GG genotype versus AA/AG genotypes ($P < 0.05$). Genetic associations were not observed for craving or withdrawal responses to nicotine versus placebo patch. These findings are consistent with previous evidence of association of this variant with smoking cessation and suggest that polymorphisms in the nicotinic acetylcholine receptor β2 subunit gene may influence therapeutic responsiveness to cessation medications.

▶ This interesting study done with GlaxoSmithKline support finds an association with ability to quit nicotine dependence using a patch with a polymorphism in the region of the nicotinic acetylcholine receptor (*CHRNB2*) β2 subunit (Fig 2). The genetics of vulnerability to addiction are likely to involve polymorphisms at a

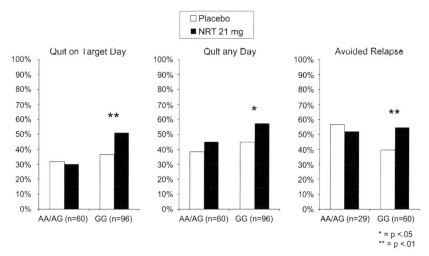

FIGURE 2.—Percentage of quitting on the target quit day, quitting any day during the patch week, and avoiding relapse if able to quit during nicotine versus placebo patch weeks by *CHRNB2* genotype groups. The main effect of nicotine patch was significant for all three outcomes. The main effect of genotype and the interaction of genotype × nicotine were significant only for quitting on the target quit day. (Reprinted from Perkins KA, Lerman C, Mercincavage M, et al. Nicotinic acetylcholine receptor β2 subunit (*CHRNB2*) gene and short-term ability to quit smoking in response to nicotine patch. *Cancer Epidemiol Biomarkers Prev.* 2009;18:2608-2612, with permission from the American Association for Cancer Research.)

number of gene locations and finding candidate locations may also tell us about the etiology and pathogenesis of addictive behaviors. These findings were not robust but are nonetheless interesting and may help us understand what helps some people quit when others have a harder time doing so. Being able to tell patients who have relatives who have successfully stopped tobacco use that this improves their odds of doing so may further strengthen motivation to do so and seek out help. Eventually tailoring pharmacologic and other treatment approaches to the specific genetic makeup of the individual is a general direction that all treatments are headed. The day when an infomatrix chip may inform which treatment to select for which disease is rapidly approaching.

R. J. Frances, MD

Cocaine Vaccine for the Treatment of Cocaine Dependence in Methadone-Maintained Patients: A Randomized, Double-blind, Placebo-Controlled Efficacy Trial

Martell BA, Orson FM, Poling J, et al (Yale Univ School of Medicine, New Haven; Baylor College of Medicine, Houston, TX; et al)

Arch Gen Psychiatry 66:1116-1123, 2009

Context.—Cocaine dependence, which affects 2.5 million Americans annually, has no US Food and Drug Administration–approved pharmacotherapy.

Objectives.—To evaluate the immunogenicity, safety, and efficacy of a novel cocaine vaccine to treat cocaine dependence.

Design.—A 24-week, phase 2b, randomized, double-blind, placebo-controlled trial with efficacy assessed during weeks 8 to 20 and follow-up to week 24.

Setting.—Cocaine- and opioid-dependent persons recruited from October 2003 to April 2005 from greater New Haven, Connecticut.

Participants.—One hundred fifteen methadone-maintained subjects (67% male, 87% white, aged 18-46 years) were randomized to vaccine or placebo, and 94 subjects (82%) completed the trial. Most smoked crack cocaine along with using marijuana (18%), alcohol (10%), and nonprescription opioids (44%).

Intervention.—Over 12 weeks, 109 of 115 subjects received 5 vaccinations of placebo or succinylnorcocaine linked to recombinant cholera toxin B-subunit protein.

Main Outcome Measure.—Semiquantitative urinary cocaine metabolite levels measured thrice weekly with a positive cutoff of 300 ng/mL.

Results.—The 21 vaccinated subjects (38%) who attained serum IgG anticocaine antibody levels of 43 µg/mL or higher (ie, high IgG level) had significantly more cocaine-free urine samples than those with levels less than 43 µg/mL (ie, low IgG level) and the placebo-receiving subjects during weeks 9 to 16 (45% vs 35% cocaine-free urine samples, respectively). The proportion of subjects having a 50% reduction in cocaine use was significantly greater in the subjects with a high IgG level than in subjects with a low IgG level (53% of subjects vs 23% of subjects, respectively) ($P = .048$). The most common adverse effects were injection site induration and tenderness. There were no treatment-related serious adverse events, withdrawals, or deaths.

Conclusions.—Attaining high ($\geq$43 µg/mL) IgG anticocaine antibody levels was associated with significantly reduced cocaine use, but only 38% of the vaccinated subjects attained these IgG levels and they had only 2 months of adequate cocaine blockade. Thus, we need improved vaccines and boosters.

Trial Registration.—clinicaltrials.gov Identifier: NCT00142857.

▶ The need for an effective prevention and/or treatment approach to cocaine and stimulant addiction, indeed for all substance abuse, is self evident, as is the fact that there have been no proven pharmacotherapies for cocaine addiction, although many promising approaches have come and gone. Every journey needs some positive first steps, and this study indicates some promise for a cocaine vaccine (see Fig 4 in the original article). While the positive effect only lasted 2 months and mostly occurred in those who had high IgG anticocaine antibody levels, more effective vaccines with more staying power could be developed. Unfortunately, if an addict is looking for a stimulant high, even if a vaccine could block a cocaine high, other amphetamine-derived substances that are as or more dangerous are available alternatives. Even incremental gains that may help some but not most cocaine addicts are welcome, and it is encouraging that researchers keep searching for biological treatments for addiction. It is also a likely bet that any effective vaccine approach would need to be accompanied by effective psychosocial behavioral treatments to have lasting results.

R. J. Frances, MD

A Double-Blind, Placebo-Controlled Trial Combining Sertraline and Naltrexone for Treating Co-Occurring Depression and Alcohol Dependence
Pettinati HM, Oslin DW, Kampman KM, et al (Univ of Pennsylvania School of Medicine, Philadelphia; Philadelphia Veterans Affairs Med Ctr, PA)
Am J Psychiatry 167:668-675, 2010

Objective.—Empirical evidence has only weakly supported antidepressant treatment for patients with co-occurring depression and alcohol dependence. While some studies have demonstrated that antidepressants reduce depressive symptoms in individuals with depression and alcohol dependence, most studies have not found antidepressant treatment helpful in reducing excessive drinking in these patients. The authors provide results from a double-blind, placebo-controlled trial that evaluated the efficacy of combining approved medications for depression (sertraline) and alcohol dependence (naltrexone) in treating patients with both disorders.

Method.—A total of 170 depressed alcohol-dependent patients were randomly assigned to receive 14 weeks of treatment with sertraline (200 mg/day [N=40]), naltrexone (100 mg/day [N=49]), the combination of sertraline plus naltrexone (N=42), or double placebo (N=39) while receiving weekly cognitive-behavioral therapy.

Results.—The sertraline plus naltrexone combination produced a higher alcohol abstinence rate (53.7%) and demonstrated a longer delay before relapse to heavy drinking (median delay=98 days) than the naltrexone (abstinence rate: 21.3%; delay=29 days), sertraline (abstinence rate: 27.5%; delay=23 days), and placebo (abstinence rate: 23.1%; delay= 26 days) groups. The number of patients in the medication combination group not depressed by the end of treatment (83.3%) approached significance when compared with patients in the other treatment groups. The serious adverse event rate was 25.9%, with fewer reported with the medication combination (11.9%) than the other treatments.

Conclusion.—More depressed alcohol-dependent patients receiving the sertraline plus naltrexone combination achieved abstinence from alcohol, had delayed relapse to heavy drinking, reported fewer serious adverse events, and tended to not be depressed by the end of treatment.

▶ This Philadelphia group has done important research on the efficacy of naltrexone in treating alcoholism and found an important role of combining antidepressants with naltrexone in treating patients with combined depression and alcoholism (Fig 2 in the original article). This important finding needs replication and indicates the value of integrating treatment approaches, including cognitive therapy, in approaching patients with dual diagnosis. These results indicate that naltrexone may be even more useful than previously thought in treating patients with dual diagnosis when combined with drugs targeted to comorbid conditions that worsen prognosis. The other most common dual diagnosis of anxiety and alcoholism is likely to benefit from the same medication combination and also needs study. The approach of adding naltrexone to whatever else helps with other psychiatric disorders, such as schizophrenia and bipolar disorder, when alcohol dependence is present also is worthy of study. Even before proof of this is fully established, these combinations are already being put into practice by clinicians.

R. J. Frances, MD

A Randomized Placebo-Controlled Clinical Trial of 5 Smoking Cessation Pharmacotherapies
Piper ME, Smith SS, Schlam TR, et al (Univ of Wisconsin School of Medicine and Public Health, Madison)
Arch Gen Psychiatry 66:1253-1262, 2009

Context.—Little direct evidence exists on the relative efficacies of different smoking cessation pharmacotherapies, yet such evidence is needed to make informed decisions about their clinical use.

Objective.—To assess the relative efficacies of 5 smoking cessation pharmacotherapy interventions using placebo-controlled, head-to-head comparisons.

Design.—A randomized, double-blind, placebo-controlled clinical trial.

Setting.—Two urban research sites.

Patients.—One thousand five hundred four adults who smoked at least 10 cigarettes per day during the past 6 months and reported being motivated to quit smoking. Participants were excluded if they reported using any form of tobacco other than cigarettes; current use of bupropion; having a current psychosis or schizophrenia diagnosis; or having medical contraindications for any of the study medications.

Interventions.—Participants were randomized to 1 of 6 treatment conditions: nicotine lozenge, nicotine patch, sustained-release bupropion, nicotine patch plus nicotine lozenge, bupropion plus nicotine lozenge, or placebo. In addition, all participants received 6 individual counseling sessions.

Main Outcome Measures.—Biochemically confirmed 7-day point-prevalence abstinence assessed at 1 week after the quit date (postquit), end of treatment (8 weeks postquit), and 6 months postquit. Other outcomes were initial cessation, number of days to lapse, number of days to relapse, and latency to relapse after the first lapse.

Results.—All pharmacotherapies differed from placebo when examined without protection for multiple comparisons (odds ratios, 1.63-2.34). With such protection, only the nicotine patch plus nicotine lozenge (odds ratio, 2.34, *P* < .001) produced significantly higher abstinence rates at 6-month postquit than did placebo.

Conclusion.—While the nicotine lozenge, bupropion, and bupropion plus lozenge produced effects that were comparable with those reported in previous research, the nicotine patch plus lozenge produced the greatest benefit relative to placebo for smoking cessation.

▶ This study found good smoking cessation in motivated quit attempters for 6 months, better than 40% for the nicotine patch plus lozenge or an odds ratio of approximately 2 compared with control placebo, and this combination did better than single treatment or another combination. The study did not include varenicline, which was not FDA approved at the time of the study, and behavior therapy generically was applied to all groups. The question of targeting the right combination of specific pharmacotherapies and behavioral therapies, including motivational and family support, to get optimal results tailored to each patient with nicotine addiction and making that sort of treatment widely available should be one of the highest public health national priorities. The relatively encouraging news is that motivated quitters have good chances of succeeding even with placebo on any given try and that if enough attempts are tried, most smokers can succeed in doing so. Providing confidence and instilling a sense of self-efficacy is a valuable tool for clinicians and families in helping the attempter to succeed at quitting.

R. J. Frances, MD

Psychosocial and Contingency Treatment

From In-Session Behaviors to Drinking Outcomes: A Causal Chain for Motivational Interviewing

Moyers TB, Martin T, Houck JM, et al (Univ of New Mexico, Albuquerque)
J Consult Clin Psychol 77:1113-1124, 2009

Client speech in favor of change within motivational interviewing sessions has been linked to treatment outcomes, but a causal chain has not yet been demonstrated. Using a sequential behavioral coding system for client speech, the authors found that, at both the session and utterance levels, specific therapist behaviors predict client change talk. Further, a direct link from change talk to drinking outcomes was observed, and support was found for a mediational role for change talk between therapist behavior and client drinking outcomes. These data provide preliminary support for the proposed causal chain indicating that client speech within treatment sessions can be influenced by therapists, who can employ this influence to improve outcomes. Selective eliciting and reinforcement of change talk is proposed as a specific active ingredient of motivational interviewing.

▶ A very important factor in treating patients with addictive disorders is motivating them for change. It is not surprising that most addicted patients are in the precontemplation stage of not being motivated to stop drinking and that without motivation actions toward change are not likely to occur. This article opens up the study of how therapists can shape sessions in such a way that can get patients to talk about change and influence them in that direction, and the effectiveness of such interventions. In my experience, the empathic, knowledgeable, and skilled addiction therapist is much like a coach using every tool possible to help the patient deal with the decisional balance of attending to the risks and the problems related to addiction and moving the patient along the path of change to take action and maintain progress as well as prevent relapses. This article begins to empirically demonstrate, albeit in small ways, that this is what actually occurs when therapists attend and respond to statements by the patient that relate to the pros and cons of change in helpful ways. The influence of therapists' well-timed comments supportive of change can make a difference in treatment outcomes.

R. J. Frances, MD

Does Precontemplation Represent a Homogeneous Stage Category? A Latent Class Analysis on German Smokers

Schorr G, Ulbricht S, Schmidt CO, et al (Ernst-Moritz-Arndt-Univ Greifswald, Germany; et al)
J Consult Clin Psychol 76:840-851, 2008

The authors examined the subtype structure of smokers classified in the precontemplation stage of change within the transtheoretical model. From a general practice-based sample of 1,499 daily smoking patients from Germany (participation rate 80%), they used a subgroup of 929 smokers who were classified in the precontemplation stage and applied latent class analysis, using the pros and cons of nonsmoking and smoking cessation self-efficacy as the defining variables. Cross-sectional validation of the emerging classes was based on smoking behavior and processes of change variables. For longitudinal validation, generalized estimation equation analyses were used on motivational and abstinence criteria from 6-, 12-, 18-, and 24-month follow-ups. A 4-class model best represented the data. Three subtypes (labeled *progressive, immotive, and disengaged pessimistic*) were similar to clusters identified in U.S. studies. The 4th (*disengaged optimistic*), by contrast, was reminiscent of a type that had previously only emerged in a Dutch study. Cross-sectional and longitudinal validation results confirmed the distinctiveness and predictive power of the classes. The findings highlight the importance of tailoring interventions for smoking behavior change to the needs of different subgroups of precontemplating smokers (Fig 1).

▶ Motivation for change and enhancing it has been an important model used in the treatment of all addictions, including smoking. This study provides evidence for tailoring smoking cessation efforts using the transtheoretical model based on subtyping rather than homogeneously categorizing smokers when they are

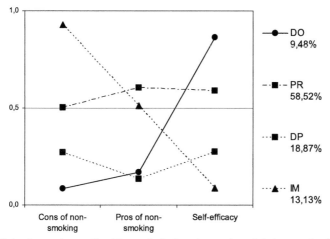

FIGURE 1.—Latent class profiles. The graph displays the transformed 0–1 expected values on the three indicator variables cons of nonsmoking, pros of nonsmoking, and smoking cessation self-efficacy that characterize the four latent classes. The conditional response probabilities for the quartiles of each indicator, which were used to compute the expected values, are given in Table 1. Percentages are probabilistic class sizes. DO = disengaged optimistic; PR = progressive; DP = disengaged pessimistic; IM = immotive. (Reprinted from Schorr G, Ulbricht S, Schmidt CO, et al. Does precontemplation represent a homogeneous stage category? A latent class analysis on German smokers. *J Consult Clin Psychol.* 2008;76:840-851, with permission from the American Psychological Association.)

in the precontemplation stage of motivation for change (Fig 1). Patients can move freely within and across stages of change, and the goal of therapists is to help these smokers, who cross-sectionally are usually in the precontemplation stage to move up the ladder of motivation and get closer to taking action. Such a ladder has been proposed for the contemplation stage, and this article posits the need to similarly see precontemplation as heterogenous and posits a benefit in tailoring approaches to subgroups within this stage. After all is said, this is just a model, and the essence of it is understanding the importance of increasing motivation in helping free patients from compulsive behavior.

R. J. Frances, MD

Genetics and Progression

Age at Regular Drinking, Clinical Course, and Heritability of Alcohol Dependence in the San Francisco Family Study: A Gender Analysis

Ehlers CL, Gizer IR, Vieten C, et al (The Scripps Res Inst, La Jolla, CA; Univ of North Carolina, Chapel Hill; California Pacific Med Ctr Res Inst, San Francisco)
Am J Addict 19:101-110, 2010

We examined gender differences in age of onset, clinical course, and heritability of alcohol dependence in 2,524 adults participating in the University of California San Francisco (UCSF) family study of alcoholism. Men were significantly more likely than women to have initiated regular drinking during adolescence. Onset of regular drinking was not found to be heritable but was found to be significantly associated with a shorter time to onset of alcohol dependence. A high degree of similarity in the sequence of alcohol-related life events was found between men and women, however, men experienced alcohol dependence symptoms at a younger age and women had a more rapid clinical course. Women were found to have a higher heritability estimate for alcohol dependence ($h^2 = .46$) than men ($h^2 = .32$). These findings suggest that environmental factors influencing the initiation of regular drinking rather than genetic factors associated with dependence may in part underlie some of the gender differences seen in the prevalence of alcohol dependence in this population.

▶ These findings have important public health implications in that onset of drinking in both sexes is not determined by heredity, and later onset or delay of alcohol use can reduce the tendency to become dependent. This finding may be especially important, as environmental influences that delay onset should be used, especially in families in which the genetic risks are high. Also interesting and important are the findings in this study that women have a higher heritability estimate for alcohol dependence than men and tend to start drinking heavily later than men, and have a more rapid clinical course. The complex gene environment of dependency unfolding helps us better understand the disease course and means to prevent and treat addiction.

R. J. Frances, MD

A genome-wide association study of alcohol dependence
Bierut LJ, as part of the Gene, Environment Association Studies (GENEVA) Consortium (Washington Univ School of Medicine, St Louis, MO; et al)
Proc Natl Acad Sci U S A 107:5082-5087, 2010

Excessive alcohol consumption is one of the leading causes of preventable death in the United States. Approximately 14% of those who use alcohol meet criteria during their lifetime for alcohol dependence, which is characterized by tolerance, withdrawal, inability to stop drinking, and continued drinking despite serious psychological or physiological problems. We explored genetic influences on alcohol dependence among 1,897 European-American and African-American subjects with alcohol dependence compared with 1,932 unrelated, alcohol-exposed, nondependent controls. Constitutional DNA of each subject was genotyped using the Illumina 1M beadchip. Fifteen SNPs yielded $P < 10^{-5}$, but in two independent replication series, no SNP passed a replication threshold of $P < 0.05$. Candidate gene *GABRA2*, which encodes the GABA receptor α2 subunit, was evaluated independently. Five SNPs at *GABRA2* yielded nominal (uncorrected) $P < 0.05$, with odds ratios between 1.11 and 1.16. Further dissection of the alcoholism phenotype, to disentangle the

TABLE 3.—SAGE Association Results for *GABRA2* Snps also Genotyped in the Family-Based COGA Sample

SNP	Position	COGA* *P*	Risk Allele	SAGE Frequency of Risk Allele Cases	Controls	Adjusted Odds Ratio (95% CI)	*P*
rs572227	45,946,150	3.80E-02	A	0.376	0.366	1.15 (1.04–1.27)	8.89E-03
rs548583	45,958,101	1.20E-02	T	0.404	0.385	1.14 (1.03–1.26)	1.05E-02
rs279858	46,009,350	8.70E-03	G	0.375	0.366	1.16 (1.05–1.28)	5.04E-03
rs279843	46,019,961	4.90E-02	T	0.444	0.421	1.11 (1.00–1.22)	4.24E-02
rs279841	46,035,520	3.80E-02	A	0.368	0.364	1.13 (1.02–1.25)	2.29E-02

Editor's Note: Please refer to original journal article for full references.
*COGA family based association from ref. 14.

influence of comorbid substance-use disorders, will be a next step in identifying genetic variants associated with alcohol dependence (Table 3).

▶ Recent years have underscored the importance of family history and genetics in the etiology and expression of alcoholism and other addictions. However, the complexity of the genetic expression of substance abuse and the mysteries of gene expression of addiction continue to confound us, even with all the advances in genome science. The promise of clinically relevant genetic applications including a targeted pharmacologic approach to mental illness, including alcoholism, based on a genetic understanding of mechanisms of the disease remains an elusive goal. The goal seemed to be within reach 10 years ago when the human genome was first sequenced and even 30 years ago, but the results including those of this well-done international effort to find genes that will give simple answers has not yet materialized (Table 3). We can expect that much basic research will be needed to get the kind of complex understanding that may lead to more fruitful treatments in the future. Building on studies such as this one are part of that effort, and the hope of increasingly less expensive gene sequencing combined with intelligent searches are likely ultimately to lead to better results, hopefully in my lifetime (age 64 at time of writing)!

R. J. Frances, MD

4 Psychiatry and the Law

Introduction

It will be interesting to see how President Obama's effort to fill Supreme Court vacancies with nominees who were picked with an effort to add compassion and sensitivity to the judicial system will effect decisions related to the mentally ill and forensic psychiatry. Our society continues to be increasingly litigious, and unfortunately rational ways to deal with direct and indirect costs of malpractice were not a major part of health care reform.

The United States' long-term involvement in wars not only affects the mental health of troops and veterans and their families, but it may contribute to our culture of violence, intimate-partner violence, and a general level of anxiety and stress. The vast cost of military expenditures has negative effects on the economy of the country and the availability of funds to advance social programs. The recent economic crisis and increases in unemployment have greater effects on those with mental illness than on the general population and adds to their suffering.

Richard J. Frances, MD

Assessment and Treatment

Gender Differences in Chronic Medical, Psychiatric, and Substance-Dependence Disorders Among Jail Inmates

Binswanger IA, Merrill JO, Krueger PM, et al (Univ of Colorado Denver; Univ of Washington, Seattle; Univ of Texas Health Science Ctr at Houston; et al)
Am J Public Health 100:476-482, 2010

Objectives.—We investigated whether there were gender differences in chronic medical, psychiatric, and substance-dependence disorders among jail inmates and whether substance dependence mediated any gender differences found.

Methods.—We analyzed data from a nationally representative survey of 6982 US jail inmates. Weighted estimates of disease prevalence were calculated by gender for chronic medical disorders (cancer, hypertension, diabetes, arthritis, asthma, hepatitis, and cirrhosis), psychiatric disorders (depressive, bipolar, psychotic, posttraumatic stress, anxiety, and personality), and substance-dependence disorders. We conducted logistic regression to examine the relationship between gender and these disorders.

Results.—Compared with men, women had a significantly higher prevalence of all medical and psychiatric conditions ($P \leq .01$ for each) and drug dependence ($P < .001$), but women had a lower prevalence of alcohol dependence ($P < .001$). Gender differences persisted after adjustment for sociodemographic factors and substance dependence.

Conclusions.—Women in jail had a higher burden of chronic medical disorders, psychiatric disorders, and drug dependence than men, including conditions found more commonly in men in the general population. Thus, there is a need for targeted attention to the chronic medical, psychiatric, and drug-treatment needs of women at risk for incarceration, both in jail and after release (Table 2).

▶ Perhaps no population suffers more than women who are not only stigmatized by being in jail but also suffer from addiction, mental illness, and/or physical illnesses that are often underdiagnosed, undertreated, and neglected in the prison system. This large US study comparing the medical and psychiatric

TABLE 2.—Percentage of Inmates Reporting Chronic Medical Conditions, Psychiatric Disorders, Substance Abuse, or Substance Dependence, by Gender: Survey of Inmates in Local Jails, 2002

	Men, Weighted %	Women, Weighted %	P
Medical condition			
Cancer	1.1	8.3	<.001
Diabetes	3.2	6.5	<.001
Hypertension	17.3	21.9	<.001
Heart problem	8.6	11.4	.002
Asthma	13.9	24.4	<.001
Arthritis	12.7	20.2	<.001
Hepatitis	4.9	9.6	<.001
Cirrhosis	1.2	2.1	.006
Any medical condition	40.0	56.8	<.001
Psychiatric disorder			
Depressive	17.4	35.5	<.001
Bipolar	8.7	20.7	<.001
Psychotic	4.4	6.0	.013
Posttraumatic stress	4.4	11.3	<.001
Other anxiety	6.1	18.5	<.001
Personality	4.7	8.7	<.001
Any psychiatric	21.6	43.6	<.001
Drug-use disorder			
Drug abuse	18.2	13.6	<.001
Drug dependence	34.5	45.7	<.001
Drug abuse or dependence	52.7	59.3	<.001
Alcohol-use disorder			
Alcohol abuse	24.6	18.0	<.001
Alcohol dependence	23.3	18.9	<.001
Alcohol abuse or dependence	47.9	36.9	<.001
History of injection drug use	17.1	24.4	<.001

disorders, including addiction in male and female prisoners, found much higher rates of these problems in women (Table 2). Striking were the high rates of cervical cancer, asthma, hypertension, and all psychiatric illnesses, including drug dependence. Perhaps it is not surprising that women with more severe life problems compared with noncriminal women were more likely to face prison terms because criminal behavior is generally less prevalent in women than in men. However, the need for services to detect, treat, and provide follow-up for these conditions has not been highlighted adequately prior to this study. High rates of morbidity and mortality for female prisoners after release also have been found, and these rates could be reduced with an improved health care system. Hopefully, some of the recent health care reforms may improve access to care for this long-neglected population.

R. J. Frances, MD

Psychosocial Predictors of Military Misconduct
Booth-Kewley S, Highfill-McRoy RM, Larson GE, et al (Naval Health Res Ctr, San Diego, CA)
J Nerv Ment Dis 198:91-98, 2010

The objective of this longitudinal study was to determine psychosocial predictors of military misconduct in a cohort of Marine Corps war veterans. The study included data from 20,746 male Marines who completed a life history questionnaire during initial basic training and were subsequently deployed to a combat zone. Associations between psychosocial variables, psychiatric diagnoses, and subsequent misconduct outcomes were analyzed using Cox proportional hazards regression. The strongest predictors of misconduct outcomes (bad conduct discharges and military demotions) were psychiatric diagnoses and young age at first combat deployment. The results indicate that combat-related psychological disorders may manifest in numerous harmful ways, including impulsive, disruptive, and antisocial behavior. We recommend that the association between misconduct and psychiatric disorders be more explicitly acknowledged in research and treatment efforts involving military war veterans and other trauma victims.

▶ This article underlines the military value, including reducing misconduct, of sending older, more experienced, better trained and better screened (for psychiatric disabilities) troops into combat zones. The fact that military persons with psychiatric problems have those problems worsen with the stress of active combat and that those problems are more likely to lead to misconduct would not be surprising to any war veteran (Table 2). The fact that war experiences can have an effect on impulsivity, morality, and antisocial behavior in those who did not show these problems before combat experience should also not be shocking but should be addressed to in programs for active duty and veteran military personnel. The courage of those who choose to serve in the military needs to be rewarded with the very best in developing ways to help combat

TABLE 2.—Distribution of Psychiatric Diagnoses, Male Marines Deployed During OEF/OIF, 2002–2007

Diagnostic Category	Precombat Diagnosis[a]	Postcombat Diagnosis[b]
All mental disorders	1457	2835
Substance-related disorders	468	816
Adjustment disorders	254	352
Mood disorders	228	384
Personality disorders	67	93
Psychotic disorders	8	12
Anxiety disorders	153	777
Panic disorder	15	27
Generalized anxiety disorder	16	35
Obsessive-compulsive disorder	0	5
Phobias	3	4
Acute stress	25	74
Posttraumatic stress disorder	62	609
Anxiety, not otherwise specified	60	151
Somatoform/dissociative/factitious disorders	7	17
Other mental disorders	272	384

OEF/OIF indicates Operation Enduring Freedom/Operation Iraqi Freedom.
[a]This column shows all 1457 precombat psychiatric diagnosis diagnoses received by 1035 Marines in a sample of 20,746.
[b]This column shows all 2835 postcombat psychiatric diagnosis diagnoses received by 1928 Marines in a sample of 20,746.

duty soldiers rehabilitate, get treatment for their combat-related exacerbation or newly emergent psychiatric problems, and readjust to the moral requirements and duties of civilian life.

R. J. Frances, MD

General Medical Problems of Incarcerated Persons With Severe and Persistent Mental Illness: A Population-Based Study

Cuddeback GS, Scheyett A, Pettus-Davis C, et al (Cecil G. Sheps Ctr for Health Services Res, Chapel Hill, NC; Univ of North Carolina at Chapel Hill)
Psychiatr Serv 61:45-49, 2010

Objective.—Persons with severe mental illness have higher rates of chronic general medical illness compared with the general population. Similarly, compared with the general population, incarcerated persons have higher rates of chronic medical illness; however, there is little information about the synergy between severe mental illness and incarceration and the general medical problems of consumers. To address this gap in the literature this study addressed the following question: are consumers with a history of incarceration at greater risk of general medical problems compared with consumers without such a history?

Methods.—Administrative data were used to compare the medical problems of 3,690 persons with severe mental illness with a history of incarceration and 2,042 persons with severe mental illness with no such history.

TABLE 2.—Probability of Any and Multiple General Medical Problems Among Persons with Severe Mental Illness[a]

Indicator	Any Medical Problem				Multiple Medical Problems			
	B	SE	OR	95% CI	B	SE	OR	95% CI
Male (reference: female)	.10	.03	1.23	1.10–1.38*	.10	.03	1.21	1.09–1.35*
Race (reference: white)								
Black	−.22	.05	.66	.58–.75*	−.21	.05	.66	.58–.75*
Other	.02	.07	.83	.68–1.02	.01	.07	.82	.67–1.00
Age	.03	.01		—	.03	.01		—
Substance use disorder (reference: no disorder)	.15	.03	1.34	1.18–1.51*	.15	.03	1.35	1.20–1.52*
Incarceration history (reference: no history)	.37	.07	1.44	1.27–1.64*	.27	.06	1.31	1.16–1.49*

[a]Logistic regression models controlled for race, gender, age, and substance use disorders.
*p<.001

Results.—Consumers with a history of incarceration were more likely than those with no such history to have infectious, blood, and skin diseases and a history of injury. Furthermore, when analyses controlled for gender, race, age, and substance use disorders, consumers with an incarceration history were 40% more likely to have any general medical problem and 30% more likely to have multiple medical problems.

Conclusions.—The findings presented here call for better communication among local public health and mental health providers and jails and better integration of primary care and behavioral health care among community mental health providers. Also, research should be accelerated on evidence-based interventions designed to divert persons with severe mental illness from the criminal justice system and facilitate community reentry for persons with severe mental illness who are released from jails and prisons (Table 2).

▶ This study found an increased odds ratio for general medical problems in those with persistent mental illness who have a history of incarceration (Table 2). This study not only highlights the need for greater attention to medical and psychiatric care of prisoners but also the need to prevent the conditions that lead to imprisonment, the need for more mental health and drug courts, diversion of nonviolent criminals to outpatient commitment or treatment, and provision of better community mental and general health resources. Parity and improved access to care have been a part of recent health reform will help, but more general medical and psychiatric services with better record-keeping and communication in the prison system should be made available.

R. J. Frances, MD

Domestic Violence

Impact of Intimate Partner Violence on Children's Well-Child Care and Medical Home

Bair-Merritt MH, Crowne SS, Burrell L, et al (Johns Hopkins Univ School of Medicine, Baltimore, MD; et al)
Pediatrics 121:e473-e480, 2008

Objectives.—Intimate partner violence has been linked to poor child health. A continuous relationship with a primary care pediatric provider can help to detect intimate partner violence and connect families with needed services. The objectives of this study were to determine the relationship between intimate partner violence and (1) maternal report of a regular site for well-child care, (2) maternal report of a primary pediatric provider, (3) well-child visits in the first year of life, (4) up-to-date immunizations at 2 years of age, (5) maternal report of medical neglect, and (6) maternal report of the pediatric provider–caregiver relationship.

Methods.—This retrospective cohort study evaluated data from 209 at-risk families participating in the evaluation of the Healthy Families Alaska program. Research staff interviewed mothers near the time of an index child's birth and again at the child's second birthday. Medical charts were abstracted for information on well-child visits and immunizations.

Results.—Mothers who disclosed intimate partner violence at the initial interview (*n* = 62) were significantly less likely to report a regular site for well-child care or a primary pediatric provider. In multivariable models, children of mothers who disclosed intimate partner violence tended to be less likely to have the recommended 5 well-child visits within the first year of life and were significantly less likely to be fully immunized at 2 years of age. Differences in medical neglect were not statistically significant. Of mothers who reported a specific primary pediatric provider, those with intimate partner violence histories trusted this provider less and tended to rate less favorably pediatric provider–caregiver communication and the overall quality of the pediatric provider–caregiver relationship.

Conclusions.—Future research should explore effective ways to link intimate partner violence–exposed children with a medical home and a primary pediatric provider and to improve relationships between pediatric providers and caregivers who face violence at home.

▶ This Alaska study looks at the effects of intimate partner violence and pediatric care and finds significant deficits in well-child care, including number of visits, immunizations, and a less trusting relationship with caregivers. Women were much more likely to be victims of the violence, and this population had high rates of substance abuse. The cycle of intimate partner violence, often combined with unemployment, substance abuse, and psychiatric problems, often also associated with criminality and poor medial care from childhood, can be hard to break. Searching for ways to improve child medical care early on can be a place to start.

R. J. Frances, MD

Association between exposure to political violence and intimate-partner violence in the occupied Palestinian territory: a cross-sectional study
Clark CJ, Everson-Rose SA, Suglia SF, et al (Univ of Minnesota, Minneapolis; Boston Univ School of Medicine, MA; et al)
Lancet 375:310-316, 2010

Background.—Intimate-partner violence might increase during and after exposure to collective violence. We assessed whether political violence was associated with male-to-female intimate-partner violence in the occupied Palestinian territory.

Methods.—A nationally representative, cross-sectional survey was done between Dec 18, 2005, and Jan 18, 2006, by the Palestinian Central Bureau of Statistics. 4156 households were randomly selected with a multistage random cluster design, from which 3815 ever-married women aged 15–64 years were identified. We restricted our analysis to presently married women (n = 3510, 92% participation rate), who completed a short version of the revised conflict tactics scales and exposure to political violence inventory. Exposure to political violence was characterised as the husband's direct exposure, his indirect exposure via his family's experiences, and economic effects of exposure on the household. We used adjusted multinomial logistic regression models to estimate odds ratios (ORs) for association between political violence and intimate-partner violence.

Findings.—Political violence was significantly related to higher odds of intimate-partner violence. ORs were $1·89$ (95% CI $1·29–2·76$) for physical and $2·23$ ($1·49–3·35$) for sexual intimate-partner violence in respondents whose husbands were directly exposed to political violence compared with those whose husbands were not directly exposed. For women whose husbands were indirectly exposed, ORs were $1·61$ ($1·25–2·07$) for physical and $1·97$ ($1·49–2·60$) for sexual violence, compared with those whose husbands were not indirectly exposed. Economic effects of exposure were associated with increased odds of intimate-partner violence in the Gaza Strip only.

Interpretation.—Because exposure to political violence is associated with increased odds of intimate-partner violence, and exposure to many traumas is associated with poor health, a range of violent exposures should be assessed when establishing the need for psychosocial interventions in conflict settings (Table 4).

▶ One of the nasty effects of war and political violence is an increase in domestic violence, which often has been the case with war veterans and has been studied in the past. Fewer studies look at civilian populations that are

TABLE 4.—Odds Ratios (95% CIs) of Intimate Partner Violence by Type of Political Violence Exposure in Separate Adjusted* Multinomial Regression Models

	Psychological IPV only	Physical IPV	Sexual IPV
Husband's exposure			
No	1·00	1·00	1·00
Yes	1·47 (1·07–2·02) p=0·0184	1·89 (1·29–2·76) p=0·0011	2·23 (1·49–3·35) p=0·0001
Family exposure			
No	1·00	1·00	1·00
Yes	1·11 (0·90–1·36) p=0·3337	1·61 (1·25–2·07) p=0·0002	1·97 (1·49–2·60) p<0·0001
Economic effect of exposure			
No	1·00	1·00	1·00
Yes	1·40 (1·19–1·65) p<0·0001	1·51 (1·22–1·87) p=0·0002	1·55 (1·21–1·99) p=0·0005

n = 3510. IPV = intimate partner violence.
*Adjusted for age, educational level, and employment status (of respondent and her husband), location (urban, rural, or camp), and region (West Bank or Gaza Strip).

under the threat of political violence, and this study was done in one of the world's hottest and most controversial spots, the Gaza Strip, which has both suffered and perpetrated violence in the Middle East. The suffering of women in the region directly and indirectly from the conflict should be taken into account by both sides, as a history of escalating violence has direct and indirect harmful effects on both Palestinians and Israelis, including increasing rates of intimate partner violence (Table 4). Respecting the needs of civilian populations (especially women and children) should increase the awareness of a need for conflict resolution and compromise in order to reduce the tragic escalation of conflict that has led to so much civilian suffering on both sides. Domestic violence, a worldwide problem, is very much affected by cultural issues including war, famine, and natural disasters and is very much a human rights issue that needs attention. Promoting education, especially for women in developing countries, may help but needs to be combined with peace-making efforts in regions like the Middle East.

R. J. Frances, MD

Markers for Intimate Partner Violence in the Emergency Department Setting
Perciaccante VJ, Carey JW, Susarla SM, et al (Emory Univ School of Medicine, Atlanta, GA; Private Practice, Canton, GA; Massachusetts General Hosp, Boston)
J Oral Maxillofac Surg 68:1219-1224, 2010

Purpose.—Intimate partner violence (IPV) is a serious, under-reported public health problem in the United States. Pilot studies suggested that injury location, that is, head, neck, or face, was a sensitive but nonspecific marker for IPV-related injuries. This study's goal was to determine whether adding a second element to the diagnostic protocol—response to an IPV-screening questionnaire—improved the specificity of the protocol.

Materials and Methods.—We used a cross-sectional study design and a sample composed of women presenting to the emergency department for evaluation and management of injuries of non-verifiable etiology. The predictor study variables were injury location (head, neck, or face vs other), responses to a verbal questionnaire (Partner Violence Screen or Woman Abuse Screening Tool), and the combination of both elements. By combining both elements, the probability for IPV-related injury was classified as high or low. The outcome variable was self-report of injury etiology (IPV or other etiology). Appropriate univariate and bivariate statistics were computed, including estimates of sensitivity, specificity, positive and negative predictive values, and relative risk.

Results.—The sample was composed of 300 women with a mean age of 36.5 years. The frequency of self-reported IPV-related injury was 32.3%. The sensitivities and specificities for injury location and the questionnaires combined ranged from 86.5% to 91.8% and 93.1% to 96.1%, respectively.

Conclusions.—The study findings suggest that combining information regarding injury location and the results of a screening questionnaire was a better predictor of a woman's likelihood to report IPV-related injuries than either modality alone.

▶ Unfortunately, most often women do not report intimate partner violence, even in an emergency room (FR) setting, where clinical staff should be alerted to the possibility and ask the right questions. ER staff need to have heightened awareness for the signs and symptoms that an injury is related to intimate partner violence, especially when the location of the injury is in the head, the neck, or the face, as found in this study. The Women Abuse Screening Tool when combined with attention to injury location led to a dramatic improvement in screening. Repeated ER visits, fear, substance abuse, depression, and signs of posttraumatic stress disorder also should raise antennas. An empathic ER staff armed with these tools can help start a referral and treatment process of immeasurable value to families. It would be interesting to know whether the same markers hold for men, who may also underreport injuries caused by their intimate partners, a less common but no less important problem.

R. J. Frances, MD

Mortality Risk Associated with Physical and Verbal Abuse in Women Aged 50 to 79
Baker MW, LaCroix AZ, Wu C, et al (Univ of Washington, Seattle; Fred Hutchinson Cancer Res Ctr, Seattle, WA; et al)
J Am Geriatr Soc 57:1799-1809, 2009

Objectives.—To investigate whether midlife and older women who reported prior-year physical abuse, verbal abuse, or both abuse types had higher mortality risk than peers who did not report prior-year abuse.

Design.—Retrospective analysis.

Setting.—Community.

Participants.—One hundred sixty-thousand six hundred seventy-six community-dwelling women ages 50 to 79 at baseline enrolled in one of two major Women's Health Initiative (WHI) study components who responded to baseline abuse questions. Observational study enrollment was $N = 93,676$ (1994–1998; 90 months average follow-up). Clinical trial enrollment was $N = 68,132$ (1993–1998; 96 months average follow-up).

Measurements.—Total mortality was measured from 1993 to 2005 using all available data sources. Blinded physician adjudicators measured cause-specific mortality. Ninety-six percent of death records were adjudicated.

Results.—Prior-year self-reported abuse prevalence was 11.3%. Women who reported physical abuse had the highest age-adjusted mortality rate, followed by women who reported both abuse types. Abuse independently predicted mortality risk after controlling for age, education, ethnicity, and WHI component. High mortality risk remained for physically abused women (hazard ratio (HR) = 1.54, 95% confidence interval (CI) = 1.09–2.18) after adjusting for demographic and health-related factors. Further adjustment for psychosocial variables diminished this association (HR = 1.40, 95% CI = 0.93–2.11), but high risk remained.

Conclusion.—Community-dwelling middle-aged and older women who reported prior-year physical, verbal, or both types of abuse had significantly higher adjusted mortality risk than women who did not report abuse. These findings highlight the need for longitudinal research into prevention of abuse in later life and accompanying excess mortality and emphasize the importance of abuse prevention in later life.

▶ This study dramatizes the need for screening for abuse in the elderly and the increase in death rates that was affected not only by physical abuse but also by verbal abuse (Fig 1 in the original article). Caregivers, whether familial or employed, can be perpetrators of this abuse, and much of the problem goes undetected. Of course the abuse can go both ways, and teaching family ways to reduce stress and de-escalate conflicts can be helpful. Medications judiciously applied may also calm situations, although in some settings they may be too heavily relied upon. Substance abuse in caretakers, partners, or family can also be a factor in committing violence or victimization.

R. J. Frances, MD

Partner Violence Before and After Couples-Based Alcoholism Treatment for Female Alcoholic Patients

Schumm JA, O'Farrell TJ, Murphy CM, et al (Harvard Med School, Boston, MA; Univ of Maryland, Baltimore County; et al)
J Consult Clin Psychol 77:1136-1146, 2009

This study examined partner violence before and in the 1st and 2nd year after behavioral couples therapy (BCT) for 103 married or cohabiting women seeking alcohol dependence treatment and their male partners; it used a demographically matched nonalcoholic comparison sample. The treatment sample received $M = 16.7$ BCT sessions over 5–6 months. Follow-up rates for the treatment sample at Years 1 and 2 were 88% and 83%, respectively. In the year before BCT, 68% of female alcoholic patients had been violent toward their male partner, nearly 5 times the comparison sample rate of 15%. In the year after BCT, violence prevalence decreased significantly to 31% of the treatment sample. Women were classified as remitted after treatment if they demonstrated abstinence or minimal substance use and no serious consequences related to substance use. In Year 1 following BCT, 45% were classified as remitted, and 49% were classified as remitted in Year 2. Among remitted patients in the year after BCT, violence prevalence of 22% did not differ from the comparison sample and was significantly lower than the rate among relapsed patients (38%). Results for male-perpetrated violence and for the 2nd year after BCT were similar to the 1st year. Results supported predictions that partner violence would decrease after BCT and that clinically significant violence reductions to the level of a nonalcoholic comparison sample would occur for patients whose alcoholism was remitted after BCT. These findings replicate previous research among men with alcoholism.

▶ Much of the attention regarding intimate partner violence in alcoholic households has focused on violence men perpetrate against women, and it has been found in the past that rehabilitation reduces the chances of future partner violence. This study finds that the same is true when women suffer from alcoholism and are violent toward men (Table 3 in the original article). What is also interesting was the high effectiveness of couples-based alcoholism treatment groups to achieve this result for female alcoholic patients and their partners. While in my experience women are more helpful to their alcoholic husbands than men are to their alcoholic or substance-abusing wives, the plight of husbands who wish to help their wives has not received adequate attention. Couples therapy, network therapy, and multiple couples groups may help these families survive intact and reduce addiction and domestic violence, all worthy goals. The treatment also helps reduce abuse and neglect that affect children in these families.

R. J. Frances, MD

Reducing Maternal Intimate Partner Violence After the Birth of a Child: A Randomized Controlled Trial of the Hawaii Healthy Start Home Visitation Program

Bair-Merritt MH, Jennings JM, Chen R, et al (Johns Hopkins Univ, Baltimore, MD; Georgetown Univ, Washington, DC)
Arch Pediatr Adolesc Med 164:16-23, 2010

Objectives.—To estimate whether home visitation beginning after childbirth was associated with changes in average rates of mothers' intimate partner violence (IPV) victimization and perpetration as well as rates of specific IPV types (physical assault, verbal abuse, sexual assault, and injury) during the 3 years of program implementation and during 3 years of long-term follow-up.

Design.—Randomized controlled trial.

Setting.—Oahu, Hawaii.

Participants.—Six hundred forty-three families with an infant at high risk for child maltreatment born between November 1994 and December 1995.

Intervention.—Home visitors provided direct services and linked families to community resources. Home visits were to initially occur weekly and to continue for at least 3 years.

Main Outcome Measures.—Women's self-reports of past-year IPV victimization and perpetration using the Conflict Tactics Scale. Blinded research staff conducted maternal interviews following the child's birth and annually when children were aged 1 to 3 years and then 7 to 9 years.

Results.—During program implementation, intervention mothers as compared with control mothers reported lower rates of IPV victimization (incidence rate ratio [IRR], 0.86; 95% confidence interval [CI], 0.73-1.01) and significantly lower rates of perpetration (IRR, 0.83; 95% CI, 0.72-0.96). Considering specific IPV types, intervention women reported significantly lower rates of physical assault victimization (IRR, 0.85; 95% CI, 0.71-1.00) and perpetration (IRR, 0.82; 95% CI, 0.70-0.96). During long-term follow-up, rates of overall IPV victimization and perpetration decreased, with nonsignificant between-group differences. Verbal abuse victimization rates (IRR, 1.14, 95% CI, 0.97-1.34) may have increased among intervention mothers.

Conclusion.—Early-childhood home visitation may be a promising strategy for reducing IPV.

▶ The study finds very positive results for home visitation after childbirth in reducing the chances of intimate partner violence. The results were fairly dramatic in the short term, but with a follow-up of 9 years the results were less dramatic (Fig 3 in the original article). However, reducing the risk early is quite important in reducing victimization and improving a child's environment at a critical period of development and growth. The value of targeting home visits to families at risk for domestic violence and child abuse is clear. When families are at highest risk, there can be risk to the clinician making the home visit, which may be best done by pairing home visitors to maximize safety.

R. J. Frances, MD

Violence

A Randomized Clinical Trial of Multisystemic Therapy With Juvenile Sexual Offenders: Effects on Youth Social Ecology and Criminal Activity
Borduin CM, Schaeffer CM, Heiblum N (Univ of Missouri, Columbia; Med Univ of South Carolina)
J Consult Clin Psychol 77:26-37, 2009

A randomized clinical trial evaluated the efficacy of multisystemic therapy (MST) versus usual community services (UCS) for 48 juvenile sexual offenders at high risk of committing additional serious crimes. Results from multiagent assessment batteries conducted before and after treatment showed that MST was more effective than UCS in improving key family, peer, and academic correlates of juvenile sexual offending and in ameliorating adjustment problems in individual family members.

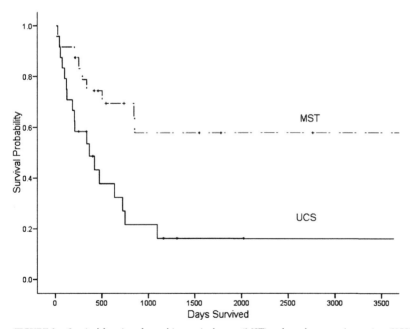

FIGURE 2.—Survival functions for multisystemic therapy (MST) and usual community services (UCS) groups for any offense. The survival probability represents the proportion of participants who were not arrested for any type of offense in each group by the length of time (in days) from the end of treatment. (Courtesy of Borduin CM, Schaeffer CM, Heiblum N. A randomized clinical trial of multisystemic therapy with juvenile sexual offenders: effects on youth social ecology and criminal activity. *J Consult Clin Psychol.* 2009;77:26-37.)

Moreover, results from an 8.9-year follow-up of rearrest and incarceration data (obtained when participants were on average 22.9 years of age) showed that MST participants had lower recidivism rates than did UCS participants for sexual (8% vs. 46%, respectively) and nonsexual (29% vs. 58%, respectively) crimes. In addition, MST participants had 70% fewer arrests for all crimes and spent 80% fewer days confined in detention facilities than did their counterparts who received UCS. The clinical and policy implications of these findings are discussed.

▶ This article finds a robust result in reducing recidivism in youthful juvenile sexual offenders using multisystemic therapy, with very good results over an almost 9-year follow-up (Fig 2). Given the significant toll that sexual offenses reap with victims, their families, the criminal justice system, and young offenders and their families, any new treatments that work and prevent abuse need to be implemented, even if the cost is higher than usual approaches, as is probably the case with multisystemic therapy. This study needs replication, as it is possible that a few dedicated therapists with talent and conviction may be able to get good results in a study like this, but reproducing these results in a large system may be difficult to achieve. With limited resources available for treatment in the criminal justice system, which is unfortunately the case, developing and targeting the most effective preventive measures requires careful consideration and evidence-based forensic research, with studies like this one being an important guide.

R. J. Frances, MD

Confectionery consumption in childhood and adult violence
Moore SC, Carter LM, van Goozen SHM (Cardiff Univ, UK)
Br J Psychiatry 195:366-367, 2009

Diet has been associated with behavioural problems, including aggression, but the long-term effects of childhood diet on adult violence have not been studied. We tested the hypothesis that excessive consumption of confectionery at age 10 years predicts convictions for violence in adulthood (age 34 years). Data from age 5, 10 and 34 years were used. Children who ate confectionery daily at age 10 years were significantly more likely to have been convicted for violence at age 34 years, a relationship that was robust when controlling for ecological and individual factors (Table 1).

▶ Wow! According to this article, eating too much candy in childhood can be a robust predictor of conviction for violence as an adult (Table 1). Awareness of this study should lend support for Michelle Obama's drive to improve the dietary consumption of American youth and give pause to parents who over-indulge their children with candy. The mechanism and understanding of the relationship found in this study are not clear and should be the subject of further research. Is it the effects of the sugar or the overindulgence that leads to later

TABLE 1.—Results from a Rare Events Logistic Multiple Regression Model Indicating a Significant Association Between Daily Confectionery Consumption at Age 10 Years and Conviction for Violence by 34 Years[a]

Variable	Wave	Odds Ratio	95% CI	P
Daily confectionery consumption	10 years	3.182	1.374–7.369	0.007
Male	5 years	8.927	2.526–31.549	0.001
Late birth	5 years	3.648	1.531–8.692	0.003
Health visitor screening	5 years	0.294	0.096–0.9	0.032
Child-oriented parenting	5 years	1.874	1.319–2.661	<0.001
Access to a motor car	34 years	0.224	0.11–0.456	<0.001
Rural area	34 years	1.801	0.977–3.321	0.059
Constant		0.003	0–0.022	<0.001

[a]Observations $n = 6942$.

trouble? How should society deal with this problem? Better awareness? A tax on sweets? Is candy a gateway drug? And when we get done with all these studies, what life pleasures will not be considered vices?

R. J. Frances, MD

Assessing Risk of Future Violence Among Forensic Psychiatric Inpatients With the Classification of Violence Risk (COVR)

Snowden RJ, Gray NS, Taylor J, et al (Cardiff Univ, UK; Partnerships in Care Ltd, Hertfordshire, UK)
Psychiatr Serv 60:1522-1526, 2009

Objectives.—Instruments are needed to help clinicians make decisions about a patient's risk of future violence in order to manage this risk, protect others, and allocate resources. One such actuarial instrument—the Classification of Violence Risk (COVR)—was developed from the MacArthur Violence Risk Assessment Study. The COVR has not been validated in a sample other than the one with which it was constructed or outside of the United States. The purpose of this study was to provide an independent validation of the COVR in a sample of forensic psychiatric inpatients in the United Kingdom.

Methods.—The prospective study was conducted at four medium-security forensic psychiatric units over six months. Two risk assessment instruments were completed for 52 patients: the COVR and the Violence Risk Appraisal Guide (VRAG), a well-established actuarial instrument. Incidents of verbal aggression, physical aggression toward others, and aggression against property were documented for the next six months from nursing records. Predictive accuracy of the instruments was analyzed using both correlational techniques and signal detection theory.

Results.—COVR was a good predictor of both verbal and physical aggression. Its predictive ability was similar to that of the VRAG, although the VRAG was a better predictor of violence to property.

Conclusions.—The study provides the first independent validation of the COVR and evidence of the usefulness of the COVR in predicting harmful behavior in forensic inpatient settings in the United Kingdom.

▶ This British study confirms the use of an American scale, the Classification of Violence Risk (COVR), which has been found to be a relatively effective predictive tool for verbal aggression, physical aggression toward others, and aggression against property, and has been used in forensic inpatient psychiatric settings (see Table 1 in the original article). The tool can be administered relatively easily and may help improve safety to staff and patients in these facilities when combined with use of treatment techniques to reduce violence potential. Predicting and reducing violence potential is one of the most difficult jobs clinicians and law enforcement agencies face, and any new effective assessment and prevention tools are of great value.

R. J. Frances, MD

Criminal behaviour and violent crimes in former inpatients with affective disorder
Graz C, Etschel E, Schoech H, et al (Ludwig-Maximilian-Univ, Munich, Germany)
J Affective Disord 117:98-103, 2009

Background.—Several studies have reported criminal and violent behaviour in people with schizophrenia but few have investigated the association between affective disorders and violent behaviour.

Methods.—We reviewed the national crime register for records of criminal offences committed by 1561 patients with affective disorders treated between 1990 and 1995 in the Psychiatric Hospital of the University of Munich. The sample was divided into patients with bipolar I disorder, manic disorder and major depressive disorder. Sociodemographic and other risk factors for non-violent and violent criminal behaviour were analysed.

Results.—Sixty-five (4.16%) patients had been convicted in the 7 to 12 years after discharge (307 cases). The rate of criminal behaviour and violent crimes was highest in the manic disorder group: 15.7% (14 of 89) were listed in the national crime register and 5.6% (5 of 89) were convicted of physical injury offences. Violence and criminality were comparatively rare in patients with major depressive disorder: only 1.42% (10 of 702) committed violent crimes. Male gender was a substantial risk factor for non-violent and especially violent behaviour: the rate of violent crimes was six times higher than in females. Marital status appeared to influence the prevalence of later delinquency: separated, divorced and widowed

TABLE 2.—(A) Descriptive Statistics of Affective Disorder Patients with Criminal (1.) and Violent (2.) Behaviour after Discharge for the Whole Group and the Three Subgroups (Bipolar, Manic, Major Depressive Disorder), (B) Type of Criminal Offence Committed after Discharge (1. Non-Violent Crimes, 2. Violent Crimes)

A: Criminal Offences of the 1561 patients with Affective Disorders in a 7–12 Year Period Following Discharge:

	Affective Disorder (Total)		Bipolar		Manic		Major Depressive	
	Number	%	Number	%	Number	%	Number	%
Total number of patients	1561	100	756	100	89	100	702	100
1. Criminal behaviour after discharge								
Convicted persons	65	4.16	17	2.24	14	15.73	33	4.70
Number of convictions	307		76		74		154	
Mean no. of convictions per person	4.72 pro 1/65		4.47 pro 1/17		5.29 pro 1/14		4.67 pro 1/33	
	0.20 pro 1/1561		0.10 pro 1/756		0.83 pro 1/89		0.22 pro 1/702	
2. Violent crimes after discharge								
Violent criminal persons	21	1.35	5	5.6	5	5.61	10	1.42
Number of violent crimes	49		14		9		25	
Mean no. of violent crimes per person	2.33 pro 1/21		2.80 pro 1/5		1.8 pro 1/5		2.5 pro 1/10	
	0.03 pro 1/1561		0.02 pro 1/756		0.10 pro 1/89		0.04 pro 1/702	
Legal procedures after discharge								
Lawsuits	210	100						
No criminal responsibility Proceedings were stopped (acquittal cases)	70	33.33						

B: Type of Criminal Offence Committed after Discharge (Multiple Cases per Person are Possible)	Number of Cases	%
1. Non-violent crimes		
Defalcation	36	11.73
Theft	24	7.82
Fraud	20	6.51
Verbal assault	16	5.21
Acquisition by false pretences	14	4.56
Driving while intoxicated	13	4.23
Civil disorder	7	2.28
Damage to property	6	1.95
Trespass/breach of domestic peace	5	1.63
Driving without license/insurance	5	1.63
Reckless driving	5	1.63
Falsification of documents	5	1.63
Hit-and-run accident	4	1.30
Drug offences	1	0.33
Exhibitionism	1	0.33
Arson	1	0.33
OTHER (misdemeanour)	89	28.99
2. Violent crimes		
Physical assault	21	6.84
Aggravated assault	9	2.93
Threatening/invasion of privacy	6	1.95
Constraint	6	1.95
Aggravated battery	3	0.98
Rape	2	0.65
Murder	1	0.33

patients committed offences more frequently. A history of substance use problems before clinical treatment was reported by 21.2% (329 of 1561) of the sample. A wide range of different crimes were committed, with defalcation, theft and fraud being the most frequent. Twenty-one cases of physical assault and one case of later homicide were recorded. In contrast to other forensic studies, we did not find a significant effect of substance abuse on the risk of later delinquent behaviour.

Conclusion.—The frequency of criminal behaviour and violent crimes in individuals with affective disorder depends on much more than just the diagnosis. This study may stimulate further research to identify psychopathological predictors for future violent and criminal behaviour.

▶ While postpartum depression violence has been the subject of many articles, surprisingly few study the relationship of affective disorders and crime. The fact that there are high rates of crime and violent behavior in those with manic disorder and low rates in those with depressive disorders should not come as a surprise to any clinician (see Table 2). What was unusual in this German sample was the finding that comorbid substance abuse did not increase crime in those with comorbid manic disorders, which is not what I have generally observed to be the case in practice. The additional problem of addiction, which is very common in manic disorders, increases impulsivity, worsens judgment, and tends to disinhibit in ways that increase crime, especially violence. The presence of a manic disorder needs to be diagnosed, and should be a factor in determining whether or not diminished capacity should be considered in sentencing in particular cases.

R. J. Frances, MD

A National Study of Violent Behavior in Persons With Schizophrenia
Swanson JW, Swartz MS, Van Dorn RA, et al (Duke Univ Med Ctr, Durham, NC; et al)
Arch Gen Psychiatry 63:490-499, 2006

Context.—Violent behavior is uncommon, yet problematic, among schizophrenia patients. The complex effects of clinical, interpersonal, and social-environmental risk factors for violence in this population are poorly understood.

Objective.—To examine the prevalence and correlates of violence among schizophrenia patients living in the community by developing multivariable statistical models to assess the net effects of psychotic symptoms and other risk factors for minor and serious violence.

Design.—A total of 1410 schizophrenia patients were clinically assessed and interviewed about violent behavior in the past 6 months. Data comprise baseline assessments of patients enrolled in the National Institute of Mental Health Clinical Antipsychotic Trials of Intervention Effectiveness.

TABLE 2.—Risk Factors for Serious Violence

Model	Bivariate Associations	OR (95% CI) Domain Models*	Final Model (N = 1401)
1: Demographic characteristics, social stratification, and housing			
Age	0.95 (0.93-0.98)†	0.95 (0.93-0.98)†	0.96 (0.94-0.99)‡
Male sex	1.32 (0.72-2.42)	NA	NA
Nonwhite race	1.37 (0.81-2.33)	NA	NA
Cohabitation	1.05 (0.56-1.97)	NA	NA
High monthly income	0.52 (0.30-0.89)§	NA	NA
College education	0.96 (0.58-1.60)	NA	NA
Substantial vocational activity	0.84 (0.29-2.40)	NA	NA
Housing during the past 30 d	NA	NA	NA
Extremely restrictive	1.85 (0.95-3.59)	NA	NA
Homeless	2.06 (0.79-5.35)	2.21 (0.83-5.89)	2.34 (0.80-6.82)
Low on economic scarcity	1.12 (0.52-2.42)	NA	NA
2: Household composition and social contact			
Currently live			
Alone (reference)	NA	NA	NA
With family or other relatives	1.21 (0.72-2.02)	NA	NA
With other people, not related	1.27 (0.72-2.24)	NA	NA
Frequent contact with family and friends	0.79 (0.41-1.53)	NA	NA
Feel "listened to" most of the time by family	0.75 (0.43-1.29)	NA	NA
3: Childhood risk factors			
Childhood physical abuse	2.28 (1.35-3.86)‡	NA	NA
Childhood sexual abuse	1.83 (1.06-3.16)§	NA	NA
Childhood conduct problems (≥2)	4.81 (2.69-8.62)†	4.81 (2.69-8.62)†	3.29 (1.79-6.07)†
4: Current clinical characteristics, impairment, and functioning			
Clinical Global Impression Scale score	1.22 (0.93-1.60)	NA	NA
PANSS score			
Negative (above median)	0.31 (0.17-0.56)†	0.26 (0.14-0.49)†	0.25 (0.13-0.47)†
Positive (above median)	3.00 (1.69-5.31)†	2.94 (1.63-5.30)†	2.71 (1.46-5.06)‡
Calgary Depression Scale for Schizophrenia score	1.09 (1.04-1.15)†	1.07 (1.01-1.13)§	1.08 (1.02-1.14)‡
Insight and Treatment Attitudes Questionnaire score (above median)	1.16 (0.70-1.91)	NA	NA
Years in treatment	0.98 (0.95-1.00)	0.97 (0.95-1.00)	NA
Substance use			
Abstinent (reference)	NA	NA	NA
Use	2.46 (1.09-5.60)§	2.42 (1.07-5.48)§	1.88 (0.78-4.51)
Abuse or dependence	4.11 (1.99-8.52)†	3.38 (1.61-7.10)†	2.10 (0.94-4.71)
Recent victimization (past 6 mo)			
Violently victimized	4.88 (1.99-11.93)†	2.57 (0.96-6.92)‡	NA
Nonviolently victimized	3.84 (2.08-7.09)†	2.87 (1.48-5.55)†	2.27 (1.12-4.61)§
QOL Scale score			
Common objects and activities subscale	1.08 (0.88-1.34)	NA	NA
Instrumental role subscale	0.97 (0.83-1.12)	NA	NA
Intrapsychic foundations subscale	1.11 (0.90-1.37)	NA	NA
Interpersonal relations subscale	1.11 (0.92-1.34)	NA	NA
Leisure activities (past week)	1.19 (0.60-2.36)	NA	NA
Instrumental ADLs (past week)	NA	NA	NA
General life satisfaction	0.83 (0.46-1.51)	NA	NA
5: Institutional contact			
Total prior hospitalizations			
Lifetime, ≥4	0.93 (0.57-1.53)	NA	NA
Past year, ≥2	1.44 (0.86-2.40)	NA	NA
			(*Continued*)

TABLE 2. (*continued*)

Model	Bivariate Associations	OR (95% CI) Domain Models*	Final Model (N = 1401)
Arrested or picked up for crime (past 6 mo)	5.85 (3.18-10.76)†	5.85 (3.18-10.76)†	3.45 (1.74-6.85)†

Abbreviations: See Table 1.
*N = 1405 for model 1, N = 1406 for model 3, N = 1348 for model 4, and N = 1407 for model 5.
†P<.001.
‡P<.01.
§P<.05.

Setting and Patients.—Adult patients diagnosed as having schizophrenia were enrolled from 56 sites in the United States, including academic medical centers and community providers.

Main Outcome Measures.—Violence was classified at 2 severity levels: minor violence, corresponding to simple assault without injury or weapon use; and serious violence, corresponding to assault resulting in injury or involving use of a lethal weapon, threat with a lethal weapon in hand, or sexual assault. A composite measure of any violence was also analyzed.

Results.—The 6-month prevalence of any violence was 19.1%, with 3.6% of participants reporting serious violent behavior. Distinct, but overlapping, sets of risk factors were associated with minor and serious violence. "Positive" psychotic symptoms, such as persecutory ideation, increased the risk of minor and serious violence, while "negative" psychotic symptoms, such as social withdrawal, lowered the risk of serious violence. Minor violence was associated with co-occurring substance abuse and interpersonal and social factors. Serious violence was associated with psychotic and depressive symptoms, childhood conduct problems, and victimization.

Conclusions.—Particular clusters of symptoms may increase or decrease violence risk in schizophrenia patients. Violence risk assessment and management in community-based treatment should focus on combinations of clinical and nonclinical risk factors.

▶ This important national study of violent behavior in persons with schizophrenia not only gives us 6-month prevalence of minor and serious violence for this population at rates higher than other reports, but also provides risk factors associated with minor and serious violence (Table 2). Awareness of and efforts to treat positive symptoms of schizophrenia, including hallucinations and psychosis, and to treat comorbid substance abuse, has the potential to reduce violence. Awareness of grandiosity and delusions of extraordinary abilities as a risk factor for serious violence can also lead to precautionary measures with such patients. Negative symptoms had a reverse correlation to violence perhaps related to the passivity and lack of social engagement that occurs as a result. One concern I have about psychiatrists' relationship to this issue is that, although we can learn more about prediction and prevention of violence in the mentally ill, there are real limitations to our predictive ability, that all must understand, if we are to give humane least restrictive care, without overconcern about legal liability when making clinical decisions.

R. J. Frances, MD

Euthanasia

Legal Euthanasia in Belgium: Characteristics of All Reported Euthanasia Cases

Smets T, Bilsen J, Cohen J, et al (Vrije Universiteit Brussel, Belgium; et al)
Med Care 48:187-192, 2010

Objectives.—To study the reported medical practice of euthanasia in Belgium since implementation of the euthanasia law.

Research Design.—Analysis of the anonymous database of all euthanasia cases reported to the Federal Control and Evaluation Committee Euthanasia.

Subjects.—All euthanasia cases reported by physicians for review between implementation of the euthanasia law on September 22nd, 2002 and December 31, 2007 (n = 1917).

Measures.—Frequency of reported euthanasia cases, characteristics of patients and the decision for euthanasia, drugs used in euthanasia cases, and trends in reported cases over time.

Results.—The number of reported euthanasia cases increased every year from 0.23% of all deaths in 2002 to 0.49% in 2007. Compared with all deaths in the population, patients who died by euthanasia were more often younger (82.1% of patients who received euthanasia compared with 49.8% of all deaths were younger than 80, $P < 0.001$), men (52.7% vs. 49.5%, $P = 0.005$), cancer patients (82.5% vs. 23.5%, $P < 0.001$), and more often died at home (42.2% vs. 22.4%, $P < 0.001$). Euthanasia was most often performed with a barbiturate, sometimes in combination with neuromuscular relaxants (92.4%) and seldom with morphine (0.9%). In almost all patients, unbearable physical (95.6%) and/or psychological suffering (68%) were reported. A small minority of cases (6.6%) concerned nonterminal patients, mainly suffering from neuromuscular diseases.

Conclusions.—The frequency of reported euthanasia cases has increased every year since legalization. Euthanasia is most often chosen as a last resort at the end of life by younger patients, patients with cancer, and seldom by nonterminal patients (Table 2).

▶ This article characterizes the use of euthanasia in Belgium and finds it to be increasingly practiced since legalization, primarily in younger terminally ill cancer patients but sometimes in nonterminal patients mainly suffering from neuromuscular diseases (Table 2). The suffering of individuals and families

TABLE 2.—Patient Characteristics of All Reported Euthanasia Cases 2002–2007 Compared with All Deaths in Belgium (Flanders and Brussels)*

Characteristic	Reported Cases of Euthanasia* N = 1917	All Deaths[†] N = 265597	P
Sex			0.005
Men	52.7	49.5	
Women	47.3	50.5	
Age			<0.001
1–17	0.0	0.3	
18–39	3.0	2.0	
40–59	26.0	9.5	
60–79	53.1	37.9	
>79	17.9	50.2	
Diagnosis			<0.001
Cancer	82.5	23.5	
Other than cancer	17.5	76.5	
Place of death			<0.001
Hospital	51.7	52.3	
Home	42.2	22.4	
Care home	4.3	22.0	
Other	1.8	3.4	

Data presented are column percentages; p-values calculated with Fisher exact test.
Percentages may not always amount to 100% because of rounding.
*Patient characteristics of reported euthanasia cases in 2008 not yet available.
[†]Deaths statistics of persons older than one year from Flanders and Brussels (Belgium), 2003 to 2007.

faced with terminal illness is enormous and in addition to the end-of-life economic costs has led to increasing discussion and fears regarding the use and possible legalization in this country of euthanasia. Carefully evaluating the experience of other countries that have legalized euthanasia is of value. The finding here that legalization in Belgium has not led to increased euthanasia among nonterminal elderly patients should be reassuring to those who fear the practice would be abused. The concern that state-dependent decisions affected by depression and other treatable conditions could lead to unnecessary deaths is a major concern, but the question of someone's right to end their suffering needs to be taken into account in deciding public policy.

R. J. Frances, MD

Miscellaneous

Bipolar disorder as a risk factor for repeat DUI behavior
Albanese MJ, Nelson SE, Peller AJ, et al (Cambridge Health Alliance, MA; Brandeis Univ Heller School for Social Policy and Management, Waltham, MA)
J Affective Disord 121:253-257, 2010

Background.—Bipolar disorder (BD) is more prevalent among people with substance use disorders (SUD) than the general population. SUD among recidivist driving under the influence (DUI) populations are extremely prevalent; not surprisingly, recent evidence suggests that rates of BD also are elevated among DUI offenders. Studies of BD patients with SUD have found high prevalence of other psychiatric disorders and relatively low rate of treatment engagement. This study examines both the prevalence of other mental disorders and treatment status among a cohort of DUI offenders with BD and SUD.

Methods.—A consecutively selected cohort $(N = 729)$ of repeat DUI offenders attending a two-week inpatient treatment program completed a standardized diagnostic interview (the Composite International Diagnostic Interview: CIDI). The CIDI generated DSM-IV diagnoses.

Results.—This study yielded three main results for this repeat DUI offender sample: (1) BD is associated with significantly higher lifetime prevalence of alcohol, drug, and non-substance psychiatric disorders (e.g., PTSD); (2) approximately one quarter of BD participants have not discussed their mania with a professional; and (3) only half of the BD participants in this cohort have had mania treatment they consider effective and even fewer have had any treatment during the past twelve months.

TABLE 1.—Characteristics and Psychiatric Comorbidity of Repeat DUI Offenders with and without Bipolar Disorder

	Participants w/Lifetime Bipolar $n = 53$	Participants w/Out Lifetime Bipolar $n = 676$
Characteristic	% (*n*)	% (*n*)
Gender (male)*	66.0% (35)	82.5% (558)
Race (white)	92.5% (49)	87.4% (591)
Income (<$20,000)	41.5% (22)	30.9% (209)
Marital status (married)	20.8% (11)	18.3% (124)
Education (HS or less)	71.7% (38)	72.2% (488)
History of physical abuse*	35.8% (19)	12.3% (83)
Ever been in jail	20.8% (11)	24.3% (164)
	M (SD)	M (SD)
Age	39.8 (10.3)	39.6 (11.7)
# of DUI Arrests	2.6 (1.4)	2.5 (0.9)
Addiction-related disorders	% (*n*)	% (*n*)
Alcohol abuse[a]*	37.7% (20)	58.4% (395)
Alcohol dependence[a]*	58.5% (31)	39.3% (266)
Drug abuse	30.2% (16)	25.6% (173)
Drug dependence[a]*	32.1% (17)	13.3% (90)
Nicotine dependence	22.6% (12)	15.4% (104)
Other psychiatric disorders	% (*n*)	% (*n*)
Generalized anxiety[a]*	24.5% (13)	7.1% (48)
Post-traumatic stress[a]*	39.6% (21)	11.2% (76)
Conduct	17.0% (9)	17.9% (121)
Attention deficit[a§]*	30.4% (14)	6.6% (38)

*Groups differ significantly according to χ^2 or t-test, $p < .01$.
[§]Analyses based on a subset of 622 cases who received attention deficit modules – $n = 46$ for lifetime bipolar participants; $n = 576$ for participants w/out lifetime bipolar.
[a]Lifetime prevalence for participants w/ and w/out lifetime bipolar disorder significantly different according to χ^2, $p < .01$.

Limitations.—Participants were predominantly Caucasian males attending treatment as a sentencing option in a single Massachusetts DUI program.

Conclusion.—These findings suggest that clinicians in DUI treatment settings should consider both evaluating for BD and initiating therapy.

▶ This article highlights the high prevalence of dual diagnosis of bipolar disorder and substance abuse in repeat driving under the influence (DUI) offenders and the fact that these individuals often are not in treatment or co-operating with treatment (Table 1). The need for screening for dual diagnosis and encouraging bipolar patients to participate in treatment of dual diagnosis when the patients are in trouble for a DUI is clear. Coercion can help these individuals get motivated to seek out help, and probation officers can insist on treatment compliance. One result of lack of dealing with this problem is having untreated bipolar patients enter the prison system, where they are likely to remain undiagnosed and untreated and are further damaged in terms of employment, etc. They are also a high-risk group for suicide in jail.

R. J. Frances, MD

Dissipation and displacement of hotspots in reaction-diffusion models of crime
Short MB, Brantingham PJ, Bertozzi AL, et al (Univ of California, Los Angeles; et al)
Proc Natl Acad Sci 107:3961-3965, 2010

The mechanisms driving the nucleation, spread, and dissipation of crime hotspots are poorly understood. As a consequence, the ability of law enforcement agencies to use mapped crime patterns to design crime prevention strategies is severely hampered. We also lack robust expectations about how different policing interventions should impact crime. Here we present a mathematical framework based on reaction-diffusion partial differential equations for studying the dynamics of crime hotspots. The system of equations is based on empirical evidence for how offenders move and mix with potential victims or targets. Analysis shows that crime hotspots form when the enhanced risk of repeat crimes diffuses locally, but not so far as to bind distant crime together. Crime hotspots may form as either supercritical or subcritical bifurcations, the latter the result of large spikes in crime that override linearly stable, uniform crime distributions. Our mathematical methods show that subcritical crime hotspots may be permanently eradicated with police suppression, whereas super-critical hotspots are displaced following a characteristic spatial pattern.

Our results thus provide a mechanistic explanation for recent failures to observe crime displacement in experimental field tests of hotspot policing.

▶ Bringing empirical evidence and science to crime fighting has led to marked reduction of crimes in recent years. This article uses mathematical models to examine crime hotspots and consider strategies to prevent crime based on awareness of patterns of crime, risk of repeat crime, and use of targeted police suppression. I might recommend that adding forensic psychiatric sophistication to the mix in further study of these techniques might be very useful. Tracking sexual offenders is 1 example; awareness and use of outpatient commitment is another example of psychiatric patients who may pose a danger but may not be chronically committable. Cooperation and communication between law enforcement and mental health agencies may lead to sophisticated police work that may even further reduce already lowered crime rates.

R. J. Frances, MD

5 Hospital and Community Psychiatry

Epidemiology, Diagnosis, and Trends

Geographic Patterns of Frequent Mental Distress: U.S. Adults, 1993–2001 and 2003–2006
Moriarty DG, Zack MM, Holt JB, et al (CDC, Atlanta, GA)
Am J Prev Med 36:497-505, 2009

Background.—Mental illnesses and other mental health problems often lead to prolonged, disabling, and costly mental distress. Yet little is known about the geographic distribution of such mental distress in the U.S.

Methods.—Since 1993, the CDC has tracked self-perceived mental distress through the Behavioral Risk Factor Surveillance System (BRFSS). In 2007 and 2008, analysis was performed on BRFSS data reported by 2.4 million adults from 1993–2001 and 2003–2006 to map and describe the prevalence of frequent mental distress (FMD)—defined as having ≥14 mentally unhealthy days during the previous 30 days—for all states and for counties with at least 30 respondents.

Results.—The adult prevalence of FMD for the combined periods was 9.4% overall, ranging from 6.6% in Hawaii to 14.4% in Kentucky. From 1993–2001 to 2003–2006, the mean prevalence of FMD increased by at least 1 percentage point in 27 states and by more than 4 percentage points in Mississippi, Oklahoma, and West Virginia. Most states showed internal geographic variations in FMD prevalence. The Appalachian and the Mississippi Valley regions had high and increasing FMD prevalence, and the upper Midwest had low and decreasing FMD prevalence.

Conclusions.—Geographic areas were identified with consistently high and consistently low FMD prevalence, as well as areas in which FMD prevalence changed substantially. Further evaluation of the causes and implications of these patterns is warranted. Surveillance of mental distress

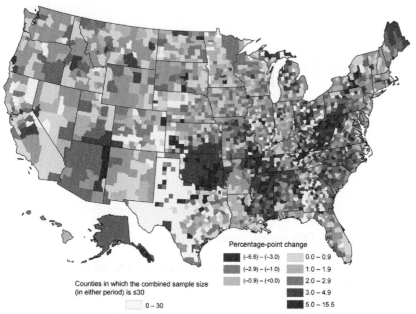

FIGURE 2.—Percentage-point change in county-level prevalence of frequent mental distress (1993–2001 to 2003–2006). (Reprinted from Moriarty DG, Zack MM, Holt JB, et al. Geographic patterns of frequent mental distress: U.S. adults, 1993–2001 and 2003–2006. *Am J Prev Med.* 2009;36:497-505, with permission from Elsevier.)

may be useful in identifying unmet mental health needs and disparities and in guiding health-related policies and interventions.

▶ Well what are we to make of this?

It's interesting and never would have occurred to me, but it's logical that there are regional differences in the mental distress felt by people living in different geographic areas.

The figures (Fig 2) that accompany the article are fascinating as well. But why and even if we could correlate these differences with income or education or geographic peculiarities (eg, idyllic islands, mine-scarred valleys, mountain areas, etc), what could we do about it?

However, the CDC thinks its important enough to look at and that counts for a lot. They suggest with such knowledge comes the possibility of targeting unmet health and social service needs and that programs in areas with such high levels should collaborate to identify and address the sources of the distress as well as promote treatment efforts.

I, for one, will watch what happens with great interest.

J. A. Talbott, MD

Generational Status and Family Cohesion Effects on the Receipt of Mental Health Services Among Asian Americans: Findings From the National Latino and Asian American Study
Ta VM, Holck P, Gee GC (Univ of Hawai'i at Mānoa; Univ of California, Los Angeles)
Am J Public Health 100:115-121, 2010

Objectives.—We investigated the relative strengths of generational status and family cohesion effects on current use of mental health services (past 12 months) among Asian Americans.

Methods.—We conducted a secondary data analysis with data from the National Latino and Asian American Study, 2002 to 2003, restricted to Asian American respondents (n = 2087). The study's outcome was current use (past 12 months) of any mental health services. Respondents included Chinese, Filipino, Vietnamese, and other Asian Americans.

Results.—Multivariate analyses suggest no significant interaction exists between second- versus first-generation Asian Americans and family cohesion. The impact of generational status on mental health service use was significant for third- or later-generation Asian Americans (versus first-generation Asian Americans) and varied with family cohesion score.

Conclusions.—Family cohesion and generational status both affect the likelihood of Asian Americans to seek mental health services. Our findings also highlight the need for primary care and other providers to consistently screen for mental health status particularly among first-generation Asian Americans. Mental health service programs should target recent immigrants and individuals lacking a strong family support system.

▶ This article reveals the schism between 2 major trends in mental health services in America: the first that pushes toward a "one size fits all" approach that reimburses and to some extent researchers and public policy makers aid and abet through evidence-based treatment guidelines; the second the pressure to be culturally competent and have services tailor-made for various ethnic, religious, and culturally-different populations.

The authors' summary conclusion, that "Mental health service programs should target recent immigrants and individuals lacking a strong family support system" is certainly logical and sound, but at this time when cutbacks in funding and services are at an all-time high, one wonders how practical it is and how well-heeded it will be.

It is unfair to criticize the authors' lack of clinical training or knowledge, but one wonders how exactly we would implement their recommendation that "primary care providers and other providers [need] to consistently screen for mental health status as it appears that those who need treatment might not be detected when we know they don't consistently screen" anyone psychiatrically?

J. A. Talbott, MD

Mental Disorders Among Homeless People Admitted to a French Psychiatric Emergency Service

Henry J-M, Boyer L, Belzeaux R, et al (La Conception Hosp, Marseille, France; La Timone Hosp, Marseille, France; et al)
Psychiatr Serv 61:264-271, 2010

Objective.—The aim of this study was to identify factors associated with homelessness status among patients admitted to the psychiatric emergency ward of a French public teaching hospital over a six-year study period (2001–2006).

Methods.—The study was based on a retrospective review of the psychiatric emergency ward's administrative and medical computer databases. Each emergency care episode had accompanying data that included demographic, financial, clinical, and management information.

Results.—During this six-year study, the psychiatric service recorded 16,754 care episodes for 8,860 different patients, of which 591 were homeless (6.7%) and 8,269 were nonhomeless (93.3%). The mean ± SD number of visits to the psychiatric emergency service was higher for homeless patients (4.9 ± 12.3) than for nonhomeless patients (1.7 ± 2.4) (p<.001). A total of 331 homeless patients (56.0%) had more than one care episode, whereas 2,180 (26.4%) of nonhomeless patients had more than one care episode. Factors associated with homelessness included being male, being single, and receiving financial assistance through government social programs. Schizophrenia (43.7%) and substance use disorders (31.0%) were the most common disorders among homeless patients. Aggressive behavior and violence were reported equally among homeless patients (3.5%) and nonhomeless patients (3.2%). Homeless patients were less likely than nonhomeless patients to be hospitalized after receiving care in the emergency ward (47.8% versus 51.1%) (p=.002).

Conclusions.—Although there is near-universal access to free mental health care in France, study findings suggest that the quality and adequacy of subsequent care are not guaranteed. Multidisciplinary and collaborative solutions are needed to improve the management of mental health care for homeless patients (Table 2).

▶ When I went on my first sabbatical in France in 1991-1992, I had already written 12 articles on the subject and was interested to learn what concerns and issues were comparable. A highly respected epidemiologist at the World Health Organization (just over the border in Geneva) told me that there was no mental illness among the homeless in France; they were all alcoholic bums. Ten years later, when these data had begun to be recorded, things had changed—granted nowhere near as bad a situation then or now as in the United States, but worse. There as here, severe mental illness, especially schizophrenia, is overrepresented, and substance abuse is slightly less. Not surprisingly, dual diagnosis is also climbing (Table 2). As a Francophile, I think of France as not only having the #1 health care system in the world but also a peerless social

TABLE 2.—Characteristics Associated with Patients' Receiving Care in a Psychiatric Emergency Ward of a French Public Hospital (2001–2006), by Homelessness Status[a]

Characteristic	Nonhomeless (N = 8,269 Patients)		Homeless (N = 591 Patients)		
	N	%	N	%	p
Sociodemographic					
Age (mean±SD years)	40.1±15.1		38.5±10.8		.029
Male	4,102	49.6	469	79.6	<.001
Marital status[b]					<.001
Married	1,815	25.2	29	6.3	
Single	5,374	74.8	431	93.7	
Children	3,438	41.6	202	34.2	<.001
Financial issues					
Unemployment benefits	543	6.6	28	4.7	.083
Financial assistance through social government programs	1,005	12.2	149	25.2	<.001
Psychiatric diagnosis					
Mental and behavioral disorders due to psychoactive substance use (*ICD-10* section F1)	978	11.8	183	31.0	<.001
Schizophrenia, schizotypal, and delusional disorders (*ICD-10* section F2)	1,971	23.8	258	43.7	<.001
Mood (affective) disorders (*ICD-10* section F3)	2,088	25.3	142	24.0	.508
Bipolar	576	7.0	28	4.7	.038
Neurotic, stress-related, and somatoform disorders (*ICD-10* section F4)	2,615	31.6	160	27.1	.021
Disorders of adult personality and behavior (*ICD-10* section F6)[c]	754	9.1	126	21.3	<.001
Cluster A	136	1.6	19	3.2	.005
Cluster B	513	6.2	104	17.6	<.001
Cluster C	120	1.5	12	2.0	.261
Other psychiatric diagnosis (*ICD-10* sections F5, F7–F9)	392	4.7	50	8.5	<.001
Dual diagnosis[d]	308	3.7	98	16.6	<.001
Number of admissions (2001–2006)					<.001
1	6,089	73.6	260	44.0	
2–3	1,622	19.6	154	26.1	
≥4	558	6.7	177	29.9	
Interval between discharge and readmission to an emergency ward (median days)	59		28		<.001

[a]Homeless patients were those who had at least one service encounter while homeless.
[b]Data were available for 7,189 nonhomeless persons and 460 homeless persons.
[c]Personality disorders defined by the *DSM-IV*. The *DSM-IV* lists ten personality disorders, grouped into three clusters: A (odd or eccentric disorders), B (dramatic, emotional, or erratic disorders), and C (anxious or fearful disorders).
[d]Substance use disorder plus any other diagnosis listed above.

security system and safety net as well as agencies that must be more coordinated than in America, so it's disheartening to see that even with all this infrastructure, we can all do a better job.

J. A. Talbott, MD

Comparing Mental Health of Francophones in Canada, France, and Belgium: 12-Month and Lifetime Rates of Mental Health Service Use (Part 2)

Tempier R, Vasiliadis H-M, Gilbert F, et al (Univ of Saskatchewan, Saskatoon; L'Université de Sherbrooke, Quebec, Canada; Univ of ParisV–René Descartes, France; et al)
Can J Psychiatry 55:295-304, 2010

Objectives.—To compare 12-month and lifetime service use for common mental disorders in 4 francophone subsamples using data from national mental health surveys in Canada, Quebec, France, and Belgium. This is the second article in a 2-part series comparing mental disorders and service use prevalence of French-speaking populations.

Methods.—Comparable World Mental Health–Composite International Diagnostic Interviews (WMH-CIDI) were administered to representative samples of adults (aged 18 years and older) in Canada during 2002 and in France and Belgium from 2001 to 2003. Two groups of francophone adults in Canada, in Quebec ($n = 7571$) and outside Quebec ($n = 500$), and respondents in Belgium ($n = 389$) and France ($n = 1436$) completed the French version of the population survey. Prevalence rates of common mental health service use were examined for major depressive episodes and specific anxiety disorders (that is, agoraphobia, social phobia, and panic disorder).

Results.—Overall, most francophones with mental disorders do not seek treatment. Canadians consulted more mental health professionals than their European counterparts, with the exception of psychiatrists.

Conclusions.—Patterns of service use are similar among francophone populations. Variations that exist may be accounted for by differences in health care resources, health care systems, and health insurance coverage.

▶ This is as close as we can get to an apples-to-apples type comparison of mental health care utilization; comparing the same genetic stock, albeit with hundreds of years of different histories, health care systems, and cultural trends. A nifty idea. I only wished they had included francophonic Switzerland, whose Huguenot status and health care system represent yet other differences. But no matter.

It is interesting to note that only half of the persons diagnosed with depression and anxiety disorders do not seek or get treatment. Granted this is better than in the United States or most seriously in China, where only 11% of persons with mental disorders received treatment, but it still shows that we all have problems of access, stigma, cultural and personal receptivity, etc. The fact that differences in utilization are in part because of the different health care systems in the 3 nations should be used in the United States as an argument for health care reform continuance but won't be because of the anticipated charges that Canada, France, and Belgium are socialist states. Finally, the fact that citizens of France get care more often from psychiatrists than those in Canada is, I believe, not only because of the systems but also because of the positive attitude about psychiatry in France, and the respect it is accorded in French intellectual circles.

J. A. Talbott, MD

Adverse Childhood Experiences and the Risk of Premature Mortality
Brown DW, Anda RF, Tiemeier H, et al (CDC, Atlanta, GA; Erasmus Univ Med Ctr, Rotterdam, The Netherlands; et al)
Am J Prev Med 37:389-396, 2009

Background.—Strong, graded relationships between exposure to child-hood traumatic stressors and numerous negative health behaviors and outcomes, healthcare utilization, and overall health status inspired the question of whether these adverse childhood experiences (ACEs) are associated with premature death during adulthood.

Purpose.—This study aims to determine whether ACEs are associated with an increased risk of premature death during adulthood.

Methods.—Baseline survey data on health behaviors, health status, and exposure to ACEs were collected from 17,337 adults aged >18 years during 1995–1997. The ACEs included abuse (emotional, physical, sexual); witnessing domestic violence; parental separation or divorce; and growing up in a household where members were mentally ill, substance abusers, or sent to prison. The ACE score (an integer count of the eight categories of ACEs) was used as a measure of cumulative exposure to traumatic stress during childhood. Deaths were identified during follow-up assessments (between baseline appointment date and December 31, 2006) using mortality records obtained from a search of the National Death Index. Expected years of life lost (YLL) and years of potential life lost (YPLL) were computed using standard methods. The relative risk of death from all causes at age ≤65 years and at age ≤75 years was estimated across the number of categories of ACEs using multivariable-adjusted Cox proportional hazards regression. Analysis was conducted during January–February 2009.

Results.—Overall, 1539 people died during follow-up; the crude death rate was 91.0 per 1000; the age-adjusted rate was 54.7 per 1000. People with six or more ACEs died nearly 20 years earlier on average than those without ACEs (60.6 years, 95% CI = 56.2, 65.1, vs 79.1 years, 95% CI = 78.4, 79.9). Average YLL per death was nearly three times greater among people with six or more ACEs (25.2 years) than those without ACEs (9.2 years). Roughly one third ($n = 526$) of those who died during follow-up were aged ≤75 years at the time of death, accounting for 4792 YPLL. After multivariable adjustment, adults with six or more ACEs were 1.7 (95% CI = 1.06, 2.83) times more likely to die when aged ≤75 years and 2.4 (95% CI = 1.30, 4.39) times more likely to die when aged ≤65 years.

Conclusions.—ACEs are associated with an increased risk of premature death, although a graded increase in the risk of premature death was not observed across the number of categories of ACEs. The increase in risk was only partly explained by documented ACE-related health and social problems, suggesting other possible mechanisms by which ACEs may contribute to premature death.

▶ Goodness gracious, this is a scary article. Let me start with the principal finding: that "people with six or more ACEs died nearly 20 years earlier on average than those without ACEs (60.6 years,... vs 79.1 years,...)." Now let's recall that adverse childhood experiences (ACEs) include: "abuse (emotional, physical, sexual); witnessing domestic violence; parental separation or divorce; and growing up in a household where members were mentally ill, substance abusers, or sent to prison." OK. Two questions immediately occurred to me: (1) what on earth is the explanation for ACEs having such a powerful influence on life expectancy, and (2) isn't this a public health threat every bit as powerful as AIDS, plagues, or nuclear war?

To answer (1)—the authors state that "the strongest associations exist between ACEs and mental health or psychosocial-related risk behaviors and outcomes... and there are strong relationships between ACEs and alcohol abuse, illicit drug use, sexual promiscuity, and suicide." They thus conclude that "some of this increase in risk is explained by ACE-related health and social problems... but lend further support to the collective body of evidence suggesting that childhood traumatic stressors represent a common pathway to a variety of long-term behavioral, health, and social problems." So if I understand the sequence ACEs lead to risk behaviors that can result in poor outcomes ranging from suicide to cancer.

To address (2) for exposure to ACEs to be in the authors' words, so "common" I find it amazing that no one in the world of public health has raised the alarm and called for a reduction in their occurrence.

J. A. Talbott, MD

Mortality Risk Associated with Physical and Verbal Abuse in Women Aged 50 to 79

Baker MW, LaCroix AZ, Wu C, et al (Univ of Washington, Seattle; Fred Hutchinson Cancer Res Ctr, Seattle, WA; et al)
J Am Geriatr Soc 57:1799-1809, 2009

Objectives.—To investigate whether midlife and older women who reported prior-year physical abuse, verbal abuse, or both abuse types had higher mortality risk than peers who did not report prior-year abuse.

Design.—Retrospective analysis.

Setting.—Community.

Participants.—One hundred sixty-thousand six hundred seventy-six community-dwelling women ages 50 to 79 at baseline enrolled in one of two major Women's Health Initiative (WHI) study components who responded to baseline abuse questions. Observational study enrollment was N = 93,676 (1994–1998; 90 months average follow-up). Clinical trial enrollment was N = 68,132 (1993–1998; 96 months average follow-up).

Measurements.—Total mortality was measured from 1993 to 2005 using all available data sources. Blinded physician adjudicators measured cause-specific mortality. Ninety-six percent of death records were adjudicated.

Results.—Prior-year self-reported abuse prevalence was 11.3%. Women who reported physical abuse had the highest age-adjusted mortality rate, followed by women who reported both abuse types. Abuse independently predicted mortality risk after controlling for age, education, ethnicity, and WHI component. High mortality risk remained for physically abused women (hazard ratio (HR) = 1.54, 95% confidence interval (CI) = 1.09–2.18) after adjusting for demographic and health-related factors. Further adjustment for psychosocial variables diminished this association (HR = 1.40, 95% CI = 0.93–2.11), but high risk remained.

Conclusion.—Community-dwelling middle-aged and older women who reported prior-year physical, verbal, or both types of abuse had significantly higher adjusted mortality risk than women who did not report abuse. These findings highlight the need for longitudinal research into prevention of abuse in later life and accompanying excess mortality and emphasize the importance of abuse prevention in later life.

▶ Here at the other end of the age span, we see that abuse of various sorts reduces longevity. The finding that "women who reported prior-year physical abuse (with or without verbal abuse) had significantly higher age-adjusted mortality rates and higher mortality risk than women who reported no abuse" is disturbing to say the least. Two other statements are of note: First, that "...the severity and significance of psychological abuse (which includes verbal abuse) has been underestimated or ignored....," which I've never understood, because battered women's programs and elder abuse have received so much attention in the press, and the second, that "psychological abuse is a much stronger predictor of fear than physical abuse, often precedes physical abuse, and is associated with chronic disease and poor health....," suggests that verbal mistreatment leads to more psychological effects leading to more physical (eg, cardiovascular) problems that result in death more often than physical abuse does. While the authors call for "...longitudinal research into mechanisms and prevention of abuse in later life and accompanying excess mortality for women and men..." it would seem to me that rather than wait for more research, this should be seen as constituting another public health emergency, worthy of taking steps to identify, treat, and prevent such abuse from leading to death.

J. A. Talbott, MD

State-Level Policies and Psychiatric Morbidity In Lesbian, Gay, and Bisexual Populations

Hatzenbuehler ML, Keyes KM, Hasin DS (Yale Univ, New Haven, CT; Columbia Univ, NY; et al)
Am J Public Health 99:2275-2281, 2009

Objectives.—We investigated the modifying effect of state-level policies on the association between lesbian, gay, or bisexual status and the prevalence of psychiatric disorders.

Methods.—Data were from wave 2 of the National Epidemiologic Survey on Alcohol and Related Conditions (NESARC), a nationally representative study of noninstitutionalized US adults (N = 34653). States were coded for policies extending protections against hate crimes and employment discrimination based on sexual orientation.

Results.—Compared with living in states with policies extending protections, living in states without these policies predicted a significantly stronger association between lesbian, gay, or bisexual status and psychiatric disorders in the past 12 months, including generalized anxiety disorder ($F = 3.87$; $df = 2$; $P = .02$), post-traumatic stress disorder ($F = 3.42$; $df = 2$; $P = .04$), and dysthymia ($F = 5.20$; $df = 2$; $P = .02$). Living in states with policies that did not extend protections also predicted a stronger relation between lesbian, gay, or bisexual status and psychiatric comorbidity ($F = 2.47$; $df = 2$; $P = .04$).

Conclusions.—State-level protective policies modify the effect of lesbian, gay, or bisexual status on psychiatric disorders. Policies that reduce discrimination against gays and lesbians are urgently needed to protect the health and well-being of this population.

▶ This is an astounding study with startling, albeit logical results. Just as the gay marriage argument in Iowa (and probably California) was framed as a civil rights/equality issue, the gay, lesbian, bisexual protection discrimination issue may now fruitfully be portrayed to the general citizenry as a real problem with real bad effects if we can show, as these authors did, that discrimination results in poor mental health (as evidenced by increases in generalized anxiety disorders, posttraumatic stress disorders, and dysthymia). Of course, the zealots and discriminators may well be the same folks who believe these are lifestyle choices, works of the devil, and evil practices as much as they may believe mental illnesses are due to a lack of willpower or paucity of religious faith, or witchcraft, in which case reason will play no role in changing their actions. But for many, this sort of epidemiological study should result in changes in public policy.

J. A. Talbott, MD

Economic Issues

Economic impact of early Intervention in people at high risk of psychosis
Valmaggia LR, McCrone P, Knapp M, et al (Inst of Psychiatry, King's College London, UK; et al)
Psychol Med 39:1617-1626, 2009

Background.—Despite the increasing development of early intervention services for psychosis, little is known about their cost-effectiveness. We assessed the cost-effectiveness of Outreach and Support in South London (OASIS), a service for people with an at-risk mental state (ARMS) for psychosis.
Method.—The costs of OASIS compared to care as usual (CAU) were entered in a decision model and examined for 12- and 24-month periods, using the duration of untreated psychosis (DUP) and rate of transition to psychosis as key parameters. The costs were calculated on the basis of services used following referral and the impact on employment. Sensitivity analysis was used to test the robustness of all the assumptions made in the model.
Results.—Over the initial 12 months from presentation, the costs of the OASIS intervention were £1872 higher than CAU. However, after 24 months they were £961 less than CAU.
Conclusions.—This model suggests that services that permit early detection of people at high risk of psychosis may be cost saving.

▶ It is always a pleasure to encounter work from the creative group at the Institute of Psychiatry in London and London School of Economics, because they have an uncanny ability to ask the right questions and provide wonderful, clear answers. And here they've done it again.

I think in our heart of hearts we all believe we should (1) try to identify severe mental illnesses as soon as possible, (2) treat them equally early, and (3) do so even at increased costs—that the social justice end justifies the cost means.

The finding that in the short-term the costs are higher for the intervention group is logical and expected, but that the 2-year costs are less is very heartening. Certainly, the authors suggest these costs may rise as time continues to go on and they must ascertain whether they are indeed intervening or merely postponing the day of reckoning (ie, frank psychosis), and in the United States at least, payors are loath to fund services that lose money even if it is gained later on. Despite all these caveats, both the intervention and research groups bear watching further.

J. A. Talbott, MD

Costs Associated With Changes in Antidepressant Treatment in a Managed Care Population With Major Depressive Disorder

Schultz J, Joish V (Univ of Minnesota; Dept of Health Outcomes, Bridgewater, NJ)
Psychiatr Serv 60:1605-1611, 2009

Objective.—This study determined whether persons with major depressive disorder who switch or augment antidepressant therapy have higher health care costs and productivity losses than those who do not.

Methods.—Data from July 1, 2002, through June 30, 2006, were taken from a national employment-based medical and pharmacy claims database. Participants were required to have filled an antidepressant prescription, be treatment naïve six months before the index prescription, be continuously enrolled in the benefits plan at least six months before and 12 months after the index prescription, and have at least one outpatient-based medical claim for major depressive disorder. Participants were categorized according to whether they switched, augmented, or maintained (that is, neither switched nor augmented) their antidepressant therapy in the 12 months after the index prescription. Productivity losses were defined as days absent from work for medical visits multiplied by average daily wage. Multivariate analyses (generalized linear models) were used to compare costs per person in the year after the index prescription, and univariate analyses (Wilcoxon tests) were used to compare productivity losses per person.

Results.—Of the 7,273 individuals who met study criteria, 40.3% switched, 1.5% augmented, and 58.2% maintained the index antidepressant therapy. After the analyses controlled for baseline characteristics, mean total and depression-related health care costs, respectively, in the year after the index prescription were significantly greater for switchers ($9,288 and $1,388 per person) and for augmenters ($9,350 and $1,027) than for maintainers ($6,151 and $723). Mean total and depression-related productivity losses, respectively, were significantly greater for switchers ($2,081 and $680) and augmenters ($2,010 and $587) than for maintainers ($1,424 and $437).

Conclusions.—Persons with major depressive disorder who switched or augmented antidepressant therapy within 12 months of treatment initiation had higher resource costs and productivity losses than those who did not.

▶ At first blush, my response to this study was to think, "Why were patients switched or augmented?" Unless one knows that, cost comparisons are meaningless, because switching or augmenting of the initial antidepressant's ineffectiveness or partial effectiveness should make economic sense. Later in their contribution, although the authors agreed that modifying treatment might be cost-saving relative to ineffective treatment, their primary recommendation is that patients who begin therapy with an antidepressant that is tolerable and effective for them will incur fewer costs than patients who require a change.

Well, of course. The secret here that these 2 nonclinicians don't reveal, although, is how to match every patient who comes through our doors with a treatment that is guaranteed to be tolerable and effective for that particular patient. If I knew how to do that with 100% of my patients, I'd not only save the system tons of money, I'd be a millionaire.

J. A. Talbott, MD

Health Status of People Undergoing Foreclosure in the Philadelphia Region
Pollack CE, Lynch J (Univ of Pennsylvania, Philadelphia)
Am J Public Health 99:1833-1839, 2009

Objectives.—We assessed the health status of people undergoing mortgage foreclosure in the Philadelphia region to determine if there was a relationship between foreclosure and health.

Methods.—Participants were recruited in partnership with a mortgage counseling agency. Participants' health status and health care use were compared with a community sample from the 2008 Southeastern Pennsylvania Household Health Survey. We used publicly filed foreclosure records to assess response bias.

Results.—Of the 250 people recruited, 36.7% met screening criteria for major depression. The foreclosure sample was significantly more likely than the community sample to not have insurance coverage (adjusted odds ratio [AOR] = 2.28; 95% confidence interval [CI] = 1.49, 3.48) and to not have filled a prescription because of cost in the preceding year (AOR = 3.44; 95% CI = 2.45, 4.83). Approximately 9% of the participants reported that their own or a family member's medical condition was the primary reason they were undergoing foreclosure. More than a quarter of those in foreclosure (27.7%) stated that they owed money to medical creditors.

Conclusions.—Foreclosure affects already-vulnerable populations. Public health practitioners may be able to leverage current efforts to connect homeowners with mortgage counseling agencies to improve health care access.

▶ While the foreclosure flood is something this country has never before seen and probably will not see within our remaining lifetimes, this article should be archived for future reference. Several things are of psychiatric interest. First, the high rate of depression and other psychiatric conditions (double the rate of a community) indicate that there are direct psychiatric consequences of foreclosing on someone's house. Second, the fact that 8.6% of the sample was behind on their mortgage payments because of medical costs, illness or hospitalization should be a scandal instead of a statistic. And third, the high rate of those who owed money to medical creditors is shameful. As I write this, the United States Senate and House of Representatives are on the brink of some sort of health care reform. One can only hope that whatever it is, it will preclude the sort of results this study shows. Social acts and omissions have health, including psychiatric, consequences.

J. A. Talbott, MD

The Long-Term Impact of Employment on Mental Health Service Use and Costs for Persons With Severe Mental Illness
Bush PW, Drake RE, Xie H, et al (Dartmouth Psychiatric Res Ctr, Lebanon, NH)
Psychiatr Serv 60:1024-1031, 2009

Objective.—Stable employment promotes recovery for persons with severe mental illness by enhancing income and quality of life, but its impact on mental health costs has been unclear. This study examined service cost over ten years among participants in a co-occurring disorders study.

Methods.—Latent-class growth analysis of competitive employment identified trajectory groups. The authors calculated annual costs of outpatient services and institutional stays for 187 participants and examined group differences in ten-year utilization and cost.

Results.—A steady-work group (N = 51) included individuals whose work hours increased rapidly and then stabilized to average 5,060 hours per person over ten years. A late-work group (N = 57) and a no-work group (N = 79) did not differ significantly in utilization or cost outcomes, so they were combined into a minimum-work group (N = 136). More education, a bipolar disorder diagnosis (versus schizophrenia or schizoaffective disorder), work in the past year, and lower scores on the expanded Brief Psychiatric Rating Scale predicted membership in the steady-work group. These variables were controlled for in the outcomes analysis. Use of outpatient services for the steady-work group declined at a significantly greater rate than it did for the minimum-work group, while institutional (hospital, jail, or prison) stays declined for both groups without a significant difference. The average cost per participant for outpatient services and institutional stays for the minimum-work group exceeded that of the steady-work group by $166,350 over ten years.

Conclusions.—Highly significant reductions in service use were associated with steady employment. Given supported employment's well-established contributions to recovery, evidence of long-term reductions in the cost of mental health services should lead policy makers and insurers to promote wider implementation.

▶ OK, let's cut to the chase: The Drake Group's conclusion about stable employment versus minimum-work is that the average cost per participant for outpatient services and institutional stays for the minimum-work group exceeded that of the steady-work group by $166 350 over 10 years or $16 635 a year. Therefore, they say, that their findings (in addition to previously having shown that stable employment "enhanc[es] income and quality of life...") should lead "policy makers and insurers to promote [its] wider implementation." They'll get no argument from me, but I'm pessimistic about it happening. Why? Because policy makers and insurers are penny wise/pound foolish, see only to the next election or budget or open-enrollment cycle, and they almost never spend money to get even more money back. This study, note study, was supported by the NIDRR (The National Institute on Disability and Rehabilitation Research), without which I'm afraid such patients would never receive such training from your average policy makers or insurers.

J. A. Talbott, MD

Financial Incentives and Accountability for Integrated Medical Care in Department of Veterans Affairs Mental Health Programs
Kilbourne AM, Greenwald DE, Hermann RC, et al (Serious Mental Illness Treatment Res and Evaluation Ctr, Ann Arbor, MI; VA Pittsburgh Ctr for Health Equity Res and Promotion; VA Boston Healthcare System Ctr for Organization, Leadership, and Management Res, MA; et al)
Psychiatr Serv 61:38-44, 2010

Objective.—This study assessed the extent to which mental health leaders perceive their programs as being primarily accountable for monitoring general medical conditions among patients with serious mental illness, and it assessed associations with modifiable health system factors.

Methods.—As part of the Department of Veterans Affairs (VA) 2007 national Mental Health Program Survey, 108 mental health program directors were queried regarding program characteristics. Perceived accountability was defined as whether their providers, as opposed to external general medical providers, were primarily responsible for specific clinical tasks related to serious mental illness treatment or high-risk behaviors. Multivariable logistic regression was used to determine whether financial incentives or other system factors were associated with accountability.

Results.—Thirty-six percent of programs reported primary accountability for monitoring diabetes and cardiovascular risk after prescription of second-generation antipsychotics, 10% for hepatitis C screening, and 17% for obesity screening and weight management. In addition, 18% and 27% of program leaders, respectively, received financial bonuses for high performance for screening for risk of diabetes and cardiovascular disease and for alcohol misuse. Financial bonuses for diabetes and cardiovascular screening were associated with primary accountability for such screening (odds ratio=5.01, p<.05). Co-location of general medical providers was associated with greater accountability for high-risk behavior screening or treatment.

Conclusions.—Financial incentives to improve quality performance may promote accountability in monitoring diabetes and cardiovascular risk assessment within mental health programs. Integrated care strategies (co-location) might be needed to promote management of high-risk behaviors among patients with serious mental illness.

▶ In light of the Grigoletti et al's study[1] it is clear that something needs to be done to screen and treat non-psychiatric illnesses among the mentally ill, especially the chronic mentally ill. Here, the Veterans Administration gave mental health program directors financial bonuses for motivating (if that's the word) their providers, to become more accountable in screening, treating, and following-up patients suffering from diabetes and cardiovascular disease. In addition, because this population also shows the need for doing the same for hepatitis C, obesity, and alcohol abuse, those are additional targets.

As crass as it sounds to give bonuses to professionals who are supposed to "subordinate their own interests to the interests of others, ... exercise accountability for themselves ..., [and] demonstrate a continuing commitment to excellence,"[2] it may be no more kooky than bribing children to stay in school and do well. Plus it's the American (capitalistic) way.

J. A. Talbott, MD

References

1. Grigoletti L, Perini G, Rossi A. Mortality and cause of death among psychiatric patients: a 20-year case-register study in an area with a community-based system of care. *Psychol Med.* 2009;39:1875-1884.
2. Swick HM. Toward a definition of medical professionalism. *Acad Med.* 2000;75: 612-616.

Black-skies planning? Prioritising mental health services in times of austerity
McDaid D, Knapp M (London School of Economics and Political Science, UK)
Br J Psychiatry 196:423-424, 2010

During the period of austerity that we now face, the National Health Service (NHS), including mental health services, will have to make efficiency savings at a time when demand for services is likely to rise. It is critical to highlight that investment in evidence-based prevention, early intervention and treatment for mental disorders can have economic benefits that go far beyond the health sector. Many potential areas for efficiency savings, such as resources invested in management and administration, are relevant across the whole of the health system. The economic downturn may, however, also present a specific opportunity for radical innovation within the mental health system.

▶ It is an administrative/management truism that changes are best made in either hard times or boom years. The title of this Editorial presumably contrasted with planning under blue skies and it examines what to do now. Because most of the world is in an economic decline, governments all over are looking at what to cut. This article is authored by 2 astute economists at the London School of

Economics, who are open to psychiatry, having worked with psychiatrists for many years, and they have some fascinating ideas about where to look both to invest and to cut. The UK government has already committed itself to manage these hard times by: "smarter procurement practices; being more energy efficient; making better use of property; reducing staff sickness absenteeism; as well as reining back on the national health information technology programme."

On the investment side, they would invest in:

- "Preventive actions and better coordination between healthcare professionals" because individuals with comorbid physical and mental conditions cost us 50% more;
- "early intervention and better management of individuals with psychoses who come into – or are at risk of – contact with the criminal justice system";
- "mental health promotion, disorder prevention and early intervention measures across the lifespan [because they] can be cost-effective and have benefits for other sectors."

On the cost-cutting side they note that:

- "cuts in mental health services may...have adverse spillover impacts on sectors well beyond," but cuts should be considered;
- to streamline and pool "management and administrative structures";
- "further rebalance services towards cost-effective community-based care alternatives?...simplify care pathways so that individuals see a specialist early in the referral process";
- "streamline links between primary and specialist care."

In addition they "sky" ideas about "financial incentives and other rewards," "internet-delivered psychotherapy," and so forth.

This is a very interesting and positive way to look at our current situation.

J. A. Talbott, MD

Public Expenditures Related to the Criminal Justice System and to Services for Arrestees With a Serious Mental Illness
Petrila J, Andel R, Constantine R, et al (Univ of South Florida, Tampa, FL; School of Aging Studies at the Univ, Tampa; FL)
Psychiatr Serv 61:516-519, 2010

Objective.—The study identified expenditures related to criminal justice, health, mental health, and social welfare services over a four-year period for arrestees with serious mental illnesses in a large Florida county and characteristics of subgroups.

Methods.—Multiple data sets were used to identify 3,769 persons arrested in a one-year period who had serious mental illnesses. Multiple regression with all variables mutually adjusted was used to explore associations with a log of aggregate criminal justice, health, mental health, and social welfare expenditures.

Results.—Aggregate expenditures were $94,957,465, with a median per person of $15,134. Individuals with the highest expenditures were at least 40 years old with a psychotic disorder, an involuntary psychiatric examination, and more arrests and mental health contacts. Medicaid enrollees had higher expenditures than nonenrollees overall but lower criminal justice expenditures.

Conclusions.—Identifying characteristics of subgroups with higher expenditures may assist policy makers and providers in designing appropriate criminal justice and treatment responses.

▶ The numbers here are staggering. A total of $15134 per person is a lot of money to spend on someone suffering from a psychosis. It seems to me that such persons should be the easiest for correctional individuals to recognize, for the system to divert, and for the psychiatric care system to treat. The fact that 10% of persons arrested in one county in Florida had serious mental illness is another shameful fact. Also, these are not young offenders; their average age is 36. The other thing that is annoying is that, as the authors point out, most mentally ill persons are arrested for minor offenses making them more suitable for treatment in the mental health arena than incarceration. The issue of the mentally ill in the correctional system is no longer a health care issue—it is a public policy, moral, and economic one. One wonders when those in positions of public trust will wake up.

J. A. Talbott, MD

Schizophrenia

Is Early Intervention in Psychosis Cost-Effective Over the Long Term?
Mihalopoulos C, Harris M, Henry L, et al (Deakin Univ, Burwood, Australia; Univ of Queensland, Australia; Orygen Res Centre, Parkville, Australia)
Schizophr Bull 35:909-918, 2009

Objective.—This study assesses the long-term cost-effectiveness of a comprehensive model of mental health care for first-episode psychosis. The study is an extension of a previous economic evaluation of the Early Psychosis Prevention and Intervention Centre (EPPIC) that assessed the first-year costs and outcomes of treatment.

Method.—The current study used a matched, historical control group design with a follow-up of approximately 8 years. Complete follow-up data were available for 65 of the original 102 participants. Direct public mental health service costs incurred subsequent to the first year of treatment and symptomatic and functional outcomes of 32 participants initially treated for up to 2 years at EPPIC were compared with a matched cohort of 33 participants initially treated by generic mental health services. Treatment-related resource use was measured and valued using Australian published prices.

Results.—Almost 8 years after initial treatment, EPPIC subjects displayed lower levels of positive psychotic symptoms ($P = .007$), were more likely to be in remission ($P = .008$), and had a more favorable course of illness ($P = .011$) than the controls. Fifty-six percent of the EPPIC cohort were in paid employment over the last 2 years compared with 33% of controls ($P = .083$). Each EPPIC patient costs on average A\$3445 per annum to treat compared with controls, who each costs A\$9503 per annum.

Conclusions.—Specialized early psychosis programs can deliver a higher recovery rate at one-third the cost of standard public mental health services. Residual methodological limitations and limited sample size indicate that further research is required to verify this finding.

▶ Pat McGorry and his group in Australia have been persistent in both performing pioneering efforts in early intervention in psychoses (eg, schizophrenia) as well as conducting research on its effects, and they have presented their results faithfully for years to a mixed reception. The impact of this report detailing a part of their program should be resounding. First, as opposed to some critics' skepticism about how lasting their early intervention program is, they show that its effects go out at least 8 years from initiation. Second, the finding that treatment costs are 27.5% of those of controls should be music to the ears of the policy makers, funders, and reimbursers of care. And third, the extraordinary impact on paid employment—56% versus 33% for controls—shows that one of the toughest nuts to crack in the rehabilitation business has yielded fine results to their efforts. A nice bonus for the reader is their meticulous attention to biases and objections.

J. A. Talbott, MD

Early intervention in psychosis
Singh SP (Univ of Warwick, Coventry, UK)
Br J Psychiatry 196:343-345, 2010

Early intervention in psychosis services produce better clinical outcomes than generic teams and are also cost-effective. Clinical gains made within such services are robust as long as the interventions are actively provided. Longer-term data show that some of these gains are lost when care is transferred back to generic teams. This paper argues that sustaining these early gains requires both a reappraisal of generic services and an understanding of the active ingredients of early intervention, which can be tailored for longer input in cases with poorer outcome trajectories.

▶ Although this reappraisal is a summary of 2 other articles in the same issue, it is much more than that: it is an attempt to synthesize the results of a great number of studies about early intervention in psychosis. I do not quite understand the opposition to the practice; some is based on the belief (in my opinion) that we may overtreat and stigmatize individuals who may not have serious illness, some (in my opinion) is based on the whole opposition to primary or even prompt secondary prevention, and some seems to stem from the fact that many studies have shown that the results do not persist after cessation of the intervention. The latter, however, is a problem we face with many interventions with severe and persistent mental disorders. The author's conclusion that there is mounting and continuing evidence that early intervention is both cost-effective and clinically effective seems convincing, and even though, as he points out, the United Kingdom (and the United States) faces increasing budgetary pressures, we need to use every means possible if cost and outcomes are what we and governments care about.

J. A. Talbott, MD

Neurocognitive change, functional change and service intensity during community-based psychosocial rehabilitation for schizophrenia

Brekke JS, Hoe M, Green MF (Univ of Southern California, Los Angeles; Univ of California at Los Angeles)
Psychol Med 39:1637-1647, 2009

Background.—This study examined the magnitude of neurocognitive change during 1 year of community-based psychosocial intervention, whether neurocognitive change and functional change were linked, and how neurocognitive change combined with service intensity to facilitate functional change.

Method.—A total of 130 individuals diagnosed with schizophrenia were recruited upon admission to four community-based psychosocial rehabilitation programs. Subjects were assessed at baseline, 6 and 12 months on role functioning and symptom measures. Neurocognition was measured at baseline and 12 months. Service intensity was the number of days of treatment attendance during the study period. Latent mean difference tests and Latent Growth Curve Models (LCGMs) were used to examine the study hypotheses.

Results.—There was statistically and clinically significant functional improvement over 12 months. Neurocognition improved significantly over time. Seventy-six (58%) of the sample showed neurocognitive improvement and 54 (42%) did not. There was a significant rate of functional enhancement in the neurocognitive improver group. There was a non-significant rate of functional change in the neurocognitive non-improver group. Neurocognitive improvers showed functional improvement that was 350% greater than neurocognitive non-improvers. Service intensity did not vary between neurocognitive improvers and non-improvers but there was a strong interaction between neurocognitive improvement, service intensity and rate of functional improvement such that service intensity was strongly related to functional improvement for neurocognitive improvers but not for neurocognitive non-improvers. Medication usage and symptomatology did not confound these findings.

Conclusions.—These findings suggest that neurocognitive improvement may be a foundation for functional change and treatment responsiveness during community-based psychosocial rehabilitation for individuals with schizophrenia.

▶ This is interesting stuff. This study reminded me of the tautological arguments we used to have in days gone by as to whether tears were psychological or biological in origin. Obviously the answer is both.

The most significant finding here is that there is a positive relationship between neurocognitive improvement and psychosocial rehabilitation, and the most significant missing element is why or how responders differ from non-responders or more interestingly, those whose neurocognitive functioning declined.

The next most interesting finding is that neurocognitive improvement and functional improvement go hand in hand, again leading to the question, which causes which or more intriguingly, are both influenced by an "as yet unidentified predisposition," which the authors speculate could be a "change readiness factor"?

The authors quite correctly point out that someone needs to compare this sort of group with persons not receiving psychosocial rehabilitation or cognitive remediation, and that could range from psychotherapy (including cognitive-behavioral therapy) to vocational rehabilitation to psychoeducation.

As I said, "This is interesting stuff."

J. A. Talbott, MD

Depression

The Influence of Past Unemployment Duration on Symptoms of Depression Among Young Women and Men in the United States

Mossakowski KN (Univ of Miami, Coral Gables, FL)
Am J Public Health 99:1826-1832, 2009

Objectives.—I examined whether unemployment while looking for a job and being out of the labor force while not seeking work have distinct effects on symptoms of depression among young women and men in the United States. I also investigated whether past unemployment duration predicts depressive symptoms.

Methods.—I used ordinary least squares regression to analyze data from the 1979–1994 National Longitudinal Survey of Youth.

Results.—Cross-sectional results suggested that current unemployment status and out-of-the-labor-force status were significantly associated with depressive symptoms at ages 29 through 37 years. The association between being out of the labor force and depressive symptoms was stronger for men. Longitudinal results revealed that past unemployment duration across 15 years of the transition to adulthood significantly predicted depressive symptoms, net of demographics, family background, current socioeconomic status, and prior depressive symptoms. However, duration out of the labor force did not predict depressive symptoms.

Conclusions.—Longer durations of unemployment predict higher levels of depressive symptoms among young adults. Future research should measure duration longitudinally and distinguish unemployment from being out of the labor force to advance our understanding of socioeconomic mental health disparities.

▶ I found that the link between depression and long-term unemployment shown so clearly in this article was compelling and disturbing. Am I being naive? Have I missed the photos of the dustbowl by Dorothy Lange and of Wall Street brokers selling apples in the *New York Times* during the Great Depression; not read or fully appreciated the impact of farm foreclosures; not seen almost all nations' unemployment steadily increase over the past 2 years? Of course not. But like we no longer see the homeless man who lives on our block, we have become inured to the current crisis. Is it because we cannot do anything? After all, even in Socialist European States unemployment has risen and "creating jobs" is not easy to do. As psychiatrists and public health physicians, however, we can diagnose and treat; we can also suggest that the "fierce urgency of now," as stated by Dr Martin Luther King, Jr, must take into consideration not just economic factors but emotional consequences.

J. A. Talbott, MD

Long-Term Mental Health Resource Utilization and Cost of Care Following Group Psychoeducation or Unstructured Group Support for Bipolar Disorders: A Cost-Benefit Analysis
Scott J, Colom F, Popova E, et al (Univ of Newcastle Upon Tyne, UK; Hosp Clinic, Barcelona, Spain; et al)
J Clin Psychiatry 70:378-386, 2009

Objective.—To explore the short- and long-term mental health resource utilization and cost of care in a sample of 120 individuals with bipolar disorders who participated in a randomized controlled efficacy trial of group psychoeducation versus unstructured group support.

Method.—Prospective, independent monitoring of DSM-IV bipolar disorder type I or II patients aged 18 to 65 years was conducted during the intervention phase (6 months) and follow-up phase (5-year postintervention) of a randomized controlled trial reporting clinical outcomes and inpatient and outpatient mental health service utilization, with estimation of cost of treatment per patient. The study was conducted from October 1997 through October 2006.

Results.—Compared with individuals with bipolar disorder receiving the control intervention, psychoeducated patients had twice as many planned outpatient appointments, but the estimated mean cost of emergency consultation utilization was significantly less. There were trends for psychoeducated patients to opt for self-funded psychotherapy after completing group psychoeducation and to utilize more medications. However, inpatient care accounted for 40% estimated total cost in the control group but only about 15% in the psychoeducation group.

Conclusions.—This study demonstrates the importance of taking a long-term overview of the cost versus benefits of adjunctive psychological therapy in bipolar disorders. If viewed only in the short-term, the psychoeducation group used more mental health care resources without clear additional health gain. However, extended follow-up demonstrated a long-term advantage for psychoeducated individuals, such that, compared to an unstructured support group intervention, group psychoeducation is less costly and more effective.

▶ This study is useful for several reasons:

- It shows that psychoeducation, at least with bipolar patients, is effective,
- It shows that psychoeducation cuts down on emergency consultation utilization, at least with patients suffering from bipolar illnesses,
- It shows that psychoeducation reduces expenditures for inpatient care, at least with patients suffering from bipolar illnesses, and
- It shows that there is often a difference between short-term and long-term economic impacts, at least with patients suffering from bipolar illnesses.

One of the downsides of our current model of evaluating treatment efficacy is its dependence on seeing every intervention as if it were psychopharmacological and thus subject to short-term trials. We know, with mood disorders especially, that a combination of psychopharmacological and psychosocial treatments are twice as effective as just one intervention. And it often takes longer to see the effects of the latter.

Let us hope that this and other such studies bring more reason and patience to our attempts to assess all treatment efficacy.

J. A. Talbott, MD

Barriers to Care

Dropout From Outpatient Mental Health Care in the United States
Olfson M, Mojtabai R, Sampson NA, et al (Columbia Univ, NY; Johns Hopkins Bloomberg School of Public Health, Baltimore; Harvard Med School, Boston, MA; et al)
Psychiatr Serv 60:898-907, 2009

Objective.—Although mental health treatment dropout is common, patterns and predictors of dropout are poorly understood. This study explored patterns and predictors of mental health treatment dropout in a nationally representative sample.

Methods.—Data were from the National Comorbidity Survey Replication, a nationally representative household survey. Respondents who had received mental health treatment in the 12 months before the interview (N = 1,664) were asked about dropout, which was defined as quitting treatment before the provider wanted them to stop. Cross-tabulation and discrete-time survival analyses were used to identify predictors.

Results.—Approximately one-fifth (22%) of patients quit treatment prematurely. The highest dropout rate was from treatment received in the general medical sector (32%), and the lowest was from treatment received by psychiatrists (15%). Dropout rates were intermediate from treatment in the human services sector (20%) and among patients seen by nonpsychiatrist mental health professionals (19%). Over 70% of all dropout occurred after the first or second visits. Mental health insurance was associated with low odds of dropout (odds ratio = .6, 95% confidence interval = .4–.9). Psychiatric comorbidity was associated with a trend toward dropout. Several patient characteristics differentially predicted dropout across treatment sectors and in early and later phases of treatment.

Conclusions.—Roughly one-fifth of adults in mental health treatment dropped out before completing the recommended course of treatment. Dropout was most common in the general medical sector and varied by patient characteristics across treatment sectors. Interventions focused on high-risk patients and sectors that have higher dropout rates will likely be required to reduce the large proportion of patients who prematurely terminate treatment.

▶ The authors, all distinguished and impressive experts, some of whom I consider friends, start off with an unstated assumption that stopping treatment before a provider is ready to call it completed is bad. Says who? Leaving aside what used to be called "flights into health," studies have shown that sometimes very brief courses of treatment, indeed, even extensive workups and evaluations, often produce enough good feeling that patients leave treatment.

But, setting that aside, there are some findings that are startling. For instance, why are the dropout rates of those treated in the general medical sector, where, after all, most psychiatric patients receive treatment, double that of psychiatrists? Is it that we're better at assessing and using transference, avoiding destructive countertransference, providing answers and/or support, shifting gears between modalities of treatment, etc, spending time (as they suggest) or are the groups treated in the 2 sectors different sorts of animals?

I also was interested in the protective factor of use of complementary alternative medicine. I originally interpreted that as acupuncture and herbal/etc stuff and was puzzled, but I can readily see how self-help group participation would enhance continuance in psychiatric treatment.

Why do those with more comorbidity drop out more at the beginning? The authors attribute this to the fact that general practitioners may have less experience (and implied less expertise) in treating those with shifting symptoms and diagnoses, and this inflexibility certainly could account for higher early dropout rates.

Finally, the fact that previous use predicts future stick-to-it-ness may not only be because of decreased stigma and embarrassment but a sense that psychiatric treatment is no longer mysterious and potentially menacing.

J. A. Talbott, MD

A Delphi Study of Problems in Providing Community Care to Patients With Nonpsychotic Chronic Mental Illness
Koekkoek B, Meijel BV, Schene A, et al (Brinkveld Outpatient Community Care, Altrecht Mental Health Care, Netherlands; INHOLLAND Univ for Applied Sciences, Amsterdam; Univ of Amsterdam; et al)
Psychiatr Serv 60:693-697, 2009

Objective.—The study identified problems that professionals perceive in community care of patients with nonpsychotic chronic mental illness.

Methods.—Eight national experts from the Netherlands participated in a four-phase modified Delphi procedure to identify and rate the urgency of problems in patient care and the extent to which problems were amenable to change.

Results.—A total of 39 problems were identified in five categories: patients, professionals, their interactions, the family and social system, and the mental health system. Participants noted the many social problems of these patients and their unusual help-seeking behavior. They often perceived these patients as able but unwilling to get better. They also noted that their diagnoses tend to be unclear and shifting and that more precise classifications would help in development of treatments.

Conclusions.—Elucidating the distinction between the psychiatric symptoms of these patients and their unusual help-seeking behavior may improve diagnosis and patient care.

▶ This study raises some absolutely fascinating questions and issues as related to the real world of psychiatry and our patients.

Just the day before this was written, I was supervising a resident about a psychotherapy case. The patient certainly qualifies as someone who has a nonpsychotic chronic mental illness and in supervision I raised a question about how discouraging it must be to treat someone who seemingly rejects all forms of looking at her situation other than her extremely negative one.

The resident is attempting to work with her patient to break her patient's negative thinking patterns through cognitive behavioral interventions, but the patient steadfastly refuses to examine her thinking patterns, her emotional spiral patterns, and to do any homework. Everything is met with negativity, even when it's clear the patient has some capacity for improvement and some diurnal variation that suggests she is not always at the bottom of the well of despond. I can, therefore, see how these Dutch experts regard some of these patients as able but unwilling to get better.

On my part, I found myself suggesting tossing out a myriad of ideas, suggestions, hypotheses, and interventions, trying to "flood" the patient with stimuli, and seeing if her opposition could be harnessed in the service of a push back into health.

I guess what I'm saying is that we all know patients such as are described in the study; we often want to throw up our hands, but our medical oaths and professionalism and humanism force us to keep trying. But it is often frustrating, indeed more frustrating to treat nonpsychotic chronic mental illnesses than psychotic ones; as an old colleague/mentor of mine once said—the difference between psychotic and nonpsychotic patients is simple, one group gets better (meaning the psychotic group).

J. A. Talbott, MD

Negative Attitudes Toward Help Seeking for Mental Illness in 2 Population–Based Surveys From the United States and Canada
Jagdeo A, Cox BJ, Stein MB, et al (Univ of Manitoba, Winnipeg; Psychology and Community Health Sciences, Winnipeg; Univ of California San Diego; et al)
Can J Psychiatry 54:757-766, 2009

Objectives.—To determine the prevalence and sociodemographic correlates of negative attitudes toward help seeking for mental illness among the general population in the United States and Ontario.

Methods.—Two contemporaneous population-based surveys (aged 15 to 54 years) were analyzed: the US National Comorbidity Survey (NCS) ($n = 5877$) and the Ontario Health Survey (OHS) ($n = 6902$). Multiple logistic regression analyses were used to examine the correlates of a derived negative attitudes composite variable obtained from questions assessing probability, comfort, and embarrassment related to help seeking for mental illness.

Results.—Negative attitudes toward help seeking for mental illness were prevalent in both countries. Fifteen percent of OHS and 20% of NCS respondents stated they probably or definitely would not seek treatment if they had serious emotional problems. Almost one-half of recipients in both surveys stated they would be embarrassed if their friends knew about their use of mental health services. Negative attitudes toward help seeking were highest among socioeconomically challenged young, single, lesser-educated men in Ontario and the United States. In both countries, substance abuse or dependence and antisocial personality disorder were associated with greater negative attitudes, as was not having sought treatment in the past.

Conclusions.—Negative attitudes toward mental health service use are prevalent in Ontario and the United States. They are most common in young adults, especially those with lower education and socioeconomic resources, and those with substance abuse or dependence problems. This information can be used to target educational efforts aimed at improving willingness to seek care for mental health problems.

▶ I do not think that 20% or so of the population who are resistant to seeking care for mental illness is so bad; I think it is rather good, in fact. With all the time and money we have spent in the northern hemisphere in the last few decades on antistigma research and campaigns, the fact that 80% to 85% of Americans and Canadians would seek help seems to me to be much more significant and a much more accurate way to state their conclusions.

Of course, as H. Richard Lamb's famous study[1] of young men in California board and care homes showed, the demographic group Jagdeo et al (these authors) singled out (young, single, and socioeconomically challenged men) as having the most negative attitudes, sounds rather like the group Lamb identified as restless and moving around rather than sticking within treatment or care settings.

It would seem to me that an obvious public health action follows from these findings, specifically, that this younger, poorer, less educated group be targeted in antistigma, outreach, and identification efforts—through television, games, and social networks—in other words, media they use as opposed to traditional print or educational media.

J. A. Talbott, MD

Reference

1. Lamb HR. Board-and-care home wanderers. *Arch Gen Psychiatry*. 1980;37: 135-137.

The Psychiatric Rehabilitation of African Americans With Severe Mental Illness
Whitley R, Lawson WB (Dartmouth Psychiatric Res Ctr, Lebanon, NH; Howard Univ, Washington, DC)
Psychiatr Serv 61:508-511, 2010

African Americans make up approximately 12% of the U.S. population, a total of around 36 million people. Evidence suggests that African Americans suffer from significant and persistent disparities within the mental health system. African Americans with severe mental illness are less likely than Euro-Americans to access mental health services, more likely to drop out of treatment, more likely to receive poor-quality care, and more likely to be dissatisfied with care. Dominant patterns of treatment for African Americans with psychiatric disabilities are often least suited to long-term rehabilitation. To be successful, interventions must simultaneously target three levels: macro, provider, and patient. Five domains are posited that cut across these levels. These are cross-cultural communication, discrimination, explanatory models, stigma, and family involvement. These need appropriate research and action to enhance the psychiatric rehabilitation of African Americans. Potential solutions to overcome barriers raised within these domains are suggested.

▶ Over the last few decades, the issue of health care disparities in this country has become so obvious to everyone that the United States Government's initiative in the 1990s was a welcome response. Psychiatrists have participated in the research on the issue and have, as Whitley and Lawson report in this contribution to the literature, shown how African Americans with severe mental illness are less likely than Euro-Americans to access mental health services, more likely to drop out of treatment, more likely to receive poor-quality care, and more likely to be dissatisfied with care. The authors' focus is on psychiatric rehabilitation, where once again African-Americans use services less and are more dissatisfied with such services. They examine 5 areas: cross-cultural communication, that is, seeing the rehabilitation facility as a threat and not an opportunity; discrimination, that is, such services have a nefarious purpose (like the Tuskegee syphilis study); explanatory models (of illness), that is, distress is seen as moral or religious rather than medical or psychiatric; stigma, that leads them to see primary care physicians not specialists; and family involvement, where close-knit families make decisions for individuals or the fact that many vanilla (my word) mental health services do not include families. This thoughtful open forum deserves wide attention.

J. A. Talbott, MD

The REACT Study: Cost-Effectiveness Analysis of Assertive Community Treatment in North London

McCrone P, Killaspy H, Bebbington P, et al (Inst of Psychiatry, London, UK; Univ College London)
Psychiatr Serv 60:908-913, 2009

Objective.—Assertive community treatment (ACT) is a key component of mental health care, but recent information on its cost-effectiveness is limited. This article provides a cost-effectiveness analysis of assertive community treatment and usual care from community mental health teams (CMHTs) in the United Kingdom.

Methods.—Participants who had difficulties engaging with community services were randomly assigned to ACT (N = 127) or continued usual care from CMHTs (N = 124). Costs were measured at baseline and 18 months later and compared between the two groups. In the analysis, cost data were linked to information on satisfaction, which had been shown to be significantly higher with ACT.

Results.—Total follow-up costs over 18 months were higher for the ACT group by £4,031 ($6,369), but this was not statistically significant (95% confidence interval of −£2,592 to £10,690 [−$4,095 to $16,890]). A one-unit improvement in satisfaction was associated with extra costs in the ACT group of £473 ($747).

Conclusions.—The costs of ACT were not significantly different from usual care. ACT did, however, result in greater levels of client satisfaction and engagement with services and as such may be the preferred community treatment option for patients with long-term serious mental health problems.

▶ When the first assertive community treatment study (ACT/PACT) was published in 1980 with a sophisticated economic analysis performed by economist Burton Weisbrod,[1] we were confronted by a puzzling contradiction; namely, that while such programs cost a bit more per patient than usual treatment, when you factor in all the costs to society, they are actually a bit cheaper. The problem is that no legislator will spend more in mental health to get more back to the rest of the economy. It's as if they refused to subsidize motorcycle helmets from Highway Safety funds because cost savings would accrue to Trauma Units in the health system. So for 30 years we've seen lots of analyses and lots of evidence that ACT/PACT is liked better by patients, but we cannot show it saves oodles of money or that the slight cost increase is valued enough by patients.

Now comes this study that once again shows ACT is $747 more expensive, which the authors argue is not statistically significant. The problem is that legislators and policy makers don't look at statistical significance—they look at absolute numbers.

So we're back in the same old spot.

J. A. Talbott, MD

Reference

1. Weisbrod BA, Test MA, Stein LI. Alternative to mental hospital treatment: II. Economic benefit-cost analysis. *Arch Gen Psychiatry.* 1980;37:400-405.

Community Care

Cost, Effectiveness, and Cost-Effectiveness of a Collaborative Mental Health Care Program for People Receiving Short-Term Disability Benefits for Psychiatric Disorders

Dewa CS, Hoch JS, Carmen G, et al (Centre for Addiction and Mental Health, Toronto, Ontario; St Michael's Hosp, Toronto, Ontario; Global Business and Economic Roundtable on Addiction and Mental Health, Toronto, Ontario; et al)
Can J Psychiatry 54:379-388, 2009

Objective.—To examine the cost, effectiveness, and cost-effectiveness of a collaborative mental health care (CMHC) pilot program for people on short-term disability leave for psychiatric disorders.

Method.—Using a quasi-experimental design, the analyses were conducted using 2 groups of subjects who received short-term disability benefits for psychiatric disorders. One group ($n = 75$) was treated in a CMHC program during their disability episode. The comparison group ($n = 51$) received short-term disability benefits related to psychiatric disorders in the prior year but did not receive CMHC during their disability episode. People in both groups met screening criteria for the CMHC program. Differences in cost and days absent from work were tested using Student t tests and confirmed using nonparametric Wilcoxon rank sum tests. Differences in return to work and transition to long-term disability leave were tested using chi-square tests. The cost-effectiveness analysis used the net benefit regression framework.

Results.—The results suggest that with CMHC, for every 100 people on short-term disability leave for psychiatric disorders, there could be $50 000 in savings related to disability benefits along with more people returning to work ($n = 23$), less people transitioning to long-term disability leave ($n = 24$), and 1600 more workdays.

Conclusions.—CMHC models of disability management based on our Canadian data may be a worthwhile investment in helping people who are receiving short-term disability benefits for psychiatric disorders to receive adequate treatment.

▶ I like this study's recommendation.

I was all set to either not review this contribution to the literature or to minimize its importance because (once again) I figured that there was no way that policy makers and legislators would expend more funds even if it comes back plus interest in the long run after you calculate all costs (cf, assertive community treatment, depression screening, day hospitalization, etc).

Then I read the recommendation.

These authors, from Canada mind you, that socialist state up north, didn't say government should fund such programs to persons with psychiatric disability; no, they say that employers, acting in their own enlightened best interests, should in order to save money, return workers to work more quickly, and reduce the number of sick days.

I guess that before that happens here, though, researchers in the United States had better replicate their findings so they are not seen as "not translatable south."

J. A. Talbott, MD

Effectiveness and Outcomes of Assisted Outpatient Treatment in New York State
Phelan JC, Sinkewicz M, Castille DM, et al (Columbia Univ, NY; Univ of Michigan, Ann Arbor; et al)
Psychiatr Serv 61:137-143, 2010

Objective.—Outpatient commitment has been heralded as a necessary intervention that improves psychiatric outcomes and quality of life, and it has been criticized on the grounds that effective treatment must be voluntary and that outpatient commitment has negative unintended consequences. Because few methodologically strong data exist, this study evaluated New York State's outpatient commitment program with the objective of augmenting the existing literature.

Methods.—A total of 76 individuals recently mandated to outpatient commitment and 108 individuals (comparison group) recently discharged from psychiatric hospitals in the Bronx and Queens who were attending the same outpatient facilities as the group mandated to outpatient commitment were followed for one year and compared in regard to psychotic symptoms, suicide risk, serious violence perpetration, quality of life, illness-related social functioning, and perceived coercion and stigma. Propensity score matching and generalized estimating equations were used to achieve the strongest causal inference possible without an experimental design.

Results.—Serious violence perpetration and suicide risk were lower and illness-related social functioning was higher ($p < .05$ for all) in the outpatient commitment group than in the comparison group. Psychotic symptoms and quality of life did not differ significantly between the two groups. Potential unintended consequences were not evident: the outpatient commitment group reported marginally less ($p < .10$) stigma and coercion than the comparison group.

Conclusions.—Outpatient commitment in New York State affects many lives; therefore, it is reassuring that negative consequences were not observed. Rather, people's lives seem modestly improved by outpatient commitment. However, because outpatient commitment included treatment and other enhancements, these findings should be interpreted in terms of the overall impact of outpatient commitment, not of legal coercion per se. As such, the results do not support the expansion of coercion in psychiatric treatment.

▶ I'm not sure why the authors and others are tiptoeing around this issue. They speak of outpatient civil commitment having "been criticized on the grounds that effective treatment must be voluntary" and a potential harm of "restrictions on personal freedom." The former seems to be an untrue view of psychoanalytic and 12-step philosophies and the latter something that the American Civil Liberties Union would say to rev up their base. They looked at 2 "possible unintended negative consequences (perceived coercion and stigma)" and found them absent. So given the fact that patients who were in the outpatient civil commitment category showed suicide risk and violent behavior that were less frequent and higher illness-related social functioning, why are they so seemingly ashamed of their results? Do they think they will be seen as politically incorrect? Are they afraid to challenge the National Mental Heath Association? Serious mental illness is a serious public health, public safety, and economic problem. Even a modest improvement from a tool such as outpatient civil commitment should be viewed with admiration and imitation and yes, expansion, which they counsel against.

J. A. Talbott, MD

A Randomized Trial of Medical Care Management for Community Mental Health Settings: The Primary Care Access, Referral, and Evaluation (PCARE) Study
Druss BG, von Esenwein SA, Compton MT, et al (Emory Univ, Atlanta, GA; Emory Univ School of Medicine, Atlanta, GA)
Am J Psychiatry 167:151-159, 2010

Objective.—Poor quality of healthcare contributes to impaired health and excess mortality in individuals with severe mental disorders. The authors tested a population-based medical care management intervention designed to improve primary medical care in community mental health settings.

Method.—A total of 407 subjects with severe mental illness at an urban community mental health center were randomly assigned to either the medical care management intervention or usual care. For individuals in the intervention group, care managers provided communication and advocacy with medical providers, health education, and support in overcoming system-level fragmentation and barriers to primary medical care.

Results.—At a 12-month follow-up evaluation, the intervention group received an average of 58.7% of recommended preventive services compared with a rate of 21.8% in the usual care group. They also received a significantly higher proportion of evidence-based services for cardiometabolic conditions (34.9% versus 27.7%) and were more likely to have a primary care provider (71.2% versus 51.9%). The intervention group showed significant improvement on the SF-36 mental component summary (8.0% [versus a 1.1% decline in the usual care group]) and a nonsignificant improvement on the SF-36 physical component summary. Among subjects with available laboratory data, scores on the Framingham Cardiovascular Risk Index were significantly better in the intervention group (6.9%) than the usual care group (9.8%).

Conclusions.—Medical care management was associated with significant improvements in the quality and outcomes of primary care. These findings suggest that care management is a promising approach for improving medical care for patients treated in community mental health settings.

▶ Medical illnesses in psychiatric patients are a serious matter. As the authors point out in detail, they are underdetected, undertreated, and result in premature death. Therefore, an intervention that addresses conditions such as myocardial infarction, diabetes, and asthma would not only be the right thing to do but also would be life saving or life extending.

Wanting to know how the authors achieved this huge 3-fold difference from usual care (Fig 2), I went immediately to the Method section where they describe the care management intervention: "Two full-time registered nurses followed a manualized protocol for care based on standardized approaches documented in the care management literature. The program was designed to help overcome patient, provider, and system-level barriers to primary medical

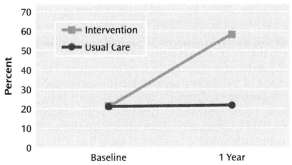

FIGURE 2.—Quality of preventive health services in mentally ill community patients randomly assigned to medical care management intervention or usual care. (Reprinted from Druss BG, von Esenwein SA, Compton MT, et al. A randomized trial of medical care management for community mental health settings: the Primary Care Access, Referral, and Evaluation (PCARE) study. *Am J Psychiatry.* 2010;167:151-159, with permission from the American Psychiatric Association. Copyright 2010.)

care experienced by persons with mental disorders...by providing information to the patient about 1) his or her medical conditions, 2) available medical providers in the community, and 3) upcoming appointments....Motivational interviewing techniques...were used to help support patients' self-management skills. Action plans involving goals for medical care or lifestyle change were used to foster health behavior change as well as to help patients become more active participants in their healthcare." They then describe how they helped overcome barriers. "Usual care" (which almost seems to constitute malpractice) was to give patients "a list with contact information for local primary care medical clinics that accept uninsured and Medicaid patients."

Knowing the senior author's expertise, I expect future contributions will discuss economic issues, including the cost and benefits of such an intervention.

J. A. Talbott, MD

Provision of Mental Health Services in U.S. Nursing Homes, 1995–2004
Li Y (Univ of Iowa)
Psychiatr Serv 61:349-355, 2010

Objective.—This study tracked the ability of U.S. nursing homes to provide on-site mental health services after the Omnibus Budget Reconciliation Act (OBRA) of 1987 mandated the detection and treatment of mental illness among nursing home patients. The study also determined cross-sectional correlates of service availability and models of services.

Methods.—Retrospective analyses were done using National Nursing Home Surveys from 1995, 1997, 1999, and 2004 (the most recent survey). The surveys are periodically conducted by the Centers for Disease Control and Prevention and represent the nation's approximately 17,000 nursing homes. The longitudinal trend of mental health service provision was analyzed for all facilities and for subgroups of facilities. Multivariate regression determined facility and geographic correlates in 2004.

Results.—Roughly 80% of facilities provided on-site mental health services each survey year. In 2004, 25% of facilities provided mental health services regularly or at routinely scheduled times (regular basis), 24% provided them in an on-call manner (or as needed), and 28% provided them on both a regular and on-call basis. The remaining 22% of facilities provided no on-site mental health services. Multivariate analyses found that largest facilities ($\geq$200 beds) were more able than small facilities (<100 beds) to serve persons with mental illness (odds ratio=3.80, p=.024); compared with their counterparts, facilities were more likely to provide on-site services if they had a larger proportion of residents covered by Medicare or Medicaid programs, were in the Northeast region, or were in metropolitan areas. Similar correlates were found when the types of service provision models (regular basis, on-call basis, both a regular and on-call basis) were examined.

Conclusions.—The overall availability of nursing home–based mental health services did not improve over time during the post-OBRA era. Service availability is more problematic for certain facilities, such as small or rural ones. Financial, regulatory, and system-level efforts are needed to address this issue.

▶ I've discussed elsewhere in my reviews about the scandalous situation in the United States where jails and prisons are now accepted as legitimate sites for delivering psychiatric treatment. The second most scandalous site for the mentally ill is/are nursing homes, intended for patients who need more time to recover from medical or surgical problems than an acute hospital will allow but are not designed, nor funded, nor staffed for caring for the severely and chronically mentally ill. Granted, some persons with serious medical or surgical problems develop dementia as they age but the fact that "between 60% and 90% of nursing home residents have diagnosable mental disorders," but "22% of facilities provided no on-site mental health services" is horrible. The Omnibus Budget Reconciliation Act of 1987 was intended to remedy this situation but clearly, 23 years afterward, has not. It makes you wonder who the members of the House of Representatives represent—not those in nursing homes apparently.

J. A. Talbott, MD

Influence of perceived organisational factors on job burnout: survey of community mental health staff

Lasalvia A, on behalf of the PICOS-Veneto Group (Univ of Verona, Italy; et al)
Br J Psychiatry 195:537-544, 2009

Background.—Staff burnout is a critical issue for mental healthcare delivery, as it can lead to decreased work performance and, ultimately, to poorer treatment outcomes.

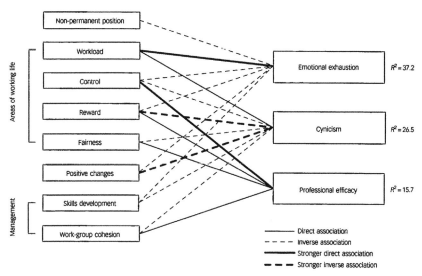

FIGURE 1.—Relation between significant predictors (individual and perceived contextual factors) and the three dimensions of burnout on the Maslach Burnout Inventory-General Survey. (Reprinted from Lasalvia A, on behalf of the PICOS-Veneto Group. Influence of perceived organisational factors on job burnout: survey of community mental health staff. *Br J Psychiatry.* 2009;195:537-544.)

Aims.—To explore the relative weight of job-related characteristics and perceived organisational factors in predicting burnout in staff working in community-based psychiatric services.

Method.—A representative sample of 2000 mental health staff working in the Veneto region, Italy, participated. Burnout and perceived organisational factors were assessed by using the Organizational Checkup Survey.

Results.—Overall, high levels of job distress affected nearly two-thirds of the psychiatric staff and one in five staff members suffered from burnout. Psychiatrists and social workers reported the highest levels of burnout, and support workers and psychologists, the lowest. Burnout was mostly predicted by a higher frequency of face-to-face interaction with users, longer tenure in mental healthcare, weak work group cohesion and perceived unfairness.

Conclusions.—Improving the workplace atmosphere within psychiatric services should be one of the most important targets in staff burnout prevention strategies. The potential benefits of such programmes may, in turn, have a favourable impact on patient outcomes.

▶ At the beginning of my tenure as editor of the *Hospital and Community Psychiatry* journal in 1978, I was overwhelmed by the number of articles on the subject of burnout among psychiatric staff members. I personally had never felt that the organizations I was in had large numbers of disaffected staff, but at times I wondered what happened to all these burned out professionals and ancillary staff members—did they leave (for where), did they stay and turn more cynical, or did they adapt?

The authors of the large study do not answer these questions, but they do reveal several findings not evident in the articles I saw and/or published.

First, psychiatry and psychiatrists are at high risk for burnout primarily, the authors posit, because of their high level of interpersonal contact, high workload, and high job demands coupled with low job resources.

Second, a cohesive work force or lack of it is highly important in preventing or prompting burnout, and cohesiveness is enhanced by the group's performance.

And third, fairness or lack thereof is the second main predictor.

In an intriguing Venn-like diagram, they show how the 8 key predictors (temp status, workload, control, reward, fairness, positive changes, skills development, and cohesion) result in 3 critical outcomes (exhaustion, cynicism, or efficiency) (Fig 1).

Lastly, while they recommend striving for a favorable team climate, they temper it by saying that individual strategies are ineffective and programs are not easy to implement. But they note that there are trade-offs, for instance, "People may be able to tolerate greater workload[s] if they value their work and feel they are doing something important or if they feel well-rewarded for their efforts."

J. A. Talbott, MD

Burnout in Nonhospital Psychiatric Residential Facilities
Pedrini L, Magni LR, Giovannini C, et al (Istituto di Ricovero e Cura a Carattere Scientifico, Italy; et al)
Psychiatr Serv 60:1547-1551, 2009

Objective.—This study evaluated levels and risk factors of burnout in a sample of mental health professionals employed in nonhospital psychiatric residential facilities of northern Italy.

Methods.—Nurses, nurse assistants, and educators completed a questionnaire evaluating demographic variables, burnout (Maslach Burnout Inventory), job characteristics (Job Diagnostic Survey), workload, relationships with colleagues, and support from supervising coordinators. A total of 202 (83% response rate) questionnaires were analyzed. Logistic linear regressions were used to estimate predictors of burnout dimensions.

Results.—Burnout risk was widespread. Low feedback about job performance, poor support from coordinators, and young age predicted emotional exhaustion. Low feedback about job performance predicted feelings of depersonalization. Low task identity and young age predicted reduced feelings of personal accomplishment.

Conclusions.—Interventions to prevent burnout among employees should be developed. These include providing feedback about performance, clearly identifying the tasks of the job, and providing support.

▶ When I was first appointed the editor of the journal in which this study was recently published—*Psychiatric Services*—in 1980, I was staggered by the number of submissions each month on burnout. I therefore developed a whole cohort of expert peer reviewers in the field who had done research, performed training, and made recommendations about how to prevent burnout to help me assess the value of further research, training, and recommendations about prevention. It seemed to me that burnout among people working with the mentally ill was widespread, ubiquitous and unsuccessfully addressed. After 28 years of further research, policies, and interventions, I read this article with a sense of foreboding, especially its conclusion that burnout risk was widespread and that it occurs in nonhospital psychiatric residential facilities just as it had been shown to exist in both acute psychiatric care hospital wards and community-based mental health care. The authors recommend providing feedback about performance, clearly identifying the tasks of the job, and providing support, and I have no quibble with them—but what have we been doing for 28 years?

J. A. Talbott, MD

The Role of Patient Activation in Psychiatric Visits
Salyers MP, Matthias MS, Spann CL, et al (Indiana Univ-Purdue Univ Indianapolis; Butler Univ, Indianapolis, Indiana; Howard Univ, Washington, DC; et al)
Psychiatr Serv 60:1535-1539, 2009

Objective.—This study identified ways that consumers of mental health services are active participants in psychiatric treatment.

Methods.—Four providers (three psychiatrists and one nurse practitioner) were recruited, and ten consumers with severe mental illness were recruited per provider (40 total). Consumers completed questionnaires on patient activation, illness self-management, and medication attitudes on the day of a psychiatric visit. The visit was audiotaped, transcribed, and thematically analyzed. Providers gave information on diagnosis, substance use disorder, and medication adherence.

Results.—Consumer-rated patient activation was positively related to illness self-management and negatively related to substance use disorder. Transcripts of the psychiatric visit showed that consumers were active in partnership building, seeking and displaying competence, and directing treatment; however, the relationship was weak between consumer-reported activation and observed activation behaviors.

Conclusions.—Consumers were found to be active participants in treatment in a variety of ways, but similar to other populations, the relationship between observed patient activation and consumer-reported desire for involvement was not direct.

▶ This contribution to the literature starts off, "Living successfully with chronic health conditions requires active collaboration in managing illness—that is, the consumer and health care provider working together to help the consumer identify problem areas, set goals, learn self-management skills, and participate in actions and behaviors that will improve chances of recovery. An active partnership is critical because the majority of time spent managing chronic illnesses takes place when the consumer is on his or her own in the community rather than in the provider's office." Makes sense.

Then they show that they can measure active participation and conclude that consumer-rated patient activation was positively related to illness self-management and negatively related to substance use disorder. OK.

Where's step 3? Meaning—how do the authors propose to increase patients' interest, active participation, and involvement in their treatment in their enlightened self-interest? It seems that the authors get halfway to the goal and then give up; or are they merely reflecting their patients/subjects' behavior?

J. A. Talbott, MD

Assessment of Physical Illness by Mental Health Clinicians During Intake Visits
Carson N, Katz AM, Gao S, et al (Ctr for Multicultural Mental Health Res, Cambridge Health Alliance, Somerville, MA)
Psychiatr Serv 61:32-37, 2010

Objectives.—This study explored how mental health clinicians assess and respond to physical illness among patients presenting for mental health intake evaluations.

Methods.—A total of 129 adults were seen for a mental health intake visit. The intake visits were videotaped and involved 47 mental health clinicians from eight clinics who provided outpatient mental health and substance abuse treatment. A total of 120 videos of patient-provider interactions were coded using an information checklist containing 21 physical illness items. Twenty-eight intake visits exemplifying in-depth physical illness assessments were selected and transcribed for qualitative analysis.

Results.—Physical health was discussed in most intake visits (87%). Clinicians elicited information on physical health in 79 visits (66%), and patients volunteered such information in 80 visits (67%). Frequency of assessment differed by clinician discipline ($p < .05$) and by patient ethnicity ($p = .06$). Qualitative analysis revealed characteristics of appropriate assessments, such as formulating the contribution of physical conditions in the psychiatric differential diagnosis, noting physical side effects of medications, adjusting treatment plans, encouraging patient contact with primary care providers, and promoting physical health care.

Conclusions.—Assessment of physical illness is relatively common among mental health clinicians but was lacking in one-third of the cases in this study, until raised by patients. Because frequency of assessment differed by clinician discipline and patient ethnicity, innovations in patient assessment and clinician education are needed to address disparities in management of physical illness among individuals with mental illness.

▶ We are well aware that persons with severe mental illness have heightened morbidity and mortality from non-psychiatric illnesses, of the increase in metabolic syndromes in the mentally ill, and of studies showing that medical illnesses are often not complained about by patients nor inquired about by providers. Thus, at least over the past few decades there has been an increased emphasis on looking for and treating non-psychiatric medical disorders. How well have we done responding to this public health crisis/problem?

Well, this study suggests a good news and bad news response. The good news is that a "majority" of clinicians at least discussed non-psychiatric medical disorders. The bad news was that such an assessment was missing in one-third of the patients. The authors suggest the reason for the latter may be that clinicians are "following the patients" lead and asking open-ended, not focused questions.

There has been much interest of late in the checklist approach touted by Dr Peter Provonost[1] at Johns Hopkins and Dr Atul Gawande[2] at Harvard. Much as I tend to look down on psychiatrists who merely move machine-gun like through their lists of questions when interviewing new patients, maybe some items—physical health, family history, suicidal thoughts, pain, and so forth—lend themselves to a check list approach, while others—history of the present illness, environmental situation, and interpersonal relationships—do not. Something to consider.

J. A. Talbott, MD

References

1. Pronovost P, Needham D, Berenholtz S, et al. An intervention to decrease catheter-related bloodstream infections in the ICU. *N Engl J Med.* 2006;355:2725-2732.
2. Gawande A. *The Checklist Manifesto: How to Get Things Right.* New York: Henry Holt; 2009.

Mortality and cause of death among psychiatric patients: a 20-year case-register study in an area with a community-based system of care
Grigoletti L, Perini G, Rossi A, et al (Univ of Verona, Italy; et al)
Psychol Med 39:1875-1884, 2009

Background.—Most mortality studies of psychiatric patients published to date have been conducted in hospital-based systems of care. This paper describes a study of the causes of death and associated risk factors among psychiatric patients who were followed up over a 20-year period in an area where psychiatric care is entirely provided by community-based psychiatric services.

Method.—All subjects in contact with the South Verona Community-based Mental Health Service (CMHS) over a 20-year period with an ICD-10 psychiatric diagnosis were included. Of these 6956 patients, 938 died during the study period. Standardized mortality ratios (SMRs) and Poisson multiple regressions were used to assess the excess of mortality in the sample compared with the general population.

Results.—The overall SMR of the psychiatric patients was 1.88. Mortality was significantly high among out-patients [SMR 1.71, 95% confidence interval (CI) 1.6–1.8], and higher still following the first admission (SMR 2.61, 95% CI 2.4–2.9). The SMR for infectious diseases was higher among younger patients and extremely high in patients with diagnoses of drug addiction (216.40, 95% CI 142.5–328.6) and personality disorders (20.87, 95% CI 5.2–83.4).

Conclusions.—This study found that psychiatric patients in contact with a CMHS have an almost twofold higher mortality rate than the general population. These findings demonstrate that, since the closure of long-stay psychiatric hospitals, the physical health care of people with mental health problems is often neglected and clearly requires greater attention by health-care policymakers, services and professionals.

▶ This is a stunning figure: never or deinstitutionalized psychiatric patients have twice the mortality rate of the general population.

I recall that in my years as Editor of *Psychiatric Services* (previously called *Hospital and Community Psychiatry* and *H&CP*) we published several articles by Lawrence Koran and colleagues that spanned the years 1984-2002, and all highlighted the high incidence of non-psychiatric illnesses among the mentally ill, the "missing" of medical diagnoses and the potential for (my words) a disaster if we did not attend to the identification, treatment, and follow-up care of this population.[1]

Now granted, Italy did something that many experts in the field felt was revolutionary (some revolutionarily good and some revolutionarily stupid) in shutting down their long-term hospitals in favor of general hospitals and "rehabilitation centers." And, granted that a lot of this early morality in this study seems to be the result of alcohol and drug abuse that go with living in the big wide world instead of sheltered "warehouses." But if by deinstitutionalizing the chronic mentally ill we're killing them off faster, the movement needs a serious reexamination.

J. A. Talbott, MD

Reference

1. Koran LM, Sheline Y, Imai K, et al. Medical disorders among patients admitted to a public-sector psychiatric inpatient unit. *Psychiatr Serv.* 2002;53:1623-1625.

Toward Successful Postbooking Diversion: What Are the Next Steps?
Ryan S, Brown CK, Watanabe-Galloway S (Univ of Nebraska Med Ctr, Omaha)
Psychiatr Serv 61:469-477, 2010

Objective.—The authors reviewed studies of U.S. postbooking jail diversion programs for adults with serious mental illness. Questions regarding clients who are most appropriate for diversion, types of existing programs, progress in substantiating beneficial outcomes, and factors that might predict successful diversion are addressed.

Methods.—PsycINFO and MEDLINE databases were searched for articles published between 1999 and 2008; the following keywords were used: jail diversion, mental health diversion, serious mental illness, and criminal justice.

Results.—Although accumulated data do not give a complete picture, clients served by postbooking diversion programs are diverse in demographic and clinical characteristics and criminal history; their needs, which are great, are driven by this diversity. Programs use several approaches, including assertive community treatment, intensive case management, intensive psychiatric probation and parole, mental health courts, and residential support. Much of the outcome evidence is at the client level, such as a reduction in criminal justice contacts and, over the longer term, in hospitalizations. At the system level, effects such as greater use of mental health services and changes in the distribution of use have been documented, although research on cost-effectiveness is needed. Data on outcomes at the community and the broader societal levels are scarce or non-existent. Definitive evidence is lacking on factors predicting successful diversion; however, mandated treatment may increase the likelihood of program completion.

Conclusions.—Many strategies have been developed for diverting clients with serious mental illness from the justice system, but more research is needed, especially on how to enhance positive outcomes of diversion programs.

▶ It is evident from my remarks about other articles I have selected that I consider the problem of transinstitutionalizing persons with severe and persistent mental illnesses from psychiatric auspices to the correctional system one of the great scandals of our era. This contribution to the literature is an encyclopedia of information on what is the state of the art of trying to cope with this problem by redirecting these persons back into mental health care. The fact that there is no simple solution, no gold standard, and no evidence-based best practice regarding postbooking diversion demonstrates to me that states and dedicated experts are doing everything they can and trying everything they can and know that they are dealing with tough illnesses to treat. One finding from their summary of the studies that I find disturbing is the lack of data on cost factors. When this country spends so much on incarceration and so little on mental health care, you would think the powers that be would want to know.

J. A. Talbott, MD

Oil and Water or Oil and Vinegar? Evidence-Based Medicine Meets Recovery

Davidson L, Drake RE, Schmutte T, et al (Yale Univ School of Medicine, New Haven, CT)

Community Ment Health J 45:323-332, 2009

With the increasing prominence of the notions of "recovery" and "recovery-oriented practice," practitioners, program managers, and system leaders are increasingly asking about the relationship between "evidence-based practices" and recovery. After reviewing the concepts of recovery from mental illness, being in recovery with a mental illness, recovery-oriented care, and evidence-based medicine, the authors argue for a complementary relationship between recovery and evidence-based practices. This relationship is neither simple nor straightforward, but results in a whole that is greater than the sum of its parts through which each element benefits from the influence of the other.

▶ Ever since the field of mental health and/or psychiatry has adopted the "recovery" model as its summum bonum, many of us have struggled with a number of dilemmas. First is whether there is substance behind the assertion that making services "recovery oriented" improves outcome, because if it's just a slogan or politically correct rhetoric, it would constitute not much more than a "big lie." Second is whether the differences and similarities between recovery of persons with substance abuse and those suffering from mental illnesses are crisp enough to make the concept useful. And third is whether the recovery model is in conflict with evidence-based medicine or evidence-based practices or whether they are compatible. The authors have chosen to deal with the latter, and I must say it is one of the most sensible articles written on the topic of recovery. I am all in favor of having patients set goals and state preferences, having everyone become more comfortable seeking care rather than cure and realizing that we are dealing with a spectrum phenomenon, not a one size fits all disease or treatment approach. However, I've found that a very old model, the consultation-liaison (C/L) one, that takes an approach that whether it's cancer or schizophrenia, doctors and patients must struggle together against the illness, using whatever coping and scientific skills they have, rather than seeing the illness or disability as the controlling factor, is a very useful one.

J. A. Talbott, MD

Hospital Care

Approval Ratings of Inpatient Coercive Interventions in a National Sample of Mental Health Service Users and Staff in England

Whittington R, Bowers L, Nolan P, et al (Univ of Liverpool, UK; City Univ, London; Staffordshire Univ, UK; et al)
Psychiatr Serv 60:792-798, 2009

Objective.—This study sought to ascertain the degree to which psychiatric inpatients and staff approved of various coercive measures commonly used in acute inpatient care.

Methods.—A cross-sectional design was adopted. The Attitudes to Containment Measures Questionnaire (ACMQ) was completed by 1,361 service users and 1,226 staff (68% nurses) in acute care mental health services from three regions of England. This provided evaluation of 11 coercive measures (for example, seclusion) on six dimensions of approval (for example, whether the coercive measure is seen as being acceptable or safe to use) in a large national sample. Comparisons between groups were tested with independent samples t tests, chi square analysis, or Spearman correlations.

Results.—Service users and staff strongly disapproved of net beds and mechanical restraint. The three methods that received the most approval by the service user group were intermittent observation, time out, and PRN (as needed) medication; for the staff group, the three methods that were most approved of were transfer to a psychiatric intensive care unit, PRN medication, and observation. Male staff, older service users, and staff who had been involved in implementing coercion expressed greater approval of coercive measures.

Conclusions.—There are clear gender differences in how coercive measures that are used in inpatient settings are viewed. Personal involvement in deploying coercive interventions was linked to greater acceptance, suggesting a link between experience and attitudinal changes.

▶ There are a couple of things that spring to my mind on reading this study. First is the essentially high degree of concordance between patients and providers when it comes to the top 3 methods they most endorse. That is, intermittent observation and PRN (as needed) medication were much preferred to other interventions.

It is also interesting that consensual PRN (one presumes oral) medication was preferred over intramuscular (IM) injections; the question that popped into my head was how often a refusal to consent moves over to the nonconsensual IM category in real life.

The other thing I was interested in was the relegation to the bottom of the list of seclusion rather than physical restraint by both groups (albeit it was 3 up from the bottom on the part of patients). In addition, I am puzzled and there is no explanation for the dislike of patients of transfer to an ICU (the most unpopular of all choices). Is this because it is seen as a rebuke/punishment, because experience with ICU staffs was bad or because it more severely limits one's freedom and independence?

How much these results from England would hold in the United States is unclear.

J. A. Talbott, MD

Coercion and Treatment Satisfaction Among Involuntary Patients
Katsakou C, Bowers L, Amos T, et al (Queen Mary Univ of London, UK; City Univ London, UK; Univ of Bristol, UK; et al)
Psychiatr Serv 61:286-292, 2010

Objective.—This study aimed to assess involuntary inpatients' satisfaction with treatment and explore how coercion and other factors are associated with satisfaction.

Methods.—An observational prospective study was conducted in 67 acute wards in 22 hospitals in England. A total of 778 in-voluntary inpatients were recruited, and their satisfaction with treatment was assessed a week after admission and at the one-month, three-month, and one-year follow-ups. Perceived and documented coercion at admission and during hospital treatment, sociodemographic and clinical characteristics, and clinical improvement were tested as potential predictors of satisfaction.

Results.—Mean scores on the Client's Assessment of Treatment Scale measuring satisfaction with treatment ranged from 5.5 to 6.0 (on a scale with possible scores ranging from 0 to 10) at different time points and improved significantly from admission to the follow-ups. Patients who perceived less coercion at admission and during hospital treatment were more satisfied overall, whereas coercive measures documented in the medical records were not linked to satisfaction. Patients with more symptom improvement expressed higher levels of treatment satisfaction.

Conclusions.—Satisfaction with treatment among involuntary patients was associated with perceptions of coercion during admission and treatment, rather than with the documented extent of coercive measures. Interventions to reduce patients' perceived coercion might increase overall treatment satisfaction.

▶ Few subjects in psychiatry generate as much heat among professionals, family members, and patients as coercive treatment. Alan Stone is credited with the "thank you theory" of involuntary treatment satisfaction by Alexander et al.[1] The contention is that in the end, many patients thank us for having had them treated, even against their will(s). But coercive treatment is not merely that which happens with civil commitment but is used both as a carrot (providing, say, housing in return for compliance with medication taking) and a stick. ("If you don't sign in voluntarily, I'll commit you anyway.") The conclusions of this study are another example of good news/bad news or glasses half-empty or half-full. Yes, patients often saw involuntary commitment in a positive light after the fact but might have been even more satisfied if not coerced. But then, would they have been treated "properly?"

J. A. Talbott, MD

Reference

1. Alexander V, Bursztajn HJ, Brodsky A, Gutheil TG. Deciding for others; autonomy and protection in tension. In: Gutheil TG, Bursztajn HJ, Brodsky A, Alexander V, eds. *Decision Making in Psychiatry and the Law.* Baltimore, MD: Williams & Wilkins; 1991:133-152.

Characteristics of Inpatients With a History of Recurrent Psychiatric Hospitalizations: A Matched-Control Study

Schmutte T, Dunn C, Sledge W (Yale Univ School of Medicine, New Haven, CT)
Psychiatr Serv 60:1683-1685, 2009

Objective.—This study examined the association between patient characteristics and inpatient hospitalization among patients with a history of recurrent psychiatric hospitalizations (two or more hospitalizations in the 18 months before the index hospitalization) (N = 75) and patients without such a history (N = 75).

Methods.—Characteristics at the time of the index hospitalization and 48-month inpatient utilization rates (24 months before and 24 months after the index hospitalization) were extracted from medical records. Backwards stepwise regression models were used to identify characteristics independently associated with inpatient utilization.

Results.—Psychotic disorder and unemployment at the time of index hospitalization were independently associated with higher inpatient utilization over the 48 months. Only the number of hospitalizations in the prior 24 months predicted the number of readmissions after the index hospitalization.

Conclusions.—Psychosis and unemployment seem to have an independent effect on the number of hospitalizations.

▶ After reading that only psychosis and unemployment were associated with recurrent hospitalizations, I immediately assumed that people who were psychotic couldn't usually hold a job and of course they were readmitted. But as the authors show, these 2 findings are independent. My next reaction was to think about what has to be done to prevent rehospitalization, and the authors' response is refreshingly new: work on getting them employed, and to accomplish this they have a special program. For so many years, research has shown that getting severely mentally ill persons into employment was the toughest task among our goals, that I think as a field we've sort of abandoned that in favor of rehabilitation and/or day care. But apparently, at Yale, they're not so discouraged. The authors promise to tell us about their program and its results in future contributions, and I'm looking forward to that. I'd also be interested in their efforts to tackle psychosis earlier on or more aggressively because that accounts for 11% of the variance.

J. A. Talbott, MD

Weekend Prescribing Practices and Subsequent Seclusion and Restraint in a Psychiatric Inpatient Setting
Goldbloom DL, Mojtabai R, Serby MJ (Beth Israel Med Ctr, NY; Johns Hopkins Bloomberg School of Public Health, Baltimore, MD)
Psychiatr Serv 61:193-195, 2010

Objective.—This case-control study examined the role of early medication management in preventing seclusion and restraint.

Methods.—Data were extracted from the medical records, including whether standing medication was increased, decreased, or left unchanged during the first 48 hours of hospitalization.

Results.—Compared with inpatients who did not experience seclusion or restraint (N = 39), those who did (N = 39) were younger (p = .01) and more likely to be male (p = .023) and to have a primary discharge diagnosis of bipolar disorder, mixed or manic episode, schizophrenia, or schizoaffective disorder (p < .001). Patients whose standing medication was not changed during the first 48 hours of hospitalization had 5.5 times as many restraints as patients whose dose was increased or who received new prescriptions (p = .027).

Conclusions.—Early use of medication can reduce the incidence of seclusion and restraint among high-risk patients early in their hospitalization.

▶ We do not usually think of medication as a method of prevention of psychiatric problems, but here it is clear. The authors begin by stating the magnitude of the problem and reference the National Alliance for the Mentally Ill report[1] citing an "alarming number of deaths of individuals in seclusion or restraint across the United States...."

The finding that those patients admitted with adequate medication orders have a 5-fold reduction in seclusion and restraint versus those admitted by physicians who took a watch and wait approach to anticipate trouble is a cautionary tale. From my own experience making weekend rounds at a university teaching service, I'm aware that the physician who parachutes into a strange ward is reluctant to change medication regimens, and this may be partly responsible for clinicians not starting "new standing medications or increas[ing] the dosage of the patient's current medications." However, with this study I think it is time to urge more aggressive treatment on weekends.

J. A. Talbott, MD

Reference

1. Policy Research Institute: Seclusion and Restraints Task Force Report. Arlington, VA: National Alliance for the Mentally Ill; May 2003. nami.org/Template. cfm?Section=Issue_Spotlights&template=/ContentManagement/ContentDisplay. cfm&ContentID=18522. Accessed June 10, 2010.

Factors Associated With Success of Smoke-Free Initiatives in Australian Psychiatric Inpatient Units
Lawn S, Campion J (Flinders Univ, Adelaide, South Australia, Australia; St George's Univ of London, UK)
Psychiatr Serv 61:300-305, 2010

Objective.—Smoking is the largest cause of preventable illness in the United States, the United Kingdom, Canada, Australia, and many other countries. Smokers with mental illness smoke significantly more than those without mental illness and therefore experience even greater smoke-related harm. Internationally, there is increasing pressure on psychiatric inpatient settings to adopt smoke-free policies. This study examined smoke-free policies across psychiatric inpatient settings in Australia and thereby identified factors that may contribute to the success or failure of smoke-free initiatives in order to better inform best practice in this important area.

Methods.—Semistructured in-depth telephone interviews were conducted with 60 senior administrators and clinical staff with direct day-to-day experience with smoking activities in 99 adult psychiatric inpatient settings across Australia. Quantitative data were analyzed using descriptive statistical analysis and Pearson's chi square correlations measure of association.

Results.—Factors associated with greater success of smoke-free initiatives were clear, consistent, and visible leadership; cohesive teamwork; extensive training opportunities for clinical staff; fewer staff smokers; adequate planning time; effective use of nicotine replacement therapies; and consistent enforcement of a smoke-free policy.

Conclusions.—A smoke-free policy is possible within psychiatric inpatient settings, but a number of core interlinking features are important for success and ongoing sustainability.

▶ On my way from the garage to my office, I pass the State Medical Examiner's office outside which persons who have just been exposed to the blackened lungs of the deceased are busy lighting up, and hospital personnel (from doctors to construction workers) are all smoking on the university sidewalk because it is forbidden on the hospital side. So I have concluded that neither scare tactics nor forbidding smoking proximal to a building works. What does? Well, we know that class is a factor (high-income earners, including tobacco industry CEOs, do not), peer habits are another (couples and groups quit more easily than individuals), and different strokes (hypnosis, patches, Smoke Enders) work for different folks at different points in time. But none of these involves the factors unearthed here in hospital units, which are administrative-managerial ones, that is, leadership, communication, team cohesiveness, and consistent enforcement of rules. It will be interesting to see if some of these can be applied in a nonmental health, nonhospital, civilian setting because as the authors rightly point out, "Smoking is the largest cause of preventable illness …" and a high-ticket item economically.

J. A. Talbott, MD

The Influence of Neighborhood Environment on Treatment Continuity and Rehospitalization in Dually Diagnosed Patients Discharged From Acute Inpatient Care
Stahler GJ, Mennis J, Cotlar R, et al (Temple Univ, Philadelphia, PA)
Am J Psychiatry 166:1258-1268, 2009

Objective.—Environmental contingencies inherent in neighborhoods and communities have been shown to affect individual behavior. The authors analyzed neighborhood and individual factors predicting initial outpatient treatment attendance and rehospitalization within 1 year among patients who were dually diagnosed with at least one mental disorder and a substance use disorder and discharged from an acute psychiatric inpatient care unit.

Method.—Stepwise-forward logistic regression modeling and a geographic information system were utilized to assess data extracted from the medical records of 380 patients who, upon hospital admission, had one or more mental health disorders and a positive urine drug screen for prototypical illicit drugs. Geographic data on patients' neighborhood environment were obtained from public sources. Outcome variables were whether a patient attended the first outpatient treatment appointment within 30 days of hospital discharge and whether a patient was readmitted to the inpatient unit within 1 year of discharge. Predictor variables were features relating to individual-level patient characteristics and features associated with neighborhood environment.

Results.—Factors that decreased the likelihood of attending the initial outpatient treatment were returning home following hospitalization (versus returning to an institutional setting), residing in an area with a high vacant housing rate, residing in an area far from an Alcoholics Anonymous meeting location, having the chief complaint of bizarre behavior (i.e., grossly inappropriate behavior), and having a urine drug screen positive for heroin. The likelihood of being rehospitalized within 1 year was greater for Hispanic patients, patients who had at least one prior hospital admission, and patients who lived in close proximity to a Narcotics Anonymous meeting location. Patients living in areas with higher educational attainment had a reduced likelihood of rehospitalization.

Conclusions.—A more explicit focus on the neighborhood and community context represents an important area in psychiatry, in terms of both research and clinical practice, which can potentially enhance long-term care and treatment planning for psychiatric patients. Future research is needed to better understand the influence of the neighborhood environment to help predict important clinical outcomes.

▶ Let me cherry-pick a few points here:

First, currently, hospital discharge planning treatment staff rarely take into account the overall quality of a patient's neighborhood or proximity to certain environmental features that might trigger relapse and rehospitalization. Really? As a third-year medical student I recall the most widely respected clinical internist in my medical school quizzing a cardiac patient about the number of stairs, location of her washing machine, and exertion necessary to carry-out the tasks of everyday living in her living situation.

Second, patients were more likely to be rehospitalized when they were residing in an area far from an Alcoholics Anonymous meeting location, and paradoxically lived in close proximity to a Narcotics Anonymous meeting location. The authors address this paradox sensibly as indicative of the need for access to AA to ensure community tenure but access to high drug availability areas as facilitating repeat drug use.

In any event, if my revered internist professor knew the importance of environment to recovery, how come mental health experts don't take such factors into account?

J. A. Talbott, MD

Post-Traumatic Stress Disorder (PTSD) and Stress

Severity of injury does not have any impact on posttraumatic stress symptoms in severely injured patients
Quale AJ, Schanke A-K, Frøslie KF, et al (Sunnaas Rehabilitation Hosp/Univ of Oslo, Norway; Rikshospitalet-Radiumhospitalet Med Ctr, Oslo, Norway; et al)
Injury 40:498-505, 2009

Background.—Due to improved surgical techniques and more efficient decision making in treating severely injured patients, survival rates have increased over the years. This study was initiated to evaluate the incidence and identify risk factors for developing posttraumatic stress symptoms, using both extensive trauma-related data and data assessing the psychological trauma, in a population of severely injured patients.

Patients and Methods.—79 patients admitted to the Department of Multitrauma and Spinal Cord Injury at Sunnaas Rehabilitation Hospital from 2003 to 2005, prospectively completed semistructured psychological interviews and questionnaires, such as Impact of Event Scale-Revised. In addition, extensive injury-related data, such as injury severity score (ISS), new injury severity score (NISS), and probability of survival (PS) were collected.

Results.—39% had multiple trauma, 34% had multiple injuries including spinal cord injuries, and 27% had isolated spinal cord injuries. Mean NISS was 31.5 (S.D. 13.7). 6% met diagnostic criteria for posttraumatic stress disorder (PTSD) and 9% met the criteria for subsyndromal PTSD. Injury-related data did not influence the prevalence of posttraumatic stress symptoms, however, some psychosocial variables did have a significant impact.

Conclusions.—We found a low incidence of PTSD and subsyndromal PTSD. No significant differences were found between the patients suffering from posttraumatic stress symptoms and the non-symptoms group in relation to injury-related data such as ISS/NISS, PS, or multiple trauma versus spinal cord injury. The most evident risk factors for developing posttraumatic stress symptoms were symptoms of anxiety, female gender and negative attitudes toward emotional expression.

▶ This is one of those rare articles where a single finding is very important and thus there is very little to discuss.

I recall interviewing 2 Vietnam combat veterans as part of the "Legacies" study[1] of which Arthur Egendorf was a leading force in the 1970s. One had severe posttraumatic stress disorder years after an incident where he was the "point man" on a night patrol, who lit a cigarette, dropped his lighter and when stooping to pick it up saw the #2 man get shot in the head where his had been only seconds before; he had no physical injuries. The second was a multiple amputee who had undergone so many surgeries, he was a criss cross of scars and plastic surgeons' efforts; he had very slight problems sleeping but no flashbacks, startle reaction, depression, etc.

I often refer to these 2 individuals when discussing the relationship between physical and emotional trauma, but they are after all, a study of 2; and thus not subject to generalization. But here we have a much larger sample size and much more impressive conclusions.

J. A. Talbott, MD

Reference

1. Egendorf A, Kadushin C, Laufer R, Rothbart G, Sloan L. *Legacies of Vietnam: Comparative Adjustment of Veterans and their Peers.* Washington, D.C.: U. S. Government Printing Office; 1981. A study prepared for the Veterans' Administration (pursuant to Public Law 95-202, the GI Improvement Act of 1977); submitted to the Committee on Veterans' Affairs U.S. House of Representatives.

The Impact of Repression, Hostility, and Post-Traumatic Stress Disorder on All-Cause Mortality: A Prospective 16-Year Follow-up Study
Boscarino JA, Figley CR (Ctr for Health Res, Danville, PA; Tulane Univ, New Orleans, LA; et al)
J Nerv Ment Dis 197:461-466, 2009

A common assumption is that repression of traumatic memories is harmful to health. To assess this, we examined all-cause mortality among a national random sample of 4462 male US Army veterans evaluated in 1985 and followed up in 2000. Our hypothesis was that repression on the Welsh R scale would be associated with increased future mortality. We also expected to find a repression × post-traumatic stress disorder (PTSD) interaction effect. Multivariate Cox regression results for all veterans and for theater veterans (Vietnam service) and era veterans (no Vietnam service) separately, revealed that while PTSD was significant in all models, no main or interaction effect was found for repression. In addition, for era veterans, higher repression symptoms were protective for future mortality (HR = 0.95, $p = 0.03$). For hostility symptoms, although no interaction effect was found by PTSD, a positive main effect was detected for hostility, but only for theater veterans (HR = 1.04, $p = 0.034$). Disease-specific results were nonsignificant. Similar to a recent study, we also found that repression symptoms were negatively correlated with PTSD symptoms (r = −0.109, $p < 0.001$), suggesting repression might be protective. Our study found no evidence that repression had an adverse health impact on men exposed to psychological trauma.

▶ One of the legacies of the 1960s and 1970s psychoanalytic and self-indulgent/hippie era was the notion that psychiatric problems and symptoms all represented repressed stuff and if you "let it all out," you'd get better and we'd all be healthier and happier.[1] Well, that led to Bion, Encounter, and other Group excesses that caused brutal office warfare and broke up long-term friendships.

So, now we have this careful 16-year study by 2 of America's leading experts in posttraumatic stress disorder (PTSD) showing clearly that not only does repression not lead to PTSD but also it's protective. It's also of interest that the authors found that mortality was the same no matter what defenses or mental mechanisms were used.

Maybe it's simplistic, but it's possible to conclude that we've gone from the 1960s "let it all out" to the 2000s "just get over it" for a reason.

J. A. Talbott, MD

Reference

1. Wolfe T. The me decade and the third great awakening. In: *Mauve Gloves & Madmen, Clutter & Vine.* New York: Bantam; 1977.

Injury-specific predictors of posttraumatic stress disorder

MacGregor AJ, Corson KS, Larson GE, et al (Naval Health Res Ctr, San Diego, CA; et al)
Injury 40:1004-1010, 2009

Objective.—Posttraumatic stress disorder (PTSD) is an important source of morbidity in military personnel, but its relationship with characteristics of battle injury has not been well defined. The aim of this study was to characterise the relationship between injury-related factors and PTSD among a population of battle injuries.

Patients and Methods.—A total of 831 American military personnel injured during combat between September 2004 and February 2005 composed the study population. Patients were followed through November 2006 for diagnosis of PTSD (ICD-9 309.81) or any mental health outcome (ICD-9 290-319).

Results.—During the follow-up period, 31.3% of patients received any type of mental health diagnosis and 17.0% received a PTSD diagnosis. Compared with minor injuries those with moderate (odds ratio [OR], 2.37; 95% confidence interval [CI], 1.61–3.48), serious (OR, 4.07; 95% CI, 2.55–6.50), and severe (OR, 5.22; 95% CI, 2.74–9.96) injuries were at greater risk of being diagnosed with any mental health outcome. Similar results were found for serious (OR, 3.03; 95% CI, 1.81–5.08) and severe (OR, 3.21; 95% CI, 1.62–6.33) injuries with PTSD diagnosis. Those with gunshot wounds were at greater risk of any mental health diagnosis, but not PTSD, in comparison with other mechanisms of injury (OR 2.07; 95% CI, 1.35, 3.19). Diastolic blood pressure measured postinjury was associated with any mental health outcome, and the effect was modified by injury severity.

Conclusions.—Injury severity was a significant predictor of any mental health diagnosis and PTSD diagnosis. Gunshot wounds and diastolic blood pressure were significant predictors of any mental health diagnosis, but not PTSD. Further studies are needed to replicate these results and elucidate potential mechanisms for these associations.

▶ In a previously discussed article[1] the title screams out that severity of injury does not have any impact on posttraumatic stress symptoms in severely injured patients, whereas these authors conclude that, "Injury severity was a significant predictor of any mental health diagnosis and PTSD diagnosis."

So, what's going on here?

Well, the Quale study concerned severely injured civilians and this study dealt with military personnel who suffered a range of severity of injuries.

I assumed that even though the Quale study was published in the journal *Injury: The International Journal of Care Injured* in March 2009 and the above study in September 2009, there would be an editorial explaining the seeming contradiction or a reference in one of the other; but I can find none such.

Thus, I am left for the moment unsure of the reasons for the differences and will await further clarification.
But it is certainly interesting.

J. A. Talbott, MD

Reference

1. Quale AJ, Schanke A-K, Frøslie KF, Røise O. Severity of injury does not have any impact on posttraumatic stress symptoms in severely injured patients. *Injury*. 2009;40:498-505.

A National US Study of Posttraumatic Stress Disorder, Depression, and Work and Functional Outcomes After Hospitalization for Traumatic Injury
Zatzick D, Jurkovich GJ, Rivara FP, et al (Univ of Washington School of Medicine, Seattle; et al)
Ann Surg 248:429-437, 2008

Objective.—To examine factors other than injury severity that are likely to influence functional outcomes after hospitalization for injury.

Summary Background Data.—This study used data from the National Study on the Costs and Outcomes of Trauma investigation to examine the association between posttraumatic stress disorder (PTSD), depression, and return to work and the development of functional impairments after injury.

Method.—A total of 2707 surgical inpatients who were representative of 9374 injured patients were recruited from 69 hospitals across the US. PTSD and depression were assessed at 12 months postinjury, as were the following functional outcomes: activities of daily living, health status, and return to usual major activities and work. Regression analyses assessed the associations between PTSD and depression and functional outcomes while adjusting for clinical and demographic characteristics.

Results.—At 12 months after injury, 20.7% of patients had PTSD and 6.6% had depression. Both disorders were independently associated with significant impairments across all functional outcomes. A dose-response relationship was observed, such that previously working patients with 1 disorder had a 3-fold increased odds of not returning to work 12 months after injury odds ratio = 3.20 95% (95% confidence interval = 2.46, 4.16), and patients with both disorders had a 5–6 fold increased odds of not returning to work after injury odds ratio = 5.57 (95% confidence interval = 2.51, 12.37) when compared with previously working patients without PTSD or depression.

Conclusions.—PTSD and depression occur frequently and are independently associated with enduring impairments after injury hospitalization.

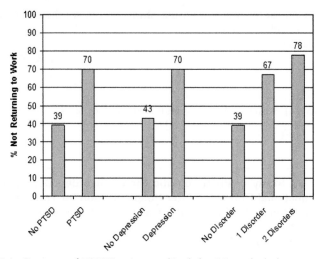

FIGURE 1.—Percentage of NSCOT patients working before injury who had not returned to work 12 months after injury. Two disorders indicate PTSD and depression; 1 disorder, PTSD or depression; 0 disorders, no PTSD or depression. Symptoms consistent with a diagnosis of PTSD were assessed with the PCL.[16] Symptoms consistent with a diagnosis of depression were assessed with the Center for Epidemiologic Studies Depression Scale Revised.[21] Editor's Note: Please refer to original journal article for full references. (Courtesy of Zatzick D, Jurkovich GJ, Rivara FP, et al. A national US study of posttraumatic stress disorder, depression, and work and functional outcomes after hospitalization for traumatic injury. *Ann Surg.* 2008;248:429-437.)

Early acute care interventions targeting these disorders have the potential to improve functional recovery after injury.

▶ Almost 3 decades ago, I was hit by a taxi running a red light while standing on the sidewalk after buying a newspaper; as soon as I was out of surgery and fully conscious I telephoned my good friend and colleague who ran the Consultation-Liaison Service and said I wanted to contract with him to treat me, the goal being that I would never develop a startle reaction, have flashbacks, avoid taxis, or develop any other symptoms of posttraumatic stress disorder.

Okay, granted that I was a psychiatrist who had studied combat related posttraumatic stress disorder, granted that I had the connections and insurance to get superb care, and granted I acted immediately, long before I got out of the hospital, out of casts and completed physical therapy. But if 20% of surgical inpatients develop posttraumatic stress disorder and their risk of not returning to work (Fig 1) is 6-fold, the personal, family, and global economic impacts are enormous and must be addressed.

Thus, it is heartening to read that: (1) this article was given and published to surgical audiences, (2) Level 1 Trauma Centers must have on-site alcohol screening and brief intervention services for accreditation, and (3) that the American College of Surgeons' manual recommends posttraumatic stress disorder assessments.

PS—My psychiatrist fulfilled his contract with glory.

J. A. Talbott, MD

Morphine Use after Combat Injury in Iraq and Post-Traumatic Stress Disorder

Holbrook TL, Galarneau MR, Dye JL, et al (Naval Health Res Ctr, San Diego, CA)
N Engl J Med 362:110-117, 2010

Background.—Post-traumatic stress disorder (PTSD) is a common adverse mental health outcome among seriously injured civilians and military personnel who are survivors of trauma. Pharmacotherapy in the aftermath of serious physical injury or exposure to traumatic events may be effective for the secondary prevention of PTSD.

Methods.—We identified 696 injured U.S. military personnel without serious traumatic brain injury from the Navy–Marine Corps Combat Trauma Registry Expeditionary Medical Encounter Database. Complete data on medications administered were available for all personnel selected. The diagnosis of PTSD was obtained from the Career History Archival Medical and Personnel System and verified in a review of medical records.

Results.—Among the 696 patients studied, 243 received a diagnosis of PTSD and 453 did not. The use of morphine during early resuscitation and trauma care was significantly associated with a lower risk of PTSD after injury. Among the patients in whom PTSD developed, 61% received morphine; among those in whom PTSD did not develop, 76% received morphine (odds ratio, 0.47; P<0.001). This association remained significant after adjustment for injury severity, age, mechanism of injury, status with respect to amputation, and selected injury-related clinical factors.

Conclusions.—Our findings suggest that the use of morphine during trauma care may reduce the risk of subsequent development of PTSD after serious injury.

▶ Researchers and clinicians have long looked for psychological and physiological factors that could bolster resistance to the development of posttraumatic stress disorders, particularly among soldiers. Now we have evidence that one of man's oldest pharmacological agents—morphine—plays just such a role. This immediately raises for me a question about complicating factors—that is, why did some soldiers receive morphine? For pain? For what? Physical injury one supposes. Doesn't that make the 2 groups noncomparable? Matthew Friedman,[1] in an accompanying editorial, raises other issues:

- Could persons "with minor injuries or no injuries in the aftermath of major trauma who do not need morphine to attenuate physical pain ...[be protected by] ...the routine administration of morphine ...from subsequent PTSD,"?

- Could "adrenergic antagonists, such as propranolol and clonidine (an 2-adrenergic agonist) [be a sort of] ...morning-after pill to prevent the later development of PTSD among persons after major trauma,"?

- But he cautions that "it is unlikely that this could become acceptable in clinical practice [and it raises] ...theoretical and practical questions that require rigorous follow-up."

This is fascinating stuff and deserves ample follow-up studies to clarify these questions in the pursuit of what is often a crippling illness all too common in our long wars in Iraq and Afghanistan.

J. A. Talbott, MD

Reference

1. Friedman M. Prevention of psychiatric problems among military personnel and their spouses. *NEJM.* 2010;362:168-169.

Psychosocial buffers of traumatic stress, depressive symptoms, and psychosocial difficulties in veterans of Operations Enduring Freedom and Iraqi Freedom: The role of resilience, unit support, and postdeployment social support
Pietrzak RH, Johnson DC, Goldstein MB, et al (Natl Ctr for Posttraumatic Stress Disorder, West Haven, CT; Univ of California San Diego School of Medicine; Central Connecticut State Univ, New Britain, CT)
J Affect Disord 120:188-192, 2010

Background.—Little research has examined the role of protective factors such as psychological resilience, unit support, and postdeployment social support in buffering against PTSD and depressive symptoms, and psychosocial difficulties in veterans of Operations Enduring Freedom (OEF) and Iraqi Freedom (OIF).

Materials and Methods.—A total of 272 OEF/OIF veterans completed a survey containing PTSD and depression screening measures, and questionnaires assessing resilience, social support, and psychosocial functioning.

Results.—Lower unit support and postdeployment social support were associated with increased PTSD and depressive symptoms, and decreased resilience and psychosocial functioning. Path analyses suggested that resilience fully mediated the association between unit support and PTSD and depressive symptoms, and that postdeployment social support partially mediated the association between PTSD and depressive symptoms and psychosocial functioning.

Limitations.—Generalizability of results is limited by the relatively low response rate and predominantly older and reserve/National Guard sample.

Conclusions.—These results suggest that interventions designed to bolster unit support, resilience, and postdeployment support may help protect against traumatic stress and depressive symptoms, and improve psychosocial functioning in veterans.

▶ A major problem with studies such as these is that they depend on self-report and not objective assessment. Therefore, while interesting, they are not definitive. In addition, I am surprised at the lack of reference to the work of Ursano and colleagues, who have written extensively about factors that protect against development of posttraumatic stress disorder.[1]

As long ago as the war in Vietnam, we were told that unit cohesion and unit morale were important factors (community factors as it were) in reducing the rates of posttraumatic stress disorder. Indeed, the entire program in Vietnam of "command consultation" was based on the principles of civilian community psychiatry's "community consultation," which essentially attempted to deal with problems as a systems issue from the top down rather than through treatment and care of the individual. I recall 1 unit in particular whose job was to drive unarmed refrigerated trucks down to Southern Vietnam from the vegetable gardens in the mountains; the morale was horrible, the confidence in leadership and survival was nil, and the sick rate sky high.

So I'm a believer in the authors' findings and recommendations—I'm just not so certain as to how they would go about actually increasing social support and unit support and reducing loneliness, and whether the military would devote the necessary time and energy preventively rather than after the development of posttraumatic stress disorder and depression.

J. A. Talbott, MD

Reference

1. Ursano RJ, Grieger TA, McCarroll JE. Prevention of posttraumatic stress: consultation, training, and early treatment. In: Van der Kolk BA, McFarlane AC, Weisaeth L, eds. *Traumatic Stress: The Effects of Overwhelming Experience on Mind, Body, and Society.* New York: Guilford Press; 1996:441-462.

Trends and Risk Factors for Mental Health Diagnoses Among Iraq and Afghanistan Veterans Using Department of Veterans Affairs Health Care, 2002–2008

Seal KH, Metzler TJ, Gima KS, et al (San Francisco VA Med Ctr, CA)

Am J Public Health 99:1651-1658, 2009

Objectives.—We sought to investigate longitudinal trends and risk factors for mental health diagnoses among Iraq and Afghanistan veterans.

Methods.—We determined the prevalence and predictors of mental health diagnoses among 289 328 Iraq and Afghanistan veterans entering Veterans Affairs (VA) health care from 2002 to 2008 using national VA data.

Results.—Of 289 328 Iraq and Afghanistan veterans, 106 726 (36.9%) received mental health diagnoses; 62 929 (21.8%) were diagnosed with posttraumatic stress disorder (PTSD) and 50 432 (17.4%) with depression. Adjusted 2-year prevalence rates of PTSD increased 4 to 7 times after the invasion of Iraq. Active duty veterans younger than 25 years had higher rates of PTSD and alcohol and drug use disorder diagnoses compared with active duty veterans older than 40 years (adjusted relative risk = 2.0 and 4.9, respectively). Women were at higher risk for depression than were men, but men had over twice the risk for drug use disorders. Greater combat exposure was associated with higher risk for PTSD.

Conclusions.—Mental health diagnoses increased substantially after the start of the Iraq War among specific subgroups of returned veterans entering VA health care. Early targeted interventions may prevent chronic mental illness.

▶ It is pretty hard to plunge into the waters of the wars in Afghanistan and Iraq without drowning politically, but the authors negotiate the issues quite successfully, maintaining their scientific objectivity. The press has been quite sympathetic to the plight of returning military personnel and their high rates of post-traumatic stress disorder, depression, and marital problems. To my astonishment, as a veteran of the War in Vietnam, I have been pleasantly surprised by the response of the current (combat) commanders, the Surgeons General, and the Veterans Administration. Instead of covering up the problems, they have asked for help from civilian experts and the veteran community. In addition, I have a sense that there is much better training of military forces being deployed overseas as well as heightened receptivity to seeking and receiving psychiatric care and treatment. Yes, one hears of the "macho" Marine who thinks crying is a weakness, but that story is offset by a thousand about those seeking care. This is not to say "mission accomplished" because as the authors point out, the differing responses of age cohorts, genders, and rank cry out for further examination as does the question of what we do about the repeated deployment of what now seems to be a core military force that will be involved forever in both areas (rather than as in Vietnam, a group, constantly rotating in and out).

J. A. Talbott, MD

Battlemind Debriefing and Battlemind Training as Early Interventions With Soldiers Returning From Iraq: Randomization by Platoon
Adler AB, Bliese PD, McGurk D, et al (Walter Reed Army Inst of Res, Heidelberg, Germany; et al)
J Consult Clin Psychol 77:928-940, 2009

Researchers have found that there is an increase in mental heath problems as a result of military-related traumatic events, and such problems increase in the months following return from combat. Nevertheless, researchers have not assessed the impact of early intervention efforts with this at-risk population. In the present study, the authors compared different early interventions with 2,297 U.S. soldiers following a year-long deployment to Iraq. Platoons were randomly assigned to standard postdeployment stress education, Battlemind debriefing, and small and large group Battlemind training. Results from a 4-month follow-up with 1,060 participants showed those with high levels of combat exposure who received Battlemind debriefing reported fewer posttraumatic stress symptoms, depression symptoms, and sleep problems than those in stress education. Small group Battlemind training participants with high combat exposure reported fewer posttraumatic stress symptoms and sleep problems than stress education participants. Compared to stress education participants, large group Battlemind training participants with high combat exposure reported fewer posttraumatic stress symptoms and lower levels of stigma and, regardless of combat exposure, reported fewer depression symptoms. Findings demonstrate that brief early interventions have the potential to be effective with at-risk occupational groups.

▶ The current conduct of 2 longstanding wars and repetitive redeployment of troops coupled with high rates of posttraumatic stress disorder and widely reported increased suicide has led the military to a searing re-examination of its policies and procedures. The fact that one form of debriefing—called Battlemind training or debriefing—in soldiers with high combat exposure resulted in fewer posttraumatic stress symptoms (PTSD) and lower levels of stigma and, regardless of combat exposure, reported fewer depression symptoms, is indeed good news. Despite the authors' careful attempts to describe this intervention, I am still uncertain what distinguishes it from standard stress education. Groups are smaller, but what have they introduced that they (or others) don't provide in the usual stress education? What does make sense to me is avoiding the immediate debriefing after traumatic events that has been shown to aggravate PTSD, using cognitive behavioral (CBT) methods and stressing the social and psychological shift from combat to home life.

J. A. Talbott, MD

Association Between Number of Deployments to Iraq and Mental Health Screening Outcomes in US Army Soldiers
Reger MA, Gahm GA, Swanson RD, et al (National Ctr for Telehealth and Technology, Tacoma, WA)
J Clin Psychiatry 70:1266-1272, 2009

Objective.—High rates of mental health concerns have been documented in US Army soldiers deployed in support of Operation Iraqi Freedom. The goal of this study was to compare the postdeployment mental health screening results of US Army soldiers with 1 or 2 deployments to Iraq.

Method.—Routine mental health screening data collected from September 7, 2005, to April 27, 2007, in the Soldier Wellness Assessment Program were compared between soldiers evaluated after their first or second deployment to Iraq (n = 1322). Standardized measures (Primary Care Evaluation of Mental Disorders Patient Health Questionnaire, Primary Care Posttraumatic Stress Disorder Screen, Alcohol Use Disorders Identification Test) were used to screen for posttraumatic stress disorder

(PTSD), panic, other anxiety, major depression, other depression, and hazardous alcohol consumption 90 to 180 days after the soldiers returned from Iraq.

Results.—There was a significant association between number of deployments and mental health screening results such that soldiers with 2 deployments showed greater odds of screening positive for PTSD (odds ratio [OR] = 1.64, P = .001). Similar results were observed when the analyses were repeated utilizing a more conservative cut-point for PTSD (OR = 1.60, P = .001). After adjustment for demographic characteristics, the results were unchanged. There was no association between the number of deployments and other mental health screening results.

Conclusions.—These results provide preliminary evidence that multiple deployments to Iraq may be a risk factor for PTSD. However, these cross-sectional data require replication in a longitudinal study.

▶ This study holds highly disturbing implications. We already knew that multiple deployments to combat zones have a devastating effect on families and on the members of the military themselves, and given the fact that we have 2 seemingly endless wars and a totally volunteer military force, there does not appear to be an end in sight. The military and Veterans' Administration have acknowledged that they have a big problem and asked for help from organizations such as the American Psychiatric Association as well as experts in epidemiology, prevention, and treatment. Unfortunately, given the factors at hand, I fear the only solution is a political policy, not a medical/psychiatric one. While the authors thought that those with multiple deployments represented a more mature and thus resilient group, being older, better educated, stably married, etc, these factors may not function to protect individuals enough against the impact of time spent in combat areas, which we know from Vietnam increases the incidence of posttraumatic stress disorder.

J. A. Talbott, MD

Deployment and the Use of Mental Health Services among U.S. Army Wives
Mansfield AJ, Kaufman JS, Marshall SW, et al (Univ of North Carolina, Chapel Hill; et al)
N Engl J Med 362:101-109, 2010

Background.—Military operations in Iraq and Afghanistan have involved the frequent and extended deployment of military personnel, many of whom are married. The effect of deployment on mental health in military spouses is largely unstudied.

Methods.—We examined electronic medical-record data for outpatient care received between 2003 and 2006 by 250,626 wives of active-duty U.S. Army soldiers. After adjustment for the sociodemographic characteristics and the mental health history of the wives, as well as the number of deployments of the personnel, we compared mental health diagnoses according to the number of months of deployment in Operation Iraqi Freedom in the Iraq–Kuwait region and Operation Enduring Freedom in Afghanistan during the same period.

Results.—The deployment of spouses and the length of deployment were associated with mental health diagnoses. In adjusted analyses, as compared with wives of personnel who were not deployed, women whose husbands were deployed for 1 to 11 months received more diagnoses of depressive disorders (27.4 excess cases per 1000 women; 95% confidence interval [CI], 22.4 to 32.3), sleep disorders (11.6 excess cases per 1000; 95% CI, 8.3 to 14.8), anxiety (15.7 excess cases per 1000; 95% CI, 11.8 to 19.6), and acute stress reaction and adjustment disorders (12.0 excess cases per 1000; 95% CI, 8.6 to 15.4). Deployment for more than 11 months was associated with 39.3 excess cases of depressive disorders (95% CI, 33.2 to 45.4), 23.5 excess cases of sleep disorders (95% CI, 19.4 to 27.6), 18.7 excess cases of anxiety (95% CI, 13.9 to 23.5), and 16.4 excess cases of acute stress reaction and adjustment disorders (95% CI, 12.2 to 20.6).

Conclusions.—Prolonged deployment was associated with more mental health diagnoses among U.S. Army wives, and these findings may have relevance for prevention and treatment efforts.

▶ This is a huge study with significant findings and large implications for prevention, public health, and future research. The fact that so many psychiatric illnesses—depression, anxiety, sleep disorders, acute stress reactions, and adjustment disorders—were increased and that increased length of deployment increased use of mental health services demonstrates vividly the impact of these deployments. In an accompanying editorial[1] by respected posttraumatic stress disorder (PTSD) expert Matthew Friedman, he discusses the contribution far better than I, saying that: because it was not hypothesis driven nor did they have the dates of deployment, "They could not assess the temporal relationship between deployment and a mental health diagnosis. In other words, was the presence or absence of the soldier more likely to be associated with mental health problems in the wife?" which would lead to very different interventions. In addition, he raised 3 critical questions that must be answered to know how to frame policy and clinical interventions: "Is it deployment per se, with all the complications of separation and worry about loved ones, that is contributing to more mental health problems? Is the intensity of soldiers' exposure to combat during deployment the critical factor? Is the deleterious effect of deployment on spouses mediated by the presence of PTSD or some other combat-related problem such as physical injury, traumatic brain injury, another psychiatric or substance-use disorder, aggressive or violent behavior, problems expressed by children, other factors, or all of the above?" These are intriguing questions, whose answers will lead to innovative solutions in this most disturbing of war situations.

J. A. Talbott, MD

Reference

1. Friedman M. Prevention of psychiatric problems among military personnel and their spouses. *N Engl J Med.* 2010;362:168-169.

Persistence of Traumatic Memories in World War II Prisoners of War
Rintamaki LS, Weaver FM, Elbaum PL, et al (State Univ of New York at Buffalo; Ctr for Management of Complex Chronic Care, Chicago, IL; Loyola Univ Med School, Chicago, IL; et al)
J Am Geriatr Soc 57:2257-2262, 2009

Objectives.—To assess the long-term effects of the prisoner of war (POW) experience on U.S. World War II (WWII) veterans.

Design.—Exploratory study.

Setting.—Participants were recruited through the Hines Veterans Affairs Hospital; a POW reunion in Orlando, Florida; and the WWII veterans periodical, "The QUAN."

Participants.—One hundred fifty-seven American military veterans who were former WWII POWs.

Measurments.—Participants completed a mailed survey describing their POW experiences, POW effects on subsequent psychological and physical well-being, and ways in which these experiences shaped major decisions in their lives.

Results.—Participants from the European and Pacific theaters reported that their captivity during WWII affected their long-term emotional well-being. Both groups reported high rates of reflection, dreaming, and flashbacks pertaining to their POW experiences, but Pacific theater POWs did so at higher rates in the present than in the past. Large portions of both groups reported greater rumination on POW experiences after retirement. Finally, 16.6% of participants met the requirements of a current, clinical diagnosis of posttraumatic stress disorder (PTSD) based on the Mississippi PTSD scale, with PTSD rates in Pacific theater POWs (34%) three times those of European theater POWs (12%).

Conclusion.—Traumatic memories and clinical levels of PTSD persist for WWII POWs as long as 65 years after their captivity. Additionally, rumination about these experiences, including flashbacks and persistent nightmares, may increase after retirement, particularly for those held in the Pacific theater. These findings inform the current therapeutic needs of this elderly population and future generations of POWs from other military conflicts.

▶ It is not surprising that the authors found that World War II veterans, even 65 years later, had impaired long-term emotional well-being characterized by high rates of reflection, dreaming, and flashbacks pertaining to their prisoner of war (POW) experiences and suffered from diagnosable posttraumatic stress disorder. What is new here is the evidence that rumination about these experiences, including flashbacks and persistent nightmares, may increase after retirement. That is certainly reasonable given the fact that retired individuals may have both more time on their hands and less demanding, distracting work to perform. With the military and Veterans Administration's heightened concerns about the identification and treatment of suicide and posttraumatic stress disorder among veterans of the Iraq and Afghanistan wars, it will be useful to ensure that once these returning soldiers are 10 or 20 years out, we remember that many may continue to experience symptoms and may need special attention after their retirements.

J. A. Talbott, MD

The Psychiatric Sequelae of Traumatic Injury
Bryant RA, O'Donnell ML, Creamer M, et al (Univ of New South Wales, Sydney, Australia; Univ of Melbourne, Victoria, Australia; the Australian Centre for Posttraumatic Mental Health, East Melbourne, Victoria, Australia; et al)
Am J Psychiatry 167:312-320, 2010

Objective.—Traumatic injury affects millions of people each year. There is little understanding of the extent of psychiatric illness that develops after traumatic injury or of the impact of mild traumatic brain injury (TBI) on psychiatric illness. The authors sought to determine the range of new psychiatric disorders occurring after traumatic injury and the influence of mild TBI on psychiatric status.

Method.—In this prospective cohort study, patients were drawn from recent admissions to four major trauma hospitals across Australia. A total of 1,084 traumatically injured patients were initially assessed during hospital admission and followed up 3 months (N = 932, 86%) and 12 months (N = 817, 75%) after injury. Lifetime psychiatric diagnoses were assessed in hospital. The prevalence of psychiatric disorders, levels of quality of life, and mental health service use were assessed at the follow-ups. The main outcome measures were 3- and 12-month prevalence of axis I psychiatric disorders, levels of quality of life, and mental health service use and lifetime axis I psychiatric disorders.

Results.—Twelve months after injury, 31% of patients reported a psychiatric disorder, and 22% developed a psychiatric disorder that they had never experienced before. The most common new psychiatric disorders were depression (9%), generalized anxiety disorder (9%), posttraumatic stress disorder (6%), and agoraphobia (6%). Patients were more likely to develop posttraumatic stress disorder (odds ratio = 1.92, 95% CI = 1.08–3.40), panic disorder (odds ratio = 2.01, 95% CI = 1.03–4.14), social phobia (odds ratio = 2.07, 95% CI = 1.03–4.16), and agoraphobia (odds ratio = 1.94, 95% CI = 1.11–3.39) if they had sustained a mild TBI. Functional impairment, rather than mild TBI, was associated with psychiatric illness.

Conclusions.—A significant range of psychiatric disorders occur after traumatic injury. The identification and treatment of a range of psychiatric disorders are important for optimal adaptation after traumatic injury.

▶ There are several issues raised by this study by the respected McFarlane group in Australia that deserve our attention. First, the fact that while they properly focus on new disorders appearing after traumatic brain injuries (TBIs), almost 10% of persons with TBIs have a return of prior symptoms or disorders. This means that we must be on the lookout for the reappearance of illnesses in our old patients as well as new ones. Second, the fact that 22% of persons suffering TBIs have newly developed psychiatric disorders is daunting. While only 33% of all individuals seek treatment, coupled with the vast increase in utilization in the United States that will surely occur with health care reform implementation, the system and psychiatrists will certainly be strained. Finally, while our focus has been on the development of post-TBI of posttraumatic stress disorders, we should broaden that focus to include persons suffering from depression, generalized anxiety disorder, agoraphobia, panic disorder, and social phobia. Given that the soldiers fighting the 2 wars that we are involved with at present (Iraq and Afghanistan) are returning with a high rate of TBI, this study gives much cause of concern for our public health, manpower, and system deficiencies.

J. A. Talbott, MD

Witnessing Trauma in the Newsroom: Posttraumatic Symptoms in Television Journalists Exposed to Violent News Clips
Weidmann A, Papsdorf J (Humboldt-Universität zu Berlin, Germany)
J Nerv Ment Dis 198:264-271, 2010

Employees working in television newsrooms are exposed to video footage of violent events on a daily basis. It is yet unknown whether they subsequently develop symptoms of posttraumatic stress disorder as has been shown for other populations exposed to trauma through television. We conducted an internet-based survey with 81 employees. Nearly 80% of the sample reported being familiar with recurring intrusive memories. However, the sample's overall posttraumatic stress disorder symptoms were low, although participants with a prior trauma, more general work stress, and a greater exposure to footage had a tendency to show more severe symptoms. Regarding general mental health, there were no differences compared with a journalistic control group. Results suggest that the population as such is not at a particular risk of developing mental problems.

▶ As I looked at the title of this article, I said to myself, "You know, there's no experience or way of exposure to all sorts of bad events that doesn't result in posttraumatic stress disorder." And then when I read the abstract I thought

"Well now, that makes sense." But wait a minute, why such divergent reactions and how come TV news folk don't show much of a reaction to seeing bad stuff? First off, study after study has appeared showing that posttraumatic stress disorder is not confined to soldiers in battle, as was believed when it was conceived of, or to those involved in major civilian disasters, as we believed afterward, but to a host of individuals exposed to bad experiences from rape to burns to torture to refugee camps. So it is logical to assume when picking up a journal that the authors have found one more group that's vulnerable. Now to my second point. We know very little about factors that are protective against developing posttraumatic stress disorder. We've been told that a good solid life before, strong personality, lack of prior trauma, and positive outlook probably are protective as are inoculation exercises for first responders, say. And I would guess that there is a distancing that viewing TV rather than real life offers one as well as a fatigue that sets in on viewing repeated disaster scenes, be they removal of dead miners' bodies, persons blown up by car bombs, or soldiers bloodied in battle. This area of protective factors and how to increase them deserves more attention.

J. A. Talbott, MD

Violence

Schizophrenia, Substance Abuse, and Violent Crime

Fazel S, Långström N, Hjern A, et al (Univ of Oxford, England; Karolinska Institutet, Stockholm, Sweden; et al)
JAMA 301:2016-2023, 2009

Context.—Persons with schizophrenia are thought to be at increased risk of committing violent crime 4 to 6 times the level of general population individuals without this disorder. However, risk estimates vary substantially across studies, and considerable uncertainty exists as to what mediates this elevated risk. Despite this uncertainty, current guidelines recommend that violence risk assessment should be conducted for all patients with schizophrenia.

Objective.—To determine the risk of violent crime among patients diagnosed as having schizophrenia and the role of substance abuse in mediating this risk.

Design, Setting, and Participants.—Longitudinal designs were used to link data from nationwide Swedish registers of hospital admissions and criminal convictions in 1973-2006. Risk of violent crime in patients after diagnosis of schizophrenia (n = 8003) was compared with that among general population controls (n = 80 025). Potential confounders (age, sex, income, and marital and immigrant status) and mediators (substance abuse comorbidity) were measured at baseline. To study familial confounding, we also investigated risk of violence among unaffected siblings (n = 8123) of patients with schizophrenia. Information on treatment was not available.

Main Outcome Measure.—Violent crime (any criminal conviction for homicide, assault, robbery, arson, any sexual offense, illegal threats, or intimidation).

Results.—In patients with schizophrenia, 1054 (13.2%) had at least 1 violent offense compared with 4276 (5.3%) of general population controls (adjusted odds ratio [OR], 2.0; 95% confidence interval [CI], 1.8-2.2). The risk was mostly confined to patients with substance abuse comorbidity (of whom 27.6% committed an offense), yielding an increased risk of violent crime among such patients (adjusted OR, 4.4; 95% CI, 3.9-5.0), whereas the risk increase was small in schizophrenia patients without substance abuse comorbidity (8.5% of whom had at least 1 violent offense; adjusted OR, 1.2; 95% CI, 1.1-1.4; $P < .001$ for interaction). The risk increase among those with substance abuse comorbidity was significantly less pronounced when unaffected siblings were used as controls (28.3% of those with schizophrenia had a violent offense compared with 17.9% of their unaffected siblings; adjusted OR, 1.8; 95% CI, 1.4-2.4; $P < .001$ for interaction), suggesting significant familial (genetic or early environmental) confounding of the association between schizophrenia and violence.

Conclusions.—Schizophrenia was associated with an increased risk of violent crime in this longitudinal study. This association was attenuated by adjustment for substance abuse, suggesting a mediating effect. The role of risk assessment, management, and treatment in individuals with comorbidity needs further examination.

▶ Well, this issue of whether persons suffering from schizophrenia are more prone to violence has been debated for years. When deinstitutionalization began in 1955, it was often said that the mentally ill were more involved with violence, but that was because they were more likely to be the victims of violence more than its perpetrators. However, that view began to change over the years and mental health experts began to come over toward the side of the general public, which already was fearful of crazy people walking down the streets talking to themselves.

In addition, since 1955, illegal drug availability and use has increased dramatically.

Now we have this study, which while from England, is probably echoed here. Its conclusion as stated above in the abstract says, "Schizophrenia was associated with an increased risk of violent crime in this longitudinal study. This association was attenuated by adjustment for substance abuse, suggesting a mediating effect."

I do so wish instead they had used what they stated at the end of the comment section—"We demonstrate that the risk of violent crime in schizophrenia in patients without comorbid substance abuse is only slightly increased. In contrast, the risk is substantially increased among patients with comorbidity..."

That is so much clearer and more accurate and states that it is the substance abuse that is associated with increased violence and not the disease of schizophrenia.

J. A. Talbott, MD

Suicide

Posttraumatic Stress Disorder and Completed Suicide

Gradus JL, Qin P, Lincoln AK, et al (VA Boston Healthcare System, MA; Aarhus Univ, Denmark; Northeastern Univ, Boston, MA; et al)
Am J Epidemiol 171:721-727, 2010

Most research regarding posttraumatic stress disorder (PTSD) and suicide has focused on suicidal ideation or attempts; no known study of the association between PTSD and completed suicide in a population-based sample has been reported. This study examined the association between PTSD and completed suicide in a population-based sample. Data were obtained from the nationwide Danish health and administrative registries, which include data on all 5.4 million residents of Denmark. All suicides between January 1, 1994, and December 31, 2006, were included, and controls were selected from a sample of all Danish residents. Using this nested case-control design, the authors examined 9,612 suicide cases and 199,306 controls matched to cases on gender, date of birth, and time. Thirty-eight suicide cases (0.40%) and 95 controls (0.05%) were diagnosed with PTSD. The odds ratio associating PTSD with suicide was 9.8 (95% confidence interval: 6.7, 15). The association between PTSD and completed suicide remained after controlling for psychiatric and demographic confounders (odds ratio = 5.3, 95% confidence interval: 3.4, 8.1). Additionally, persons with PTSD and depression had a greater rate of suicide than expected based on their independent effects. In conclusion, a registry-based diagnosis of PTSD based on *International Statistical Classification of Diseases and Related Health Problems*, Tenth Revision, is a risk factor for completed suicide.

▶ Wow! The literature has borne out the clinical assumption that the diagnoses that carry the most risk for completed suicide include mood disorders (depression and bipolar disorder), borderline personality disorder, and schizophrenia. Even anxiety disorders constitute cause for increased vigilance. The authors, who work at the Boston Veterans Administration hospital, are rightly concerned, as they point out (reflecting the New York Times article by Goode[1]) the rate of suicide "among US Army members is currently higher than during any period on record and that researchers suspect that the increasing prevalence of PTSD among active-duty military personnel and returning combat veterans is one potential explanation...." Couple this with the knowledge that servicemen are undergoing multiple rapid redeployments and that these add to the stress, we have a very distressing situation.

J. A. Talbott, MD

Reference

1. Goode E. After combat, victims of an inner war. NY Times. August 1, 2009. http://www.nytimes.com/2009/08/02/us/02suicide.html. Accessed June 3, 2010.

Mobile Crisis Team Intervention to Enhance Linkage of Discharged Suicidal Emergency Department Patients to Outpatient Psychiatric Services: A Randomized Controlled Trial

Currier GW, Fisher SG, Caine ED (Univ of Rochester Med Ctr, NY)
Acad Emerg Med 17:36-43, 2010

Objectives.—Many suicidal patients treated and released from emergency departments (ED) fail to follow through with subsequent outpatient psychiatric appointments, often presenting back for repeat ED services. Thus, the authors sought to determine whether a mobile crisis team (MCT) intervention would be more effective than standard referral to a hospital-based clinic as a means of establishing near-term clinical contact after ED discharge. This objective was based on the premise that increased attendance at the first outpatient mental health appointment would initiate an ongoing treatment course, with subsequent differential improvements in psychiatric symptoms and functioning for patients successfully linked to care.

Methods.—In a rater-blinded, randomized controlled trial, 120 participants who were evaluated for suicidal thoughts, plans, or behaviors, and who were subsequently discharged from an urban ED, were randomized to follow-up either in the community via a MCT or at an outpatient mental health clinic (OPC). Both MCTs and OPCs offered the same structured array of clinical services and referral options.

Results.—Successful first clinical contact after ED discharge (here described as "linkage" to care) occurred in 39 of 56 (69.6%) participants randomized to the MCT versus 19 of 64 (29.6%) to the OPC (relative risk = 2.35, 95% CI = 1.55–3.56, p < 0.001). However, we detected no significant differences between groups using intention-to-treat analyses in symptom or functional outcome measures, at either 2 weeks or 3 months after enrollment. We also found no significant differences in outcomes between participants who did attend their first prescribed appointment via MCT or OPC versus those who did not. However divided (MCT vs. OPC, present at first appointment vs. no show), groups showed significant improvements but maintained clinically significant levels of dysfunction and continued to rely on ED services at a similar rate in the 6 months after study enrollment.

Conclusions.—Community-based mobile outreach was a highly effective method of contacting suicidal patients who were discharged from the ED. However, establishing initial postdischarge contact in the community versus the clinic did not prove more effective at enhancing symptomatic or functional outcomes, nor did successful linkage with outpatient psychiatric care. Overall, participants showed some improvement shortly after ED discharge regardless of outpatient clinical contact, but nonetheless remained significantly symptomatic and at risk for repeated ED presentations.

▶ Bummer.

I was sure when I printed out this article that it would show that the personal visit by one or more staff members of a Mobile Crisis Team, to someone discharged from a hospital emergency room for suicidal ideation would be more effective in having the patient(s) keep their follow-up appointments and in turn, result in better outcomes. Wrong.

Why was I so certain? Because a long time ago there was a contribution to the literature that demonstrated that a personal contact by the outpatient staff to an about to be discharged inpatient resulted in a greater "show" rate at the clinic than just handing them an appointment slip.

Well, the first part of my belief was borne out in this study; more than double the percentage of patients who received mobile team visits were connected with care than those just handed appointment slips, but the second part didn't result—the outcomes of the 2 groups were the same.

The authors raise some interesting points in their discussion, they ask: "Are there low-cost measures that could be added to enhance such effects? Should all patients be assigned an urgent outpatient appointment, consistent with our current practice, or are there subgroups for whom this approach is unnecessary or even counterproductive?" Perhaps it might be more worthwhile to offer appointments only to those who wish immediate follow-up, while providing a "ready-access" telephone contact for appointments when patients call for care. This might mitigate inappropriate reuse of the ED following index contact, and help address the challenging problem of "no-shows," while offering expedited access to care at a time of increased distress." This is "out-of-the-box" thinking that goes against what I talked about elsewhere: "one size fits all" treatment and deserves support.

Likewise, they discovered that "patients who participate in aftercare, however briefly, are likely to have better outcomes," not a new finding, because we've known for years that something as simple as a medical student "intake interview" can produce therapeutic results, but it is one that also merits our attention. The consequence is that we need not necessarily have long-term treatment, and follow-up if improvement is evident in specific patients.

J. A. Talbott, MD

Miscellaneous

Public attitudes towards people with mental illness in England and Scotland, 1994–2003

Mehta N, Kassam A, Leese M, et al (Inst of Psychiatry, London, UK)
Br J Psychiatry 194:278-284, 2009

Background.—Understanding trends in public attitudes towards people with mental illness informs the assessment of ongoing severity of stigma and evaluation of anti-stigma campaigns.

Aims.—To analyse trends in public attitudes towards people with mental illness in England and Scotland using Department of Health Attitudes to Mental Illness Surveys, 1994–2003.

Method.—We analysed trends in attitudes for 2000 respondents in each survey year (6000 respondents in 1996 and 1997) using quota sampling methods and the adapted Community Attitudes Toward the Mentally Ill scale.

Results.—Comparing 2000 and 2003, there was significant deterioration for 17/25 items in England and for 4/25 items in Scotland. Neither country showed significant improvements in items between 2000 and 2003.

Conclusions.—Public attitudes towards people with mental illness in England and Scotland became less positive during 1994–2003, especially in 2000–2003, and to a greater extent in England. The results are consistent with early positive effects for the 'see me' anti-stigma campaign in Scotland.

▶ A number of years ago I read somewhere (now untraceable) that since World War II, national surveys have been conducted that show an ever decreasing amount of stigma about the mentally ill in America; the good news being things are getting better each year; the bad news that 50% of people still harbor fears about them.

Now we have this study of attitudes showing that between 1994 and 2003 things have gotten worse despite an antistigma campaign conducted by the Royal College of Psychiatrists, which the authors attribute to tabloid newspaper exploitation of the link between violence and mental illness. Except the authors note that a better funded antistigma campaign in Scotland helped improve the public's view starting in 2002, presumably despite continued newspaper attention.

What are the implications of this study for us in the United States?

First, that antistigma campaigns do work—if well-funded and extensive.

Second, that poorly funded and limited campaigns can be undone by press attention to "hot button" issues.

And third, that newspapers will be newspapers and there's little we can do to stop their selling scandals, but we can advocate for effective antistigma efforts.

J. A. Talbott, MD

Jail Administrators' Perceptions of the Use of Psychiatric Advance Directives in Jails
Scheyett AM, Vaughn JS, Francis AM (Univ of North Carolina at Chapel Hill)
Psychiatr Serv 61:409-411, 2010

Objective.—Individuals with serious mental illnesses are at high risk of incarceration. Jails are often unable to obtain information needed to provide appropriate care. Psychiatric advance directives may be useful tools to communicate treatment information to jails. This study explored their use as a novel intervention for individuals with mental illnesses in jails.

Methods.—Eighty jail administrators in North Carolina were surveyed to determine their support for psychiatric advance directives in jails.

Relationships between respondents' job type (jail administrator or medical administrator) or jail census and support for the directives were examined by using chi square tests. Open-ended responses were analyzed using qualitative methods.

Results.—Seventy-three percent of respondents indicated they supported psychiatric advance directives. Respondents from jails at or below a median census of 120 were significantly more likely to support psychiatric advance directives than those from larger jails.

Conclusions.—Psychiatric advance directives' informational function may prove valuable in jail settings. Additional research assessing directives as interventions for individuals with mental illnesses at risk of incarceration is needed.

▶ In some ways this is an encouraging article and in other ways dismaying. I like the fact that psychiatric advance directives are receiving more attention these days and are proving effective. But I am appalled that we have become so used to jails and prisons being considered legitimate treatment sites for severely and chronically mentally ill individuals that an article like this just accepts it as a given, a fact of life that we have to get used to. Listen to these introductory sentences: "Individuals with serious mental illnesses have high incarceration rates. A recent study estimated that approximately 15% of male and 31% of female jail inmates have mental disorders. Individuals with mental illnesses often receive little treatment while incarcerated." In addition, it seems that the respondents (jail administrators) have accepted their roles as quasi psychiatrists: "Anything that establishes a course of action for us to follow … is a good idea." As I said, appalling.

J. A. Talbott, MD

State Hospital-University Collaborations: A 25-Year Follow-Up
Talbott JA, Faulkner LR, Buckley PF (Univ of Maryland School of Medicine in Baltimore; American Board of Psychiatry & Neurology, IL; Dept of Psychiatry at the Med College of Georgia in Augusta)
Acad Psychiatry 34:125-127, 2010

Objective.—A formative survey of psychiatry departments 25 years ago showed strong and valued relationships between these departments and state hospitals. The authors sought to evaluate the extent of present-day collaborative relationships.

Methods.—A repeat of a similar survey was sent in 2005 to 119 chairs of departments of psychiatry.

Results.—Fifty-eight of 119 chairs (49% response rate) participated. A sustained high level of programmatic partnership was still observed, with 75% of respondents reporting ongoing administrative relationships. Seventy-four percent of respondents reported ongoing residency training relationships.

Conclusion.—These findings suggest that strong state-university collaborations have prevailed over the past 25 years despite major changes for academic health care and psychiatry residency training during this period.

▶ I obviously have a strong conflict of interest in selecting this article and commenting on it because I am the first author and the one who actually sent out, collected, and tabulated the results of this survey. If I were coming on it as a detached editor, my assumption would be that in 25 years, the blush has come off the rose of state-university collaborations, state monies (especially for research) have dried up, and federal National Institutes of Health/National Institute of Mental Health funding expanded dramatically, resulting in vastly diminished monies for and interest in state-university collaborations. But I would be wrong because in fact things look pretty robust. More interesting to me than the fact that state-university collaborations are still numerous is the finding that they are still highly valued. And the finding that many residents receive training in state facilities is interesting to me because it is surely important in attracting and retaining highly qualified psychiatrists to state systems.

J. A. Talbott, MD

6 Clinical Psychiatry

Introduction

Similar to all recent years, there has again been marked progress in the science supporting the clinical practice of psychiatry. Once again, this section starts with articles about depression. I included several studies about the interaction of genetics, specifically the serotonin gene, but also other loci for depression, and interactions between the environment and these genes. There continues to be increasing understanding of the direct relationship between diabetes and depression, and this year I included a couple of articles documenting how that comorbid condition leads to much worse complications of diabetes, and even increased rates of dementia. Again, there are advances in brain stimulation techniques including direct stimulation of the brain, repetitive transcranial magnetic stimulation (rTMS), and the old standby, electroconvulsive therapy (ECT). The story of the beneficial effects of adding a second-generation antipsychotic (SGA) to antidepressants continues with a meta-analysis, and also included are reports of individual trials with aripiprazole and olanzapine. Despite some modern criticism of the efficacy of psychotherapy in treating psychiatric illnesses, I include articles documenting the effectiveness of mindfulness-based psychotherapy and the new Canadian algorithm for the treatment of depression in which the evidence strongly supports psychotherapy as a major aspect in the treatment of depression.

I am particularly pleased to see studies that directly address practical, frequent decisions that clinical psychiatrists have to make. For instance, this year there are studies documenting the value of using 2 antidepressants from the beginning of treatment, that early improvement in the first 2 weeks of treatment is predictive of ultimate outcome, that quickly treating depression to reduce the period of untreated illness is very beneficial, and that gradual discontinuation of antidepressants is valuable.

Similarly, in the bipolar field, I include an article documenting the value of psychotherapy, particularly psychoeducation, in this condition. There is a study discussing antidepressant discontinuation, and several reports are included that demonstrate the value of SGAs in both phases of bipolar illness, often in combination with antidepressants or lithium. I included an article about the value of anticonvulsants in reducing suicide risks, and there are reports on the value of benzodiazepines and ECT. I also included several articles about various ways to reduce suicide in our patients.

In the anxiety section, there is a large study on postpartum depression with panic disorder emerging as a risk, and another documents the increased risk of stroke among panic disorder patients. I included an article about deep brain stimulation for obsessive-compulsive disorder (OCD), and another reports on predictors of response to serotonin reuptake inhibitor (SRI) pharmacotherapy in OCD.

In the schizophrenia section, I included several articles to help us understand the value of SGAs in schizophrenia, as well as how to understand and deal with the metabolic abnormalities that are sometimes attendant with this new class. I also included an article on a promising new treatment (minocycline) for treatment of negative and cognitive symptoms. There is a large study about cognitive effects of antipsychotics and also an article demonstrating the value of psychotherapy in this condition as well.

In the general psychiatry section, there are articles touching on psychogenic nonepileptic attacks, quetiapine in delirium, cognitive behavior therapy versus paroxetine in hypochondriasis, and adult outcomes of irritability in childhood; also included is a report from a controlled trial of St John's wort for irritable bowel syndrome.

In the miscellaneous category, I included an article on a surprising study comparing brand-name versus generic formulations of antidepressants; another reports on evolving attitudes of the general public about psychiatric medicines. I included an article on the use of nortriptyline and gabapentin in chronic pain, and another reviews treatment for the behavioral disturbances of Alzheimer disease.

All in all, it is an excellent year in the basic science supporting psychiatry, but in particular, there are many important articles affecting the daily practice of clinical psychiatry.

James C. Ballenger, MD

Depression

Comorbid Depression Is Associated with an Increased Risk of Dementia Diagnosis in Patients with Diabetes: A Prospective Cohort Study
Katon WJ, Lin EHB, Williams LH, et al (Univ of Washington School of Medicine, Seattle; Group Health Res Inst, Seattle, WA)
J Gen Intern Med 25:423-429, 2010

Background.—Both depression and diabetes have been found to be risk factors for dementia. This study examined whether comorbid depression in patients with diabetes increases the risk for dementia compared to those with diabetes alone.

Methods.—We conducted a prospective cohort study of 3,837 primary care patients with diabetes (mean age 63.2 ± 13.2 years) enrolled in an HMO in Washington State. The Patient Health Questionnaire (PHQ-9) was used to assess depression at baseline, and ICD-9 diagnoses for dementia were used to identify cases of dementia. Cohort members with no previous ICD-9 diagnosis of dementia prior to baseline were followed for a 5-year period. The risk of dementia for patients with both major depression and diabetes at baseline relative to patients with diabetes alone was estimated using cause-specific Cox proportional hazard regression models that adjusted for age, gender, education, race/ethnicity, diabetes duration, treatment with insulin, diabetes complications, nondiabetes-related medical comorbidity, hypertension, BMI, physical inactivity, smoking, HbA_{1c}, and number of primary care visits per month.

Results.—Over the 5-year period, 36 of 455 (7.9%) patients with major depression and diabetes (incidence rate of 21.5 per 1,000 person-years) versus 163 of 3,382 (4.8%) patients with diabetes alone (incidence rate of 11.8 per 1,000 person-years) had one or more ICD-9 diagnoses of dementia. Patients with comorbid major depression had an increased risk of dementia (fully adjusted hazard ratio 2.69, 95% CI 1.77, 4.07).

Conclusions.—Patients with major depression and diabetes had an increased risk of development of dementia compared to those with diabetes alone. These data add to recent findings showing that depression was associated with an increased risk of macrovascular and microvascular complications in patients with diabetes.

▶ As previously stated in another selection, depression and diabetes appear to be linked to each other, and this article links those 2 and the risk for dementia. This study prospectively followed 3837 patients with diabetes, rated their level of depression at entry, and followed them for 5 years. After controlling for the many issues involved, they, in fact, did note over a 5-year period, an almost doubling of risk for patients who had both depression and diabetes (7.9%) and dementia versus those with diabetes alone (4.8%). Also, comorbid major depression had an increased risk, hazard ratio of 2.69. In another article I reviewed, diabetes and depression are associated with increased risk in both micro- and macrovascular complications of stroke, renal failure, etc, and it is clear that they presented an increased risk for dementia. This is yet another set of medical areas where pertinence of the diagnosis and treatment of depression is critically important to serious medical outcomes, including increased mortality.

J. C. Ballenger, MD

Early adversity and 5-HTT/BDNF genes: new evidence of gene–environment interactions on depressive symptoms in a general population
Aguilera M, Arias B, Wichers M, et al (Instituto de Salud Carlos III, Barcelona, Spain; Maastricht Univ, The Netherlands; et al)
Psychol Med 39:1425-1432, 2009

Background.—Adverse childhood experiences have been described as one of the major environmental risk factors for depressive disorder.

Similarly, the deleterious impact of early traumatic experiences on depression seems to be moderated by individual genetic variability. Serotonin transporter (5-HTT) and brain-derived neurotrophic factor (BDNF) modulate the effect of childhood adversity on adult depression, although inconsistencies across studies have been found. Moreover, the gene × environment (G × E) interaction concerning the different types of childhood adversity remains poorly understood. The aim of this study was to analyse the putative interaction between the 5-HTT gene (5-HTTLPR polymorphism), the BDNF gene (Val66Met polymorphism) and childhood adversity in accounting for adult depressive symptoms.

Method.—A sample of 534 healthy individuals filled in self-report questionnaires of depressive symptomatology [the Symptom Check List 90 Revised (SCL-90-R)] and different types of childhood adversities [the Childhood Trauma Questionnaire (CTQ)]. The 5-HTTLPR polymorphism (5-HTT gene) and the Val66Met polymorphism (BDNF gene) were genotyped in the whole sample.

Results.—Total childhood adversity ($\beta = 0.27$, $p < 0.001$), childhood sexual abuse (CSA; $\beta = 0.17$, $p < 0.001$), childhood emotional abuse ($\beta = 0.27$, $p < 0.001$) and childhood emotional neglect ($\beta = 0.22$, $p < 0.001$) had an impact on adult depressive symptoms. CSA had a greater impact on depressive symptoms in Met allele carriers of the BDNF gene than in the Val/Val group ($F = 5.87$, $p < 0.0001$), and in S carriers of the 5-HTTLPR polymorphism (5-HTT gene) ($F = 5.80$, $p < 0.0001$).

Conclusions.—Childhood adversity per se predicted higher levels of adult depressive symptoms. In addition, BDNF Val66Met and 5-HTTLPR polymorphisms seemed to moderate the effect of CSA on adult depressive symptoms.

▶ In many modern studies, it is clear that childhood adversities lead to significant adult difficulties, particularly with depression. We have seen evidence that the impact of childhood adverse experiences may interact with our genetic makeup. This study of 534 individuals provides very interesting and clear data in that regard. These individuals were questioned about their histories of childhood adversity, childhood sexual abuse, as well as emotional abuse and emotional neglect. All of these had clear impact on adult depressive symptoms. Not surprisingly, childhood sexual abuse had the greatest impact and was most closely related to Met allele carriers of the brain-derived neurotrophic factor (BDNF) gene, and in carriers of the 5-HTTLPR polymorphism of the 5-HTT gene. This study also contributes to the large and growing group of data indicating polymorphism of the serotonin transporter and BDNF genes in various aspects of depression, from vulnerability to potentially predicting treatment response. This whole field certainly represents an exciting evolution for our field.

J. C. Ballenger, MD

A Double-blind Randomized Controlled Trial of Olanzapine Plus Sertraline vs Olanzapine Plus Placebo for Psychotic Depression: The Study of Pharmacotherapy of Psychotic Depression (STOP-PD)

Meyers BS, for the STOP-PD Group (New York Presbyterian Hosp–Westchester)

Arch Gen Psychiatry 66:838-847, 2009

Context.—Evidence for the efficacy of combination pharmacotherapy has been limited and without positive trials in geriatric patients with major depression (MD) with psychotic features.

Objectives.—To compare remission rates of MD with psychotic features in those treated with a combination of atypical antipsychotic medication plus a serotonin reuptake inhibitor with those treated with antipsychotic monotherapy; and to compare response by age.

Design.—Twelve-week, double-blind, randomized, controlled trial.

Setting.—Clinical services of 4 academic sites.

Patients.—Two hundred fifty-nine subjects with MD with psychotic features randomized by age (<60 or ≥60 years) (mean [standard deviation (SD)], 41.3 [10.8] years in 117 younger adults vs 71.7 [7.8] years in 142 geriatric participants).

Intervention.—Target doses of 15 to 20 mg of olanzapine per day plus masked sertraline or placebo at 150 to 200 mg per day.

Main Outcome Measure.—Remission rates of MD with psychotic features.

Results.—Treatment with olanzapine/sertraline was associated with higher remission rates during the trial than olanzapine/placebo (odds ratio [OR], 1.28; 95% confidence interval [CI], 1.12-1.47; $P < .001$); 41.9% of subjects who underwent combination therapy were in remission at their last assessment compared with 23.9% of subjects treated with monotherapy ($\chi_1^2 = 9.53$, $P = .002$). Combination therapy was comparably superior in both younger (OR, 1.25; 95% CI, 1.05-1.50; $P = .02$) and older (OR, 1.34; 95% CI, 1.09-1.66; $P = .01$) adults. Overall, tolerability was comparable across age groups. Both age groups had significant increases in cholesterol and triglyceride concentrations, but statistically significant increases in glucose occurred only in younger adults. Younger adults gained significantly more weight than older subjects (mean [SD], 6.5 [6.6] kg vs 3.3 [4.9] kg, $P = .001$).

Conclusions.—Combination pharmacotherapy is efficacious for the treatment of MD with psychotic features. Future research must determine the benefits vs risks of continuing atypical antipsychotic medications beyond 12 weeks.

Trial Registration.—clinicaltrials.gov Identifier: NCT00056472.

▶ In this large trial ($N = 259$) of major depression with psychotic features with patients randomized by above or below age 60, the authors were able to demonstrate markedly better improvement with the combinations of olanzapine and sertraline versus olanzapine alone. In the trial, 41.9% of patients treated with combination therapy reached remission versus 23.9% with monotherapy. This combination therapy was equally superior in both the younger and older patient groups. Interestingly, it was the younger patients who had greater weight gain and greater increases in glucose. This trial is a modern update of the standard treatment of psychotic depression and again shows superiority of the combination of an antipsychotic (now second generation) combined with an antidepressant. These results are so clear over time that this certainly represents the standard of care in psychotic depression.

J. C. Ballenger, MD

A Randomized, Double-Blind, Placebo-Controlled Study of Testosterone Treatment in Hypogonadal Older Men With Subthreshold Depression (Dysthymia or Minor Depression)

Shores MM, Kivlahan DR, Sadak TI, et al (Veterans Affairs [VA] Puget Sound Health Care System, Seattle, WA; Univ of Washington, Seattle)
J Clin Psychiatry 70:1009-1016, 2009

Objective.—Hypogonadism and subthreshold depression are common conditions in elderly men. The objective of this study was to examine the effect of testosterone treatment in older, hypogonadal men with subthreshold depression.

Method.—A randomized, double-blind, placebo-controlled study was conducted at a university-affiliated Veterans Affairs Medical Center among men aged 50 years or older (N = 33) with screening total testosterone levels of ≤ 280 ng/dL and subthreshold depression (dysthymia or minor depression, according to DSM-IV). Recruitment for the study was conducted from November 2002 through May 2005. Participants received either 7.5 g of testosterone gel or placebo gel daily for 12 weeks, followed by a 12-week open-label extension phase during which all subjects received 7.5 g of testosterone gel. The primary outcome measure was the change in the Hamilton Rating Scale for Depression (HAM-D) score from baseline to the end of the double-blind phase. Secondary outcome measures were remission of subthreshold depression (defined a priori as a HAM-D score ≤ 7) and changes in the Hopkins Symptom Checklist depression scale, the Medical Outcomes Study 36-Item Short-Form Health Survey, and the short-form 16-item Quality of Life Enjoyment and Satisfaction Questionnaire.

Results.—At the end of the double-blind phase, testosterone-treated men had a greater reduction in HAM-D scores (p = .024) and a higher remission rate of subthreshold depression (52.9% vs. 18.8%, p = .041) than did placebo-treated men, but there were no differences in other secondary outcome measures between groups. At the end of the open-label phase, the testosterone group had sustained improvement, the control group improved, and there were no differences between groups in any outcome measures.

Conclusion.—These results suggest that testosterone replacement may be efficacious treatment for subthreshold depression in older men with hypogonadism. Larger studies are needed to corroborate these findings. *Trial Registration.*—clinicaltrials.gov Identifier:NCT00202462.

▶ It has certainly been demonstrated repeatedly that in older men, decreases in testosterone are quite common. This randomized, double-blind, placebo-controlled trial studied men 50 years or older with testosterone levels ≤280 ng/dL and subthreshold depression. They received either 7.5 g of testosterone gel or placebo for 12 weeks followed by a 12-week extension phase. The testosterone treated men did in fact have a significantly greater reduction of the Hamilton Rating Scale for Depression (HAM-D) scores and higher remission rates than the placebo group. They maintained this improvement through follow-up. This obviously needs to be followed-up. It is certainly suggestive that this should be studied and considered as a clinical treatment.

J. C. Ballenger, MD

Canadian Network for Mood and Anxiety Treatments (CANMAT) Clinical guidelines for the management of major depressive disorder in adults. II. Psychotherapy alone or in combination with antidepressant medication
Parikh SV, Segal ZV, Grigoriadis S, et al (Univ of Toronto, Canada; et al)
J Affect Disord 117:S15-S25, 2009

Background.—In 2001, the Canadian Psychiatric Association and the Canadian Network for Mood and Anxiety Treatments (CANMAT) partnered to produce evidence-based clinical guidelines for the treatment of depressive disorders. A revision of these guidelines was undertaken by CANMAT in 2008–2009 to reflect advances in the field. This article, one of five in the series, reviews new studies of psychotherapy in the acute and maintenance phase of MDD, including computer-based and telephone-delivered psychotherapy.

Methods.—The CANMAT guidelines are based on a question–answer format to enhance accessibility to clinicians. Evidence-based responses are based on updated systematic reviews of the literature and recommendations are graded according to the Level of Evidence, using pre-defined criteria. Lines of Treatment are identified based on criteria that included evidence and expert clinical support.

Results.—Cognitive-Behavioural Therapy (CBT) and Interpersonal Therapy (IPT) continue to have the most evidence for efficacy, both in acute and maintenance phases of MDD, and have been studied in combination with antidepressants. CBT is well studied in conjunction with computer-delivered methods and bibliotherapy. Behavioural Activation and Cognitive-Behavioural Analysis System of Psychotherapy have significant evidence, but need replication. Newer psychotherapies including Acceptance and Commitment Therapy, Motivational Interviewing, and

Mindfulness-Based Cognitive Therapy do not yet have significant evidence as acute treatments; nor does psychodynamic therapy.

Limitations.—Although many forms of psychotherapy have been studied, relatively few types have been evaluated for MDD in randomized controlled trials. Evidence about the combination of different types of psychotherapy and antidepressant medication is also limited despite widespread use of these therapies concomitantly.

Conclusions.—CBT and IPT are the only first-line treatment recommendations for acute MDD and remain highly recommended for maintenance. Both computer-based and telephone-delivered psychotherapy–primarily studied with CBT and IPT–are useful second-line recommendations. Where feasible, combined antidepressant and CBT or IPT are recommended as first-line treatments for acute MDD.

▶ In 2001, the Canadian Psychiatric Association, as well as the Canadian Network for Mood and Anxiety Treatments group, worked together to produce evidence-based guidelines for the treatment of depression. They recently revised their guidelines, and this article reviews the new studies of psychotherapy in both the acute and maintenance phases. It is clear that Cognitive Behavior Therapy (CBT) and interpersonal therapy (IPT) continued to have the greatest evidence of efficacy both in the acute and maintenance phases. The newer psychotherapies, including mindfulness based cognitive therapy and psychodynamic therapies have not had significant new studies. Although the number of studies for the most common treatment, ie, combination of psychotherapy and antidepressants, has not been recently studied well, they continued to recommend combination treatment as first-line treatment. These Canadian guidelines are certainly consistent with United States ones and also would represent the standard of care in this area.

J. C. Ballenger, MD

Volumetric MRI study of the insular cortex in individuals with current and past major depression
Takahashi T, Yücel M, Lorenzetti V, et al (Univ of Melbourne, Australia; et al)
J Affect Disord 121:231-238, 2010

Background.—Functional neuroimaging studies have implicated the insular cortex in emotional processing, including the evaluation of one's own emotion, as well as in the neurobiology of major depressive disorder (MDD). Nevertheless, it remains largely unknown whether MDD patients exhibit morphologic changes of the insular cortex, and whether such changes reflect state or trait markers of the disorder.

Methods.—We delineated the anterior and posterior insular cortices using magnetic resonance imaging in 29 currently depressed patients (mean age = 32.5 years, 7 males), 27 remitted depressed patients (mean age = 35.1 years, 9 males), and 33 age- and gender-matched healthy control subjects (mean age = 34.0 years, 12 males).

Results.—Both current and remitted MDD patients showed significant volume reduction of the left anterior insular cortex as compared with healthy controls, but there was no group difference in the posterior insular cortex volume. Insular volumes did not correlate with the severity of depressive symptoms. Furthermore, the presence of melancholia and co-morbidity with anxiety disorders did not affect insular cortex volumes.

Limitations.—Although there was no difference in the insular cortex volume between medicated and unmedicated patients, a comprehensive investigation of medication effects was not possible, as complete data (e.g., dose, duration) were not available.

Conclusions.—These findings suggest that the morphologic abnormality of the anterior insular cortex, which plays a major role in introspection and emotional control, may be a trait-related marker of vulnerability to major depression, supporting the notion that MDD involves pathological alterations of limbic and related cortical structures.

▶ We continue to come closer in the evolution of our knowledge to defining brain anatomy relative to major depressive disorder (MDD). We certainly know from multiple sources that the insular cortex, which is closely related to the limbic system, is involved in various aspects of emotional processing and in the neurobiology of MDD. These authors studied the anterior and posterior insular cortices with MRI in 29 currently depressed males, 27 remitted depressed males, and 33 matched controls. They were able to demonstrate that in both currently depressed and remitted MDD patients, there was significant volume reduction in the anterior but not the posterior insular cortex compared with controls. It would appear that the anterior insular cortex is a trait-related marker of vulnerability to MDD, which is consistent with other neurobiological studies of MDD. Years ago, I tasked our brain stimulation researchers to try to find where in the brain any psychiatric phenomena seem to be located. Certainly, it would be great if we could additionally locate any circuits critically involved in our major illnesses. We have come closer and closer, and this has led to some different approaches neurochemically but, in particular, has changed the field of brain stimulation. We now know more where to stimulate with the various techniques we currently have, including repetitive transcranial magnetic stimulation and most recently with deep brain stimulation. We get closer each year to a rational and more effective treatment of MDD.

J. C. Ballenger, MD

Family Problems Among Recently Returned Military Veterans Referred for a Mental Health Evaluation
Sayers SL, Farrow VA, Ross J, et al (Univ of Pennsylvania, Philadelphia; Philadelphia Veterans Affairs (VA) Med Ctr, PA)
J Clin Psychiatry 70:163-170, 2009

Context.—Existing evidence suggests that military veterans with mental health disorders have poorer family functioning, although little research has focused on this topic.

Objective.—To test whether psychiatric symptoms are associated with family reintegration problems in recently returned military veterans.

Design.—Cross-sectional survey of a clinical population. Respondents who were referred to behavioral health evaluation from April 2006 through August 2007 were considered for the survey.

Setting.—Philadelphia Veterans Affairs Medical Center, Pa.

Participants.—199 military veterans who served in Iraq or Afghanistan after 2001 and were referred for behavioral health evaluation from primary care (mean age = 32.7 years, SD = 9.1).

Main Outcome Measures.—Measures included the Mini-International Neuropsychiatric Interview for psychiatric diagnoses, the 9-item Patient Health Questionnaire for depression diagnosis and severity, and screening measures of alcohol abuse and illicit substance use. A measure of military family readjustment problems and a screening measure of domestic abuse were developed for this study.

Results.—Three fourths of the married/cohabiting veterans reported some type of family problem in the past week, such as feeling like a guest in their household (40.7%), reporting their children acting afraid or not being warm toward them (25.0%), or being unsure about their family role (37.2%). Among veterans with current or recently separated partners, 53.7% reported conflicts involving "shouting, pushing, or shoving," and 27.6% reported that this partner was "afraid of them." Depression and posttraumatic stress disorder symptoms were both associated with higher rates of family reintegration problems.

Conclusions.—Mental health problems may complicate veterans' readjustment and reintegration into family life. The findings suggest an opportunity to improve the treatment of psychiatric disorders by addressing family problems.

▶ This study is of particular importance because of the indications that veterans returning from military service in Iraq and Afghanistan are experiencing considerable psychiatric problems, typically, including posttraumatic stress disorder (PTSD) and depression. Studies of veterans returning from previous wars suggest that readjustment among this population can be extremely difficult, typically resulting in problems in family life. It is useful to begin to obtain statistics about the prevalence and nature of these difficulties.

A criticism of this study is that the authors relied on a clinical sample rather than a representative group of veterans returning from deployment. Those surveyed were veterans who were referred for behavioral health evaluation, indicating that problems were present. Thus, the reader learns only about adjustment difficulties among those who are obviously struggling.

Thus, the prevalence rates are based on a skewed sample.

Of greatest use is the report of the specific types of reactions these veterans are experiencing. For example, almost 41% reported feeling like a guest in their household. More than one-third were unsure about their family role. This type of specificity can provide a road map for the clinician in understanding the types of problems the veteran may be having. It can also be helpful in understanding the types of problems that spouses may be dealing with in trying to reintegrate the veteran who has been deployed, probably on multiple tours of duty.

Not surprisingly, the authors found that veterans with PTSD and depression had more problems associated with their roles as partners and parents. The symptoms of these disorders typically are associated with relationship issues, given symptoms such as feelings of detachment and irritability.

An advantage of this study is that problems were identified early, ie, within a year or 2 after returning from deployment. The more that is understood about the nature of the problems that these veterans experience and the more quickly the problems are identified, the greater the likelihood that interventions will be effective.

J. L. Krupnick, PhD

An Integrated Analysis of Olanzapine/Fluoxetine Combination in Clinical Trials of Treatment-Resistant Depression

Trivedi MH, Thase ME, Osuntokun O, et al (Univ of Texas Southwestern Med Ctr at Dallas; Univ of Pittsburgh School of Medicine, PA; Lilly Res Laboratories, Eli Lilly and Company, Indianapolis, IN)
J Clin Psychiatry 70:387-396, 2009

Objective.—To evaluate the efficacy of olanzapine/fluoxetine combination (OFC) versus olanzapine or fluoxetine monotherapy across all clinical trials of treatment-resistant depression sponsored by Eli Lilly and Company.

Method.—Efficacy and safety data from 1146 patients with a history of nonresponse during the current depressive episode who subsequently exhibited nonresponse during a 6- to 8-week antidepressant open-label lead-in phase and were randomly assigned to OFC (N = 462), fluoxetine (N = 342), or olanzapine (N = 342) for double-blind treatment were analyzed. All patients had a diagnosis of major depressive disorder as defined by DSM-III or DSM-IV criteria. The dates in which the trials were conducted ranged from May 1997 to July 2005.

Results.—After 8 weeks, OFC patients demonstrated significantly greater Montgomery-Asberg Depression Rating Scale improvement (mean change = −13.0) than fluoxetine (−8.6, $p < .001$) or olanzapine (−8.2, $p < .001$) patients, via a mixed-effects model repeated-measures analysis. Remission rates were 25.5% for OFC, 17.3% ($p = .006$) for fluoxetine, and 14.0% (p < .001) for olanzapine. Adverse events in ≥ 10% of OFC patients were weight gain, increased appetite, dry mouth, somnolence, fatigue, headache, and peripheral edema. Random glucose mean change (mg/dL) was +7.92 for the OFC group, +1.62 for the fluoxetine group (p = .020), and +9.91 for the olanzapine group (p = .485). Random cholesterol mean change (mg/dL) was +12.4 for OFC, +2.3 for fluoxetine (p < .001), and +3.1 for olanzapine (p < .001); incidence of treatment-emergent increase from normal to high cholesterol (baseline <200 mg/dL and ≥ 240 subsequently) was significantly higher for the OFC group (10.2%) than for the fluoxetine group (3.1%, p = .017) but not the olanzapine group (8.0%, p = .569). Mean weight change (kg) was +4.42 for OFC, −0.15 for fluoxetine (p < .001), and +4.63 for olanzapine (p = .381), with 40.4% of OFC patients gaining ≥ 7% body weight (vs. olanzapine: 42.9%, p = .515; fluoxetine: 2.3%, p < .001).

Conclusion.—Results of this analysis showed that OFC-treated patients experienced significantly improved depressive symptoms compared with olanzapine- or fluoxetine-treated patients following failure of 2 or more antidepressants within the current depressive episode. Safety results for OFC were generally consistent with those for its component monotherapies. The total cholesterol increase associated with OFC was more pronounced than with olanzapine alone.

▶ I've been personally pleased to see the increasing interest in our field and in our studies on the population of people with treatment-resistant depression. Every clinician knows that there are a large percentage of people who struggle with depression who respond poorly or not at all to most of our treatments. Lilly reanalyzed the data from its double blind trials of the olanzapine/fluoxetine combination compared with monotherapy across all of their clinical trials in 1146 patients. These patients had previously demonstrated nonresponse during their current depression, and demonstrated nonresponse to a 6- to 8-week open-label lead in phase. The combination of olanzapine and fluoxetine consistently demonstrated significantly greater improvement than either fluoxetine alone or olanzapine alone. Remission rates were 25.5% for the combination, 17.3% for fluoxetine, and 14.0% for olanzapine alone. Glucose mean changes were +7.92 mg/dL for the combination group, +9.91 for olanzapine alone, and +1.62 for fluoxetine alone. Interestingly, random cholesterol changes, mean weight change, and percentage of patients gaining ≥7% body weight, mirrored those findings, consistent with the literature demonstrating that these changes are routinely observed with olanzapine whether alone or in combination. The cholesterol increases were greater with the combination than with olanzapine alone. The efficacy results reported with combination treatment are entirely consistent with the literature demonstrating that the second generation antipsychotics have brought a real increase in our ability to treat multiple syndromes, and in particular the affective syndromes that are too often resistant to our usual treatments, including antidepressants.

J. C. Ballenger, MD

A Genomewide Association Study Points to Multiple Loci That Predict Antidepressant Drug Treatment Outcome in Depression

Ising M, Lucae S, Binder EB, et al (Max Planck Inst of Psychiatry, Munich Germany; et al)

Arch Gen Psychiatry 66:966-975, 2009

Context.—The efficacy of antidepressant drug treatment in depression is unsatisfactory; 1 in 3 patients does not fully recover even after several treatment trials. Genetic factors and clinical characteristics contribute to the failure of a favorable treatment outcome.

Objective.—To identify genetic and clinical determinants of antidepressant drug treatment outcome in depression.

Design.—Genomewide pharmacogenetic association study with 2 independent replication samples.

Setting.—We performed a genomewide association study in patients from the Munich Antidepressant Response Signature (MARS) project and in pooled DNA from an independent German replication sample. A set of 328 singlenucleotide polymorphisms highly related to outcome in both genomewide association studies was genotyped in a sample of the Sequenced Treatment Alternatives to Relieve Depression (STAR*D) study.

Participants.—A total of 339 inpatients with a depressive episode (MARS sample), a further 361 inpatients with depression (German replication sample), and 832 outpatients with major depression (STAR*D sample).

Main Outcome Measures.—We generated a multilocus genetic variable that described the individual number of alleles of the selected single nucleotide polymorphisms associated with beneficial treatment outcome in the MARS sample ("response" alleles) to evaluate additive genetic effects on antidepressant drug treatment outcome.

Results.—Multilocus analysis revealed a significant contribution of a binary variable that categorized patients as carriers of a high vs low number of response alleles in the prediction of antidepressant drug treatment outcome in both samples (MARS and STAR*D). In addition, we observed that patients with a comorbid anxiety disorder combined with a low number of response alleles showed the least favorable outcome.

Conclusion.—These results demonstrate the importance of multiple genetic factors combined with clinical features in the prediction of antidepressant drug treatment outcome, which underscores the multifactorial nature of this trait.

▶ For years I have followed the evolution of genome evaluation to try to predict treatment response or side effects. In this particular study, this German group genotyped the entire genome and used it in 2 independent replication samples. Their set of 328 single nucleotide polymorphisms was used in 339 inpatients with a depressive episode and another 361 inpatients and 832 outpatients from the Sequenced Treatment Alternatives to Relieve Depression (STAR*D) sample. They were able to find a complex relationship between multiple genes and antidepressant drug response of a multifactorial nature. When the genome will come into the clinic to help us care for patients is unclear. We will continue to follow this issue.

J. C. Ballenger, MD

Illness Risk Following Rapid Versus Gradual Discontinuation of Antidepressants

Baldessarini RJ, Tondo L, Ghiani C, et al (Harvard Med School, Boston, MA; McLean Div of Massachusetts General Hosp, Boston; Univ of Cagliari, Sardinia, Italy; et al)

Am J Psychiatry 167:934-941, 2010

Objective.—Rapid discontinuation of some psychotropic medications is followed by discontinuation symptoms as well as an increased risk of early illness recurrence. Recurrence occurs earlier after rapid than after gradual discontinuation with lithium and antipsychotics. The authors compared illness recurrence after rapid versus gradual discontinuation of antidepressants.

Method.—The authors compared 398 patients with a DSM-IV diagnosis of recurrent major depressive disorder (N=224), panic disorder (N=75), bipolar II disorder (N=62), or bipolar I disorder (N=37). Two-thirds were women, the mean age was 42 years, and patients were treated with antidepressants for a mean of 8.5 months. Antidepressants were discontinued clinically, either rapidly (over 1–7 days; N=188) or gradually (over 14 days or more; N=210), with a mean follow-up duration of 2.8 years; patients who were ill at discontinuation were excluded from the analysis. The authors compared latency to first new illness episodes using survival analysis and Cox multivariate modeling.

Results.—The latency to first illness with rapid discontinuation was 0.4 times that with gradual discontinuation, and the latency after rapid discontinuation was one-fourth the estimated average previous inter-episode interval in the same patients. The effect was similar across antidepressant classes and across years; the pace of discontinuation had less effect with drugs of prolonged half-life. The effect also varied by diagnosis (bipolar I ≥ panic > bipolar II ≥ major depressive disorder) but not by episodes per year, duration of index illness, use of concomitant treatment, or antidepressant dose or duration.

Conclusions.—The recurrence risk for depression or panic was much shorter after rapid than after gradual discontinuation of antidepressants. These findings have implications for both clinical management and the design and interpretation of clinical trials.

▶ A lot of good work in the mood disorders field comes from Italy. In this study, 398 patients were treated in a single clinic and followed after either rapid (≤7 days) or gradual (≥2 weeks) discontinuation of antidepressants. No patients were discontinued in the 8- to 14- day range. This was a fairly ill population who had been ill for an average of 14 years. About half of the patients discontinued rapidly, usually on their own initiative. These patients rapidly relapsed with an average of 3.6 months compared with 8 4 months for those who discontinued more gradually. There was also a long-term positive effect of gradual discontinuation as well. These authors have shown that discontinuing lithium and antipsychotics abruptly is also associated with more rapid relapse. They provide further evidence of what I have believed for a long time, that is, all psychotropic medicines should be gradually tapered. In my own practice, I taper even more slowly than in this article, usually taking 3 to 4 weeks and actually frequently taking even longer in some patients. This is one of the findings that I think should be immediately transferred to our clinical practices. It is my opinion that discontinuation of all psychotropics should be slow.

J. C. Ballenger, MD

Interaction between genetic polymorphisms and stressful life events in first episode depression

Drachmann Bukh J, Bock C, Vinberg M, et al (Univ Hosp of Copenhagen, Rigshospitalet, Denmark; et al)
J Affective Disord 119:107-115, 2009

Background.—A polymorphism in the serotonin transporter (5-HTT) gene seems to moderate the influence of stressful life events on depression. However, the results from previous studies of gene–environment interactions in depression are inconsistent and might be confounded by the history of depression among participants.

Method.—We applied a case-only design, including 290 ethnically homogeneous patients suffering exclusively from first episode depression. Psychiatric mo-morbidity, personality traits and disorders and stressful life events in a six months period preceding onset of depression were evaluated by means of interviews and questionnaires. Additionally, we genotyped nine polymorphisms in the genes encoding the serotonin transporter, brain derived neurotrophic factor, catechol-O-methyltransferase, angiotensin converting enzyme, tryptophane hydroxylase, and the serotonin receptors 1A, 2A, and 2C.

Results.—The low activity variants of the 5-HTT-linked polymorphic region in the serotonin transporter gene and the Met-allele of a single nucleotide polymorphism (Val66Met) in the gene encoding brain derived neurotrophic factor were independently associated with the presence of stressful life events prior to onset of depression, also when corrected for the effect of age, gender, marital status, personality disorder, neuroticism, and severity of depressive symptoms at the time of interview.

Conclusion.—Polymorphisms in the genes encoding the serotonin transporter and the brain derived neurotrophic factor interact with recent stressful life events on depression among patients with no history of previous depressive episodes.

▶ Several years ago we reviewed the landmark study in *Science* that serotonin transporter genes appeared to mediate the negative effects of stress (depression). Since that time, there have been many studies confirming this result, but many that failed to replicate this result. This has led some to believe this relationship does not exist. These authors used a methodologic refinement in that they studied only first episode depressed patients from an ethnically homogeneous population. They genotyped 9 polymorphisms in the serotonin transporter genes, brain deprived neurotrophic factors (BDNF), catechol-O-methyltransferase, angiotensin converting enzyme, and tryptophan hydroxylase, as well as the serotonin receptors 1A, 2A, and 2C. They did replicate the early positive studies in that they found that the low activity variance with the 5-HTT linked polymorphic region in the serotonin transporter gene, as well as the Met-allele polymorphism for brain neurotrophic factor, were associated with depression in response to stressful life events.

I had previously commented somewhat hyperbolically that this original study may be one of the most important studies that have come out in recent psychiatry, only to be disappointed with the checkered history of the attempts to replicate this finding. However, this study, which has some very nice methodological improvements over recent studies, does in fact again support the link between serotonin transporter alleles and BDNF genes and the effect of stress leading to depression.

J. C. Ballenger, MD

Dyadic discord at baseline is associated with lack of remission in the acute treatment of chronic depression
Denton WH, Carmody TJ, Rush AJ, et al (The Univ of Texas Southwestern Med Ctr at Dallas; et al)
Psychol Med 40:415-424, 2010

Background.—Dyadic discord, while common in depression, has not been specifically evaluated as an outcome predictor in chronic major depressive disorder. This study investigated pretreatment dyadic discord as a predictor of non-remission and its relationship to depressive symptom change during acute treatment for chronic depression.

Method.—Out-patients with chronic depression were randomized to 12 weeks of treatment with nefazodone, the Cognitive Behavioral Analysis System of Psychotherapy or their combination. Measures included the Marital Adjustment Scale (MAS) and the Inventory of Depressive Symptomatology – Self Report (IDS-SR$_{30}$). Of 681 original patients, 316 were partnered and 171 of these completed a baseline and exit MAS, and at least one post-baseline IDS-SR$_{30}$. MAS scores were analysed as continuous and categorical variables ('dyadic discord' *v.* 'no dyadic discord' defined as an MAS score >2.36. Remission was defined as an IDS-SR$_{30}$ of ≤14 at exit (equivalent to a 17-item Hamilton Rating Scale for Depression of ≤7).

Results.—Patients with dyadic discord at baseline had lower remission rates (34.1%) than those without dyadic discord (61.2%) (all three treatment groups) ($\chi^2 = 12.6$, df = 1, $p = 0.0004$). MAS scores improved significantly with each of the treatments, although the change was reduced by controlling for improvement in depression. Depression remission at exit was associated with less dyadic discord at exit than non-remission for all three groups [for total sample, 1.8 *v.* 2.4, $t(169) = 7.3$, $p < 0.0001$].

Conclusions.—Dyadic discord in chronically depressed patients is predictive of a lower likelihood of remission of depression. Couple therapy for those with dyadic discord may increase remission rates.

▶ Surprisingly, these authors were able to demonstrate in a large sample that dyadic discord in depressed patients is associated with an approximately 50% reduction in remission (34% vs 61.2%) rates. This result in depression is similar to results that we keep seeing in bipolar illness where couple therapy is associated with greater response, particularly over long term. However, this result was seen in the initial response to antidepressants combined with couple therapy.

J. C. Ballenger, MD

Effects of aripiprazole adjunctive to standard antidepressant treatment on the core symptoms of depression: A *post-hoc*, pooled analysis of two large, placebo-controlled studies

Nelson JC, Mankoski R, Baker RA, et al (Univ of California San Francisco; Bristol-Myers Squibb, Plainsboro, NJ; et al)
J Affect Disord 120:133-140, 2010

Background.—Although antipsychotic agents have a long history of use in depression, their effectiveness in treating core symptoms of depression such as loss of interest has been questioned. Adjunctive aripiprazole is beneficial for the treatment of patients with major depressive disorder but its effects on specific symptoms have not been reported. The objective of this study was to examine the effects of aripiprazole on core symptoms of depression.

Methods.—This is a *post-hoc*, pooled analysis of two trials of aripiprazole augmentation of standard antidepressants (ADT) in patients with major depression. Patients with an inadequate response to ADT received adjunctive aripiprazole ($n = 373$) or placebo ($n = 368$) for 6 weeks. Change on four subscales of the 17-item Hamilton Depression Rating Scale (HAM-D17) that capture core depression symptoms was determined and change on individual HAM-D items also was assessed. The magnitude of within-group change for the subscales and individual items was expressed as effect size (ES) and between-group significance tested with ANCOVA. The magnitude of change was also examined comparing the response rates for aripiprazole and placebo on HAM-D17 and the four subscales. Change on three composite subscales – anxiety, insomnia and drive was also examined.

Results.—Within-group change on the four core subscales was substantial (ES = 1.1–1.2) and similar to that for the 17-item HAM-D total score. Between-group comparisons indicated mean change and response rates were significantly greater with adjunctive aripiprazole than placebo for each core subscale (all $p < 0.01$). Individual HAM-D17 items showing the greatest change from baseline with adjunctive aripiprazole: depressed mood (within-group ES = 1.03) work and activities (ES = 0.86), guilt (ES = 0.77) and psychic anxiety (ES = 0.67) are the same symptoms identified by each of the core subscales and each of these items differed significantly from change on that item with placebo ($p < 0.01$). On three composite scales, adjunctive aripiprazole was significantly more effective than placebo with respect to mean change for anxiety, insomnia and drive (all $p < 0.001$).

Conclusions.—Aripiprazole augmentation of standard ADT results in significant, clinically meaningful changes in the core symptoms of depression. It is also associated with significant change in anxiety, insomnia, and drive components of the 17-item HAM-D.

▶ The results of this study you have probably already seen on television. This article reports a post hoc pooled analysis of 2 large trials of aripiprazole augmentation to standard antidepressants in major depression.

Patients who had had an inadequate response to antidepressants received adjunctive aripiprazole (n = 373) or placebo (n = 368) for 6 weeks. This study led to Food and Drug Administration approval because these studies showed large changes in the Hamilton Depression Rating Scale scores in the adjunctive aripiprazole group. Not only did depression improve but so did anxiety, insomnia, and drive. This study and other less well-controlled studies have established that one of the very best augmentation strategies in depressed patients who have not responded is to use aripiprazole and probably other second-generation antipsychotics that have not yet been so rigorously studied. This is an important change in the routine recommended treatment for nonresponsive depressed patients and one that I have certainly already adopted in my practice.

J. C. Ballenger, MD

Depression and Advanced Complications of Diabetes: A prospective cohort study
Lin EHB, Rutter CM, Katon W, et al (Group Health Res Inst, Seattle, WA; Univ of Washington School of Medicine, Seattle)
Diabetes Care 33:264-269, 2010

Objective.—To prospectively examine the association of depression with risks for advanced macrovascular and microvascular complications among patients with type 2 diabetes.

Research Design and Methods.—A longitudinal cohort of 4,623 primary care patients with type 2 diabetes was enrolled in 2000–2002 and followed through 2005–2007. Advanced microvascular complications included blindness, end-stage renal disease, amputations, and renal failure deaths. Advanced macrovascular complications included myocardial infarction, stroke, cardiovascular procedures, and deaths. Medical record review, ICD-9 diagnostic and procedural codes, and death certificate data were used to ascertain outcomes in the 5-year follow-up. Proportional hazard models analyzed the association between baseline depression and risks of adverse outcomes.

Results.—After adjustment for prior complications and demographic, clinical, and diabetes self-care variables, major depression was associated with significantly higher risks of adverse microvascular outcomes (hazard ratio 1.36 [95% CI 1.05–1.75]) and adverse macrovascular outcomes (1.24 [1.0–1.54]).

Conclusions.—Among people with type 2 diabetes, major depression is associated with an increased risk of clinically significant microvascular and macrovascular complications over the ensuing 5 years, even after adjusting for diabetes severity and self-care activities. Clinical and public health significance of these findings rises as the incidence of type 2 diabetes soars. Further research is needed to clarify the underlying mechanisms for this association and to test interventions to reduce the risk of diabetes complications among patients with comorbid depression.

▶ There is a very interesting evolving literature demonstrating a bilateral relationship between depression and diabetes. Not only does depression lead to an increase in diabetes, but diabetes appears to lead to an increased rate of depression as well. In this study, 4623 primary care patients with type II diabetes were followed for advanced macrovascular and microvascular complications like renal disease, amputations, blindness, and renal failure deaths, myocardial infarction, and stroke. After appropriate adjustments and controls, these authors did observe that major depression was associated with significantly higher risk of these outcomes during a 5-year follow-up, even after controlling for severity of diabetes. Given the high frequency of both type II diabetes and depression in the general populations, this whole area has large public health implications and is an important issue in the field to follow.

J. C. Ballenger, MD

Effects of Estradiol on Learned Helplessness and Associated Remodeling of Hippocampal Spine Synapses in Female Rats

Hajszan T, Szigeti-Buck K, Sallam NL, et al (Yale Univ School of Medicine, New Haven, CT; et al)
Biol Psychiatry 67:168-174, 2010

Background.—Despite the fact that women are twice as likely to develop depression as men, our understanding of depression neurobiology in female subjects is limited. We have recently reported in male rats that development of helpless behavior is associated with a severe loss of hippocampal spine synapses, which is reversed by treatment with the antidepressant desipramine. Considering that estradiol has a hippocampal synaptogenic effect similar to those of antidepressants, the presence of estradiol during the female reproductive life might influence behavioral and synaptic responses to stress and depression.

Methods.—With electron microscopic stereology, we analyzed hippocampal spine synapses in association with helpless behavior in ovariectomized female rats $(n = 70)$, under different conditions of estradiol exposure.

Results.—Stress induced an acute and persistent loss of hippocampal spine synapses, whereas subchronic treatment with desipramine reversed the stress-induced synaptic loss. Estradiol supplementation given either before stress or before escape testing of nonstressed animals increased the number of hippocampal spine synapses. Correlation analysis demonstrated a statistically significant negative correlation between the severity of helpless behavior and hippocampal spine synapse numbers.

Conclusions.—These findings suggest that hippocampal spine synapse remodeling might be a critical factor underlying learned helplessness and, possibly, the neurobiology of depression.

▶ This study is one of the many evolving from the concerted effort to try to understand gender differences in psychiatric illnesses. It is certainly clear that women are much more likely to have a depression during their lifetime, but the neurobiology of these differences is poorly understood. This is a follow-up on the observation that in male rats, the development of helplessness behavior is associated with marked loss in hippocampal spine synapses, which can be reversed by antidepressants. Estradiol has a hippocampal synaptogenic effect similar to the antidepressants. Their hypothesis was that the presence of estradiol might be involved in this process. They observed that stress did induce an acute lasting loss of hippocampal spine synapses again reversed by desipramine. Estradiol supplementation either before stress or escape testing of nonstressed animals did increase the number of hippocampal spine synapses. Correlational analysis showed significant negative correlation between the severity of helpless behavior and hippocampal synapses numbers. This documents a link between hippocampal spine synapse remodeling and the best animal model we have of depression, that is, learned helplessness and provides perhaps a critical piece in the neurobiology of depression, perhaps especially in women.

J. C. Ballenger, MD

A short duration of untreated illness (DUI) improves response outcomes in first-depressive episodes

de Diego-Adeliño J, Portella MJ, Puigdemont D, et al (Universitat Autònoma de Barcelona [UAB], Spain)
J Affect Disord 120:221-225, 2010

Background.—Few studies have addressed the implication of the duration of untreated illness (DUI) on the clinical outcome of mood disorders. Although not focusing on DUI, previous findings suggest that the longer it takes to start appropriate treatment, the worse will be the evolution of depressive disorder. We sought to determine the effect of the duration of untreated episode (DUE) on 1) rates of response to treatment, 2) time to attain a sustained response and 3) rates of remission of MDD, dealing specially with first-depressive episodes.

Methods.—141 patients with MDD were grouped into long DUE (>8 weeks) and short DUE (≤8). Statistical analyses were performed to determine differences in outcome variables. The same analyses were repeated by splitting the sample between first-episode and recurrent depression.

Results.—The percentage of patients who achieved a sustained response was significantly higher in the group with a short DUE [OR = 2.6; 95% CI 1.3–5.1]. Survival analyses showed that patients with a long DUE delayed longer time to attain a sustained response [39 vs. 20 days, $p = 0.012$]. Once the sample was split, these results were even more pronounced in the subsample of first-depressive episode patients.

Limitations.—Given that the sample was originally recruited for two clinical trials, the follow-up period of this study is only six weeks long.

Conclusions.—Our results indicate that response to antidepressant treatments is faster when the no-treatment interval is reduced. The earliest treatment of first-depressive episodes seems to be crucial since a shorter duration of untreated illness implies better response outcomes.

▶ There has been evidence from multiple sources that the more rapidly we treat serious psychiatric illness, the better patients do. This literature probably began in schizophrenia, but it certainly has been extended to depression. This study used 2 clinical trials to look into whether duration of untreated illness made a difference in 141 patients with major depressive disorder. Patients were grouped into 2 groups, one with a long duration of untreated episode (DUE), defined as DUE >8 weeks, and the other with a short DUE ≤8 weeks. The results were clear that a sustained response occurred significantly more frequently in the group with a short DUE, with an odds ratio of 2.6. Also survivor analysis showed that patients with a long DUE had a longer time to sustained response (39 vs 20 days). This was most pronounced in the subsample of first-episode patients. This provides further evidence that depressive illness is actually harmful to patients probably because of cumulative harmful effects to the brain. It makes clear that we should diagnose and treat as quickly as we can to prevent poorer prognosis. I hope clinicians will pay attention to this.

J. C. Ballenger, MD

Atypical Antipsychotic Augmentation in Major Depressive Disorder: A Meta-Analysis of Placebo-Controlled Randomized Trials
Nelson JC, Papakostas GI (Univ of California San Francisco; Massachusetts General Hosp, Boston; Harvard Med School, Boston, MA)
Am J Psychiatry 166:980-991, 2009

Objective.—The authors sought to determine by meta-analysis the efficacy and tolerability of adjunctive atypical antipsychotic agents in major depressive disorder.

Method.—Searches were conducted of MEDLINE/PubMed (1966 to January 2009), the Cochrane database, abstracts of major psychiatric meetings since 2000, and online trial registries. Manufacturers of atypical antipsychotic agents without online registries were contacted. Trials selected were acute-phase, parallel-group, double-blind controlled trials with random assignment to adjunctive atypical antipsychotic or placebo. Patients had nonpsychotic unipolar major depressive disorder that was resistant to prior antidepressant treatment. Response, remission, and discontinuation rates were either reported or obtained. Data were extracted by one author and checked by the second. Data included study design, number of patients, patient characteristics, methods of establishing treatment resistance, drug doses, duration of the adjunctive trial, depression scale used, response and remission rates, and discontinuation rates for any reason or for adverse events.

Results.—Sixteen trials with 3,480 patients were pooled using a fixed-effects meta-analysis. Adjunctive atypical antipsychotics were significantly more effective than placebo (response: odds ratio=1.69, 95% CI=1.46–1.95, z=7.00, N=16, p<0.00001; remission: odds ratio=2.00, 95% CI=1.69–2.37, z=8.03, N=16, p<0.00001). Mean odds ratios did not differ among the atypical agents and were not affected by trial duration or method of establishing treatment resistance. Discontinuation rates for adverse events were higher for atypical agents than for placebo (odds ratio=3.91, 95% CI=2.68–5.72, z=7.05, N=15, p<0.00001).

Conclusions.—Atypical antipsychotics are effective augmentation agents in major depressive disorder but are associated with an increased risk of discontinuation due to adverse events.

▶ These authors followed an issue that I have been interested in and reviewing for the last 4 or 5 years, that is, augmentation of antidepressants with second-generation antipsychotics. These authors analyzed all of the double-blind placebo-controlled trials at that time (N = 16). There were almost 3500 patients; the atypicals studied were olanzapine (N − 586), risperidone (N = 211), quetiapine (N = 677), and aripiprazole (N = 540), and they were compared with 1466 patients to whom placebo was administered, all in 4- to 12-week trials. Interestingly, the odds ratio with the addition of an atypical was 1.69 compared with placebo, a highly significant result (P = < .00001). The odds ratios for each of the atypicals varied from 1.9 to 2.7 and were not significantly different. The odds ratio for remission was again highly significant at 2.0, and remission rates were 31% for the atypicals and 17% for placebo. This study clearly documents the effectiveness of adding a second-generation antipsychotic to antidepressants in nonpsychotic depressed patients but again reports weight gain and the metabolic changes, which have previously been documented. These risks were what led the Texas Medication Algorithm Project to place this type of augmentation behind lithium and thyroid agents. However, in the clinic, I often find myself using this strategy before lithium and thyroid because of its increased effectiveness, and then I closely monitor patients for side effects. This appears (and is documented in the literature) to be an effective way to stay ahead of and prevent most serious side effects.

J. C. Ballenger, MD

A Randomized Controlled Trial Comparing the Memory Effects of Continuation Electroconvulsive Therapy Versus Continuation Pharmacotherapy: Results From the Consortium for Research in ECT (CORE) Study

Smith GE, for the CORE Investigators (Mayo Clinic College of Medicine, Rochester, MN; et al)

J Clin Psychiatry 71:185-193, 2010

Objective.—To compare the memory effects of continuation electroconvulsive therapy (C-ECT) versus continuation pharmacologic intervention (C-PHARM) at 12 and 24 weeks after completion of acute electroconvulsive therapy (ECT).

Method.—Eighty-five patients with Structured Clinical Interview for *DSM-IV*–diagnosed unipolar major depressive disorder, enrolled in a multisite, randomized, parallel-design trial conducted at 5 academic medical centers from 1997 to 2004, who had remitted with an acute course of bilateral ECT and remained unrelapsed through 24 weeks of continuation therapy, were included in this analysis. They were randomly assigned to C-ECT (10 treatments) or nortriptyline plus lithium (monitored by serum blood levels) for 24 weeks. Objective neuropsychological measures of retrograde and anterograde memory and subjective assessment of memory were obtained at baseline, 12 weeks, and 24 weeks. The Rey Auditory-Verbal Learning Test and the Autobiographical Memory Interview were the primary outcome measures.

Results.—The C-PHARM group showed a greater group difference (*P* < .01) for baseline to 12-week change for the Autobiographical Memory Interview. No other memory measures showed group differences for change scores from baseline to 12 weeks. Groups showed no baseline to 24-week change-score differences on any of the memory measures. For both groups, 12-week objective anterograde memory scores (eg, Auditory-Verbal Learning Test percent retention *P* = .0001; Rey-Osterrieth Complex Figure or Taylor Figure percent retention *P* < .002) and 24-week subjective memory scores were significantly improved (Squire Subjective Memory Questionnaire *P* < .02) over baseline. This result reflects the apparent resolution of a presumed decrement in anterograde memory associated with acute ECT preceding this study.

Conclusions.—The finding of no memory outcome differences between unrelapsed recipients of C-ECT and C-PHARM is consistent with clinical experience. Memory effects have only a small role in the choice between C-ECT and C-PHARM.

▶ These doctors studied 85 patients who had unipolar major depressive disorder, remitted with acute bilateral electroconvulsive therapy (ECT), and were unrelapsed through 24 weeks of combination therapy. They were randomized to continuation ECT plus nortriptyline or lithium and underwent neuropsychological testing at weeks 12 and 24. They observed that there were essentially no differences in these 2 groups on their neuropsychological scores, particularly their memory scores. They documented the resolution of the memory difficulties after acute ECT and saw no continuing memory problems with continuation ECT given at this frequency. This is not a surprising result but provides good data so that we can tell patients what to expect.

J. C. Ballenger, MD

Efficacy of the Novel Antidepressant Agomelatine on the Circadian Rest-Activity Cycle and Depressive and Anxiety Symptoms in Patients With Major Depressive Disorder: A Randomized, Double-Blind Comparison With Sertraline
Kasper S, Hajak G, Wulff K, et al (Med Univ Vienna, Austria; Univ of Regensburg, Germany; Univ of Oxford, UK; et al)
J Clin Psychiatry 71:109-120, 2010

Objective.—This study evaluates the efficacy of agomelatine, the first antidepressant to be an agonist at MT_1/MT_2 receptors and an antagonist at $5\text{-}HT_{2C}$ receptors, versus sertraline with regard to the amplitude of the circadian rest-activity cycle and depressive and anxiety symptoms in patients with major depressive disorder (MDD).

Method.—Outpatients with *DSM-IV-TR*–defined MDD received either agomelatine 25 to 50 mg (n = 154) or sertraline 50 to 100 mg (n = 159) during a 6-week, randomized, double-blind treatment period. The study was conducted from 2005 to 2006. The main outcome measure was the relative amplitude of the individual rest-activity cycles, expressed as change from baseline to week 6 and collected from continuous records using wrist actigraphy and sleep logs. Secondary outcome measures were sleep efficiency and sleep latency, both derived from actigraphy, and efficacy on depression symptoms (17-Item Hamilton Depression Rating Scale total score and Clinical Global Impressions scale scores) and anxiety symptoms (Hamilton Anxiety Rating Scale total score and subscores).

Results.—A significant difference in favor of agomelatine compared to sertraline on the relative amplitude of the circadian rest-activity cycle was observed at the end of the first week ($P = .01$). In parallel, a significant improvement of sleep latency ($P < .001$) and sleep efficiency ($P < .001$) from week 1 to week 6 was observed with agomelatine as compared to sertraline. Over the 6-week treatment period, depressive symptoms improved significantly more with agomelatine than with sertraline ($P < .05$), as did anxiety symptoms ($P < .05$).

Conclusions.—The favorable effect of agomelatine on the relative amplitude of the circadian rest-activity/sleep-wake cycle in depressed patients at week 1 reflects early improvement in sleep and daytime functioning. Higher efficacy results were observed with agomelatine as compared to sertraline on both depressive and anxiety symptoms over the 6-week treatment period, together with a good tolerability profile. These findings indicate that agomelatine offers promising benefits for MDD patients.

Trial Registration.—www.isrctn.org: ISRCTN49376288.

▶ Agomelatine is a new antidepressant, which promises to be different. It is the first to be both an agonist at the MT_1/MT_2 receptors and an antagonist at the 5-HT2C receptors. In this study, it was compared with sertraline in almost 160 patients in each cell for 6 weeks double blind. As has been observed in preliminary trials, depressive and anxiety symptoms did improve significantly on agomelatine and more than sertraline in this trial. The main outcome in the authors' minds was also a significant difference favoring agomelatine on the relative amplitude of the circadian rest activity cycle, which began at week 1. Sleep factors like sleep latency and sleep efficiency also improved from week 1 to week 6. This is obviously not surprising given that agomelatine is a melatonin agonist, but the magnitude of the improvement in the sleep and circadian areas is notable as well as the effects on daytime functioning. It also should be noted that agomelatine actually had better effects on depression and anxiety than sertraline in this particular trial.

J. C. Ballenger, MD

Combination of Antidepressant Medications From Treatment Initiation for Major Depressive Disorder: A Double-Blind Randomized Study

Blier P, Ward HE, Tremblay P, et al (Univ of Ottawa Inst of Mental Health Res, Ontario, Canada; Univ of Florida, Gainesville; Centre Hospitalier Pierre Janet, Hull, Québec, Canada)
Am J Psychiatry 167:281-288, 2010

Objective.—Various classes of antidepressant medications generally induce remission of major depressive disorder in only about one-third of patients. In a previous study using mirtazapine or paroxetine alone or in combination from treatment initiation, the rate of patients who remitted within a 6-week period was twice that of patients using either drug alone. In this double-blind study, the authors sought to produce evidence for the superiority of different combinations of antidepressant drugs from treatment initiation.

Method.—Patients (N=105) meeting DSM-IV criteria for major depressive disorder were randomly assigned to receive, from treatment initiation, either fluoxetine monotherapy (20 mg/day) or mirtazapine (30 mg/day) in combination with fluoxetine (20 mg/day), venlafaxine (225 mg/day titrated in 14 days), or bupropion (150 mg/day) for 6 weeks. The primary outcome measure was the Hamilton Depression Rating Scale (HAM-D) score.

Results.—The overall dropout rate was 15%, without notable differences among the four groups. Compared with fluoxetine monotherapy, all three combination groups had significantly greater improvements on the HAM-D. Remission rates (defined as a HAM-D score of 7 or less) were 25% for fluoxetine, 52% for mirtazapine plus fluoxetine, 58% for mirtazapine plus venlafaxine, and 46% for mirtazapine plus bupropion. Among patients who had a marked response, double-blind discontinuation of one agent produced a relapse in about 40% of cases.

Conclusions.—The combination treatments were as well tolerated as fluoxetine monotherapy and more clinically effective. The study results, which add to a growing body of evidence, suggest that use of antidepressant combinations from treatment initiation may double the likelihood of remission compared with use of a single medication.

▶ These authors were following up a previous study showing that using a combination of mirtazapine and paroxetine from initiation of treatment led to a remission rate of twice that if they used either drug alone. They followed this study with a double-blind study comparing fluoxetine alone with mirtazapine with fluoxetine, venlafaxine, or bupropion for 6 weeks. The 3 combination groups had significantly greater improvement than the fluoxetine monotherapy group. Remission rates were less than 25% for fluoxetine alone but again were more than twice that for most of the combinations, including 52% for mirtazapine plus fluoxetine, 58% for mirtazapine plus venlafaxine, and 46% for mirtazapine plus bupropion. They further demonstrated that in patients with a marked response, double-blind discontinuation of one of the agents led to a relapse in almost 40% of the cases. The combination treatments were well tolerated and obviously more clinically effective. This type of study suggests a fairly marked change in the way that we use antidepressants, and I look forward to replication of this. However, I will not be tempted to change my practice even on this kind of evidence published in *The American Journal of Psychiatry.*

J. C. Ballenger, MD

Early Improvement in the First 2 Weeks as a Predictor of Treatment Outcome in Patients With Major Depressive Disorder: A Meta-Analysis Including 6562 Patients
Szegedi A, Jansen WT, van Willigenburg APP, et al (Organon, a Part of Schering-Plough Corporation, Roseland, NJ; et al)
J Clin Psychiatry 70:344-353, 2009

Objective.—New evidence indicates that treatment response can be predicted with high sensitivity after 2 weeks of treatment. Here, we assess whether early improvement with antidepressant treatment predicts treatment outcome in patients with major depressive disorder (MDD).

Data Sources.—Forty-one clinical trials comparing mirtazapine with active comparators or placebo in inpatients and outpatients (all-treated population, N = 6907; intent-to-treat population, N = 6562) with MDD (DSM-III-R or DSM-IV Criteria) were examined for early improvement ($\geq$ 20% score reduction from baseline on the 17-item Hamilton Rating Scale for Depression [HAM-D-17] within 2 weeks of treatment) and its relationship to treatment outcome.

Study Selection.—Data were obtained from a systematic search of single- or double-blind clinical trials (clinical trials database, Organon, a part of Schering-Plough Corporation, Oss, The Netherlands). All included trials (a total of 41) employed antidepressant treatment for more than 4 weeks and a maximum of 8 weeks. The studies ranged from March 1982 to December 2003. Trials were excluded if there were no HAM-D-17 ratings available, no diagnosis of MDD, or if the study was not blinded. Trials were also excluded if HAM-D-17 assessments were not available at week 2, week 4, and at least once beyond week 4.

Data Synthesis.—Early improvement predicted stable response and stable remission with high sensitivity ($\geq$ 81% and $\geq$ 87%, respectively). Studies utilizing rapid titration vs. slow titration of mirtazapine demonstrated improved sensitivity for stable responders (98%, [95% CI = 93% to 100%] vs. 91% [95% CI = 89% to 93%]) and stable remitters (100%, [95% CI = 92% to 100%] vs. 93% [95% CI = 91% to 95%]). Negative predictive values for stable responders and stable remitters were much higher (range = 82%–100%) than positive predictive values (range = 19%–60%).

Conclusions.—These results indicate that early improvement with antidepressant medication can predict subsequent treatment outcome with high sensitivity in patients with major depressive disorder. The high negative predictive values indicate little chance of stable response or stable remission in the absence of improvement within 2 weeks. A lack of improvement during the first 2 weeks of therapy may indicate that changes in depression management should be considered earlier than conventionally thought.

▶ This remarkable trial contributes a significant piece of data, which should change clinical practice. These authors use data with the antidepressant mirtazapine from 41 clinical trials with a sample of 6562 patients. Interestingly, early improvement seen in the first 2 weeks of treatment strongly predicted a stable response and remission with high sensitivity. The negative predictive values for response and remission were even higher than the positive predictors. This suggests that if patients have not begun to respond in the first 2 weeks, there is little chance (from this dataset) that there will be a stable response or remission. It suggests that we should consider changing treatment much earlier than conventionally thought. Although we tell patients not to expect a response within the first 2 weeks, I for one routinely wait 4, and even 6 weeks, hoping to see a response if there is not one in the first 2 weeks. I may need to change my practice.

J. C. Ballenger, MD

Randomized comparison of ultra-brief bifrontal and unilateral electroconvulsive therapy for major depression: cognitive side-effects
Sienaert P, Vansteelandt K, Demyttenaere K, et al (Catholic Univ of Leuven, Kortenberg, Belgium; Catholic Univ of Leuven, Belgium)
J Affect Disord 122:60-67, 2010

Objective.—The cognitive side-effects of bifrontal (BF) and right unilateral (UL) ultra-brief pulse (0.3 ms) electroconvulsive therapy (ECT) were compared, in the treatment of patients with a depressive episode.

Method.—Neuropsychological functioning in patients with a medication refractory depressive episode, that were treated with a course of BF ultra-brief ECT at 1.5 times seizure threshold (ST) or UL ultra-brief ECT at 6 times ST, by random assignment, was assessed before treatment, and 1 and 6 weeks after the treatment course, by a blinded rater.

Results.—Of the 64 patients that were included, 32 (50%) received BF ECT, and 32 (50%) received UL ECT, by random assignment. Neuropsychological testing 1 and 6 weeks after treatment was performed by 30 (93.75%) and 19 (59.37%) patients, respectively, in the BF-group and 29 (90.62%) and 20 (62.50%), respectively, in the UL-group. There was no deterioration in any of the neuropsychological measures. Patients rated their memory as clearly improved after treatment. There were no significant differences between the patients given BF ECT and those given UL ECT.

Conclusions.—Ultrabrief pulse ECT, used either in combination with a UL electrode position and a stimulus of 6 times ST, or a BF electrode position with a stimulus of 1.5 times ST, are effective antidepressant techniques, that do not have a deleterious effect on cognitive function.

▶ This study is an example of how the administration of electroconvulsive therapy (ECT) has improved scientifically in how it is administered. In this trial, patients were either treated with bifrontal ultrabrief ECT at 1.5 times seizure threshold (ST) or by right unilateral ultrabrief (0.3 ms) ECT at 6 times ST. Patients were treated with each condition, and they were tested neuropsychologically 1 and 6 weeks after treatment. Strikingly there was no deterioration in any of the psychological measures in either group. In fact, patients rated their memory as improved with treatment. It would appear that these 2 types of ECT administration were associated with effective antidepressant response and no cognitive side effects. This is one of the multiple current modifications of ECT stimulation parameters that are being studied and shown to be better than previous bilateral treatments.

J. C. Ballenger, MD

Bilateral Epidural Prefrontal Cortical Stimulation for Treatment-Resistant Depression
Nahas Z, Anderson BS, Borckardt J, et al (Med Univ of South Carolina, Charleston)
Biol Psychiatry 67:101-109, 2010

Background.—Treatment-resistant depression presents a serious challenge to both patients and clinicians. The anterior and midlateral prefrontal cortices play complementary roles in integrating emotional and cognitive experiences and in modulating subcortical regions. Both regions offer a distinct opportunity for targeted antidepressant treatments. We chose to pilot the safety and therapeutic benefits of chronic and intermittent epidural prefrontal cortical stimulation (EpCS) in patients with treatment-resistant depression.

Methods.—We enrolled five adults with an average of 5.8 failed antidepressant treatments in their current depressive episode. All subjects underwent comprehensive clinical assessments, detailed neuropsychological testing, and presurgical magnetic resonance imaging. Four cortical stimulation paddle leads were stereotactically placed bilaterally over the anterior frontal poles and midlateral prefrontal cortex. We also acquired a postsurgical computed tomography scan and repeatedly assessed clinical outcomes over time of EpCS as an adjunctive treatment to constant medications.

Results.—All patients tolerated the therapy. At 7-month follow-up, the average improvement from preimplant baseline on the Hamilton Rating Scale for Depression and the Inventory of Depressive Symptoms—Self-Report were 54.9% (±37.7) and 60.1% (±34.1), respectively. Three implanted subjects reached remission. One patient's left hemisphere leads were explanted 12 weeks postsurgery because of a scalp infection.

Conclusions.—Bilateral EpCS over anterior and midlateral frontal cortex is a promising new technology for treatment-resistant depression. Future double-blind studies are warranted.

▶ As I have stated elsewhere, we seem to be coming closer and closer to defining the neurobiology and neuroanatomy of serious depression and finding more effective treatments. This study is an ingenious, well-founded, pilot study with promising results. The authors implanted 4 small plates for cortical stimulation paddle leads bilaterally on anterior and midlateral prefrontal cortex in 5 treatment-refractory depressed patients. These patients all had extremely severe illness patterns and no (or little) response to many previous treatments, including 5.8 failed antidepressant treatments on average in their current episodes. Remarkably, 3 out of the 5 patients actually reached remission, and there was a 55% to 65% reduction in depressive symptoms for the 5 patients. One patient did have the left hemisphere leads removed after 12 weeks because of a scalp infection. Otherwise, depression was well treated, and in the 3 of these patients, the results were remarkable. This is a promising step toward better treatment in these most difficult-to-treat patients.

J. C. Ballenger, MD

Depression relapse prophylaxis with Mindfulness-Based Cognitive Therapy: Replication and extension in the Swiss health care system
Bondolfi G, Jermann F, der Linden MV, et al (Geneva Univ Hosp, Switzerland; Univ of Geneva, Switzerland; et al)
J Affect Disord 122:224-231, 2010

Background.—Mindfulness-Based Cognitive Therapy (MBCT) is a group intervention that integrates elements of Cognitive Behavioural Therapy (CBT) with components of mindfulness training to prevent depressive relapse. The efficacy of MBCT compared to Treatment As Usual (TAU), shown in two randomized controlled trials indicates a significant decrease in 1-year relapse rates for patients with at least three past depressive episodes. The present study is the first independent replication trial comparing MBCT + TAU to TAU alone across both language and culture (Swiss health care system).

Methods.—Sixty unmedicated patients in remission from recurrent depression (≥3 episodes) were randomly assigned to MBCT + TAU or TAU. Relapse rate and time to relapse were measured over a 60 week observation period. The frequency of mindfulness practices during the study was also evaluated.

Results.—Over a 14-month prospective follow-up period, time to relapse was significantly longer with MBCT + TAU than TAU alone (median 204 and 69 days, respectively), although both groups relapsed at similar rates. Analyses of homework adherence revealed that following treatment termination, the frequency of brief and informal mindfulness practice remained unchanged over 14 months, whereas the use of longer formal meditation decreased over time.

Limitations.—Relapse monitoring was 14 months in duration and prospective reporting of mindfulness practice would have yielded more precise frequency estimates compared to the retrospective methods we utilized.

Conclusions.—Further studies are required to determine which patient characteristics, beyond the number of past depressive episodes, may predict differential benefits from this therapeutic approach.

▶ I follow with interest the evolution of the use of mindfulness-based therapies that appear to be quite promising in treating various psychiatric problems, particularly anxiety. In this study, the authors compared mindfulness-based therapy in a group setting including elements of cognitive behavioral therapy with mindfulness training in an attempt to prevent depressive relapse. This method had previously been shown to significantly reduce relapse rates at 1 year. This was the first independent replication trial of the mindfulness-based cognitive therapy (MBCT) plus treatment as usual compared with treatment as usual. The investigators observed that over the 14-month follow-up period, time to relapse was significantly longer with the MBCT combination treatment (204 vs 69 days, respectively). However, both groups did have the same rate of relapse.

J. C. Ballenger, MD

Cannabis abuse and severity of psychotic and affective disorders in Israeli psychiatric inpatients
Katz G, Durst R, Shufman E, et al (The Jerusalem Mental Health Ctr, Israel; et al)
Compr Psychiatry 51:37-41, 2010

The influence of cannabis abuse on the severity of existing psychotic and affective symptoms is still unclear. Among 470 consecutively admitted psychotic or affective patients, 54 active (in the previous month) cannabis abusers were detected via urine tests (Sure Step TM kits; Applied Biotech Inc, San Diego, Calif) and Structured Clinical Interview for DSM-IV (SCID- IV) questionnaire. In 24 cases, substances other than cannabis were abused; 392 patients were nonabusers. All patients were diagnosed according to the *Diagnostic and Statistical Manual of Mental Disorders, Fourth Edition,* criteria. The following rating scales were used: Hamilton Depression Rating Scale (HAM-D-21), Positive and Negative Syndrome Scale (PANSS), and Young Mania Rating Scale (YMRS). Cannabis abusers (n = 54) were significantly younger and more frequently males than nonuser patients. In this group, there were more schizophrenic patients and fewer affective and anxiety patients ($\chi^2 = 11.76$; $P < .01$). The double-diagnosed patients had more prominent psychotic symptoms than the nonusers (n = 392)—PANSS positive: 19.056 ± 8.30 vs 16.128 ± 8.031 ($P < .02$; $t_{446} = 2.510$). The difference was statistically significant for hallucinatory behavior, excitement, grandiosity, and hostility. General PANSS scale rate of abusers was lower: 33.012 ± 9.317 vs 37.3575 ± 11.196 ($P < .01$; $t = 2.727$), especially for depression, anxiety, somatic concern, guilt feelings, tension, motor retardation, and volition disturbances.

Rates of PANSS negative scale of abusers and nonusers were not significantly different (13.815 ± 6.868 vs 14.983 ± 6.446) except for lower rates of social withdrawal and stereotyped thinking for abusers. No significant difference in general level of manic symptoms (YMRS) between abusers and nonusers was observed (6.778 ± 10.826 vs 4.910 ± 7.754), but severity of thought/language disturbances and poor insight was found significantly higher in the abusers. Cannabis abusers are obviously less depressive (HAM-D): 5.944 ± 10.291 vs 12.896 ± 13.946 ($P < .0005$, $t = 3.535$). Such differences were observed in the high number of the subscales. Abusers' rates were higher (although not significantly) for paranoid symptoms and general somatic symptoms. Cannabis possibly produces some antidepressive and anxiolytic effect on psychotic and affective inpatients. The "price" of this effect is often an exacerbation of psychotic and some manic symptoms.

▶ In previous reviews, I have followed attempts to discern whether cannabis use or abuse leads to significant problems in psychiatric patients so that I will know what to advise my patients. Cannabis abuse is obviously very widespread in the population and especially in the seriously psychiatrically ill. These authors studied 470 consecutively admitted psychotic or affectively ill patients and found 54 who were actively abusing cannabis. These abusers were younger, were more frequently male, and more commonly had schizophrenia. In fact, those with abuse histories did have more prominent psychotic symptoms, and they were more statistically significantly prone to experience hallucinations, grandiosity, hostility, and excitement. There were no differences in the general manic symptoms of the affectively ill patients, but their thought disturbance and insight were more significantly impaired. On the other hand, there were lower scores on the negative PANSS scores and less depressive symptomatology, suggesting that there are some antidepressant and anxiolytic effects, but the price of this effect may well be exacerbation of psychosis and manic symptoms. This is a similar-type result to other studies that have shown that there is a higher rate of psychotic symptoms in patients who use cannabis versus those who do not.

J. C. Ballenger, MD

Disturbances in early parenting of depressed mothers and cortisol secretion in offspring: A preliminary study
Murray L, Halligan SL, Goodyer I, et al (Cambridge Univ, UK; Univ of Reading, UK)
J Affect Disord 122:218-223, 2010

Background.—Disturbances in cortisol secretion are associated with risk for psychiatric disorder, including depression. Animal research indicates that early care experiences influence hypothalamic-pituitary-adrenal (HPA) axis functioning in offspring. Similar effects are suggested in human development, but evidence of longitudinal associations between observed early parenting and offspring cortisol secretion is extremely limited. We studied associations between parenting disturbances occurring in the context of maternal postnatal depression (PND), and elevations in morning cortisol secretion in the adolescent offspring of PND mothers.

Methods.—We observed maternal parenting behaviour on four occasions through the first year and at five-year follow-up in postnatally depressed ($n = 29$) and well ($n = 20$) mothers. Observations were coded for maternal sensitivity and withdrawn behaviour. Basal offspring salivary cortisol secretion was measured at 13-years, using collections over 10-days.

Results.—Postnatal, but not five-year, maternal withdrawal predicted elevated mean and maximum morning cortisol secretion in 13-year-old offspring. There were no significant associations between maternal sensitivity and offspring cortisol secretion.

Limitations.—The sample size was relatively small, and effects tended to be reduced to trend level when covariates were considered. The correlational nature of the study (albeit longitudinal) limits conclusions regarding causality.

Conclusions.—Individual differences in early maternal parenting behaviour may influence offspring cortisol secretion, and thereby risk for depression. Parenting interventions that facilitate active maternal engagement with the infant may be indicated for high-risk populations.

▶ We understand many of the issues of cortisol and psychiatric problems, especially depression, as well as how early life experiences affect subsequent psychiatric illness. However, we have very little evidence of longitudinal association between these 2 factors that were studied in this study. The investigators studied maternal parenting behavior on 4 occasions during the first year, and at 5 years, in both depressed and well mothers, and the salivary cortisol secretion in offspring of these mothers at 13 years. Postnatal maternal withdrawal in the first year, but not at 5 years, did predict elevated cortisol secretion in the 13-year-old offsprings. It may be, in fact, cortisol that mediates the negative influence of early parenting by depressed mothers. These results suggest that we intervene to try to increase active maternal engagement with their infants as a high-risk group. However, it strikes me that we know already that mothers need to be involved with their infants and that we should help those who have severe problems in this area. However, this type of study, and ones like it, perhaps gives us more ammunition in the argument that is worth pursuing to convince others and ourselves.

J. C. Ballenger, MD

Antidepressants and Suicide Risk: How Did Specific Information in FDA Safety Warnings Affect Treatment Patterns?
Busch SH, Frank RG, Leslie DL, et al (Yale School of Public Health, New Haven, CT; Harvard Med School, Cambridge, MA; Pennsylvania State Univ, Hershey; et al)
Psychiatr Serv 61:11-16, 2010

Objective.—From June 2003 through October 2004, the U.S. Food and Drug Administration (FDA) released five safety warnings related to antidepressant use and the increased risk of suicidality for children. Although researchers have documented a decline in antidepressant use among children over this period, less is known about whether specific safety information conveyed in individual warnings was reflected in treatment patterns.

Methods.—Thomson Reuters MarketScan claims data (2001–2005) for a national sample of privately insured children were used to construct treatment episodes (N=22,689). For each new episode of major depressive disorder, it was determined whether treatment followed specific recommendations included in warnings released by the FDA. Treatment recommendations pertained to the use of the antidepressants paroxetine and fluoxetine and to patient monitoring. Treatment patterns were expected to change as the risk information conveyed by the FDA changed over time.

Results.—The timing of FDA recommendations was associated with trends in the use of paroxetine and fluoxetine by children with major depressive disorder who were initiating antidepressant treatment. However, no evidence of increases in outpatient visits (indicative of monitoring) among depressed children initiating antidepressant use was found.

Conclusions.—Release of specific risk and benefit information by the FDA was associated with changes in prescribing but not in outpatient follow-up. These results suggest that the FDA plays an important role in communicating information to the public and providers. Yet, although public health safety warnings were associated with changes in some practice patterns, not all recommendations conveyed in warnings were followed.

▶ One of the more significant phenomena in our field occurred after the Food and Drug Administration released safety warnings about antidepressant use, implying an increased risk for suicidality especially in children. It has been difficult for the field to develop a proper perspective for patients and physicians prescribing antidepressants in this age group, and as we feared, there was a clear decline in antidepressant use over this time period. The recommendations that made good sense to try to strike a more appropriate balance included that when children were placed on antidepressants, they be monitored more closely in the early period after treatment initiation. However, this study found no evidence of an increase in outpatient visits after treatment initiation, indicating no increased monitoring. Therefore, it appears that our patients received the worst in this scenario, actually being prescribed antidepressants less frequently but were not monitored more frequently when they were.

J. C. Ballenger, MD

Can Phase III Trial Results of Antidepressant Medications Be Generalized to Clinical Practice? A STAR*D Report
Wisniewski SR, Rush AJ, Nierenberg AA, et al (Univ of Pittsburgh, PA; Univ of Pittsburgh Med Ctr, PA; Univ of Pennsylvania School of Medicine, Philadelphia; et al)
Am J Psychiatry 166:599-607, 2009

Objective.—Phase III clinical trials for depression enroll participants with major depressive disorder according to stringent inclusion and exclusion criteria. These patients may not be representative of typical depressed patients seeking treatment. This analysis used data from the Sequenced Treatment Alternatives to Relieve Depression (STAR*D) project—which used broad inclusion and minimal exclusion criteria—to evaluate whether phase III clinical trials recruit representative depressed outpatients.

Method.—Of 2,855 participants, 22.2% met typical entry criteria for phase III clinical trials (efficacy sample) and 77.8% did not (nonefficacy sample). These groups were compared regarding baseline sociodemographic and clinical features and the characteristics and outcomes of acute-phase treatment.

Results.—The efficacy sample had a shorter average duration of illness and lower rates of family history of substance abuse, prior suicide attempts, and anxious and atypical symptom features. Despite similar medication dosing and time at exit dose, the efficacy participants tolerated citalopram better. They also had higher rates of response (51.6% versus 39.1%) and remission (34.4% versus 24.7%). These differences persisted even after adjustments for baseline differences.

Conclusions.—Phase III trials do not recruit representative treatment-seeking depressed patients. Broader phase III inclusion criteria would increase the generalizability of results to practice, potentially reducing placebo response and remission rates (reducing the risk of failed trials) but at the risk of some increase in adverse events.

▶ As readers know, FDA approval of most medications that come to the market is based on phase III clinical trials generally performed in large research trials involving multiple investigators and study sites. They also typically have multiple exclusion criteria, often making the study population unrepresentative of patients actually seen in practice. The large Sequenced Treatment Alternatives to Relieve Depression (STAR*D) trial, which had broad inclusion criteria and very little in the way of exclusion criteria, allowed a comparison of results with a more representative sample. There were 2855 participants, but only 22.2% met typical entry criteria for a phase III trial. This 22%, when compared with the 77.8% who would not have qualified, had shorter average duration of illness and lower rates of anxiety, atypical symptoms, and previous suicide attempts that generally predict poorer outcome. This 22.2% also tolerated citalopram better and had a higher response rate (51.6% vs 39.1%) and remission rates (34.4% vs 24.7%). It is an inescapable conclusion that the phase III trials are not representative of patients coming to see doctors. Most of these patients were recruited from newspaper ads and have been called "symptomatic volunteers." The authors argue that typical phase III trials should broaden their inclusion criteria, because it would make results more generalizable to the patients actually seen in clinical practice where these medicines are used. It also should reduce the placebo response and the risk of failed trials, which bedevil most development programs, particularly of new antidepressants. It would be hard to argue with their proposals given the strength of this study's methodology and the clearness of their findings.

J. C. Ballenger, MD

Effects of the Serotonin 1A, 2A, 2C, 3A, and 3B and Serotonin Transporter Gene Polymorphisms on the Occurrence of Paroxetine Discontinuation Syndrome
Murata Y, Kobayashi D, Imuta N, et al (Fukuoka Univ, Japan; Kyushu Univ, Fukuoka, Japan; et al)
J Clin Psychopharmacol 30:11-17, 2010

Paroxetine discontinuation symptoms can at times be severe enough to reduce the quality of life. However, it is currently not possible to predict the occurrence of discontinuation syndrome before the initiation or discontinuation of paroxetine treatment. In this study, we investigated the effects of genetic polymorphisms in the serotonin 1A, 2A, 2C, 3A, and 3B receptor, the serotonin transporter, and the cytochrome P450 2D6 (*CYP2D6*) genes on the occurrence of paroxetine discontinuation syndrome. A consecutive series of 56 Japanese patients who had a diagnosis of major depressive or anxiety disorder according to the *Diagnostic and Statistical Manual of Mental Disorders, Fourth Edition*, were treated with paroxetine. Paroxetine discontinuation syndrome was found in 35.7% of the patients by direct interview. Patients who stopped taking paroxetine abruptly experienced paroxetine discontinuation syndrome significantly more often than patients who had a tapering off of the dosage of medication. Patients who had the -1019C allele experienced paroxetine discontinuation syndrome more frequently than patients who had the -1019G homozygote (nominal $P = 0.0423$) of the serotonin 1A receptor gene. However, this result did not remain significant after the Bonferroni correction for multiple comparisons. The findings suggest that the abrupt stoppage of medication is a major risk factor for the occurrence of paroxetine discontinuation syndrome and that C(-1019)G polymorphism of the serotonin 1A receptor gene may be related to the occurrence of the syndrome.

▶ These Japanese authors explored a consecutive series of 56 patients with depression or anxiety who had paroxetine discontinuation. The discontinuation syndrome was observed in 35.7% of the patients and was much more frequent in the ones who had abrupt discontinuation versus tapering of the dose. They also observed preliminary results suggesting that the polymorphism of the serotonin 1A receptor gene C(-1019)G may be related to this syndrome. This is yet another example of the type of benefit we may see from the advent of the genetic era of our field. However, the value of simple slower tapering of paroxetine (and other medicines with a withdrawal syndrome) is a basic lesson that neither patients nor many doctors seem to have learned.

J. C. Ballenger, MD

Selective Serotonin Reuptake Inhibitor Exposure In Utero and Pregnancy Outcomes

Lund N, Pedersen LH, Henriksen TB (Bandim Health Project, Indepth Network, Bissau; Aarhus Univ, Denmark)
Arch Pediatr Adolesc Med 163:949-954, 2009

Objective.—To investigate the effect of intrauterine selective serotonin reuptake inhibitor (SSRI) exposure on pregnancy outcomes.

Design.—Prospective cohort study.

Setting.—Department of Obstetrics, Aarhus University Hospital, Aarhus, Denmark.

Participants.—Pregnant women receiving prenatal care in our hospital from 1989 to 2006.

Main Exposure.—Maternal SSRI use during pregnancy.

Outcome Measures.—Gestational age, birth weight, head circumference, 5-minute Apgar score, and admission to the neonatal intensive care unit.

Results.—Three hundred twenty-nine pregnant women reported treatment with SSRIs, 4902 were not treated with SSRIs but had a history of psychiatric illness, and 51 770 reported no history of psychiatric illness. Gestational age was 5 days (95% confidence interval [CI], −6 to −3) shorter and the odds ratio (OR) for preterm birth was 2.0 (95% CI, 1.3-3.2) in the women exposed to SSRIs compared with women with no history of psychiatric illness. In utero–exposed newborns had increased risk of admission to the neonatal intensive care unit (OR, 2.4; 95% CI, 1.7-3.4) and of 5-minute Apgar scores of less than 8 (OR, 4.4; 95% CI, 2.6-7.6) compared with those not exposed. Head circumference and birth weight did not differ between infants in the exposed and unexposed groups. The results were similar when compared with infants of women with a psychiatric history.

Conclusions.—Exposure to SSRIs during pregnancy was associated with an increased risk of preterm delivery, a low 5-minute Apgar score, and neonatal intensive care unit admission, which was not explained by lower Apgar scores or gestational age. The study justifies increased awareness to the possible effects of intrauterine exposure to antidepressants.

▶ We're finding out more and more about the use of antidepressants during pregnancy, and most of it is not good. We had a general sense initially with the selective serotonin reuptake inhibitor (SSRIs) that they might be safe in pregnancy, and in many ways they are. However, evidence of more subtle damage and danger continues to evolve. In this study, Danish investigators studied 329 pregnant women who were treated with SSRIs and compared them with 4902 not treated but who had a history of psychiatric illness and to over 51 000 who had no history of psychiatric illness. There were a series of difficulties associated with SSRI treatment during pregnancy. Gestational age was 5 days shorter, and there was a doubling of preterm birth. The in utero exposed newborns had a higher risk of admission to the neonatal intensive care units (OR 2.4) and of Apgar scores of less than 8 (odds ratio [OR] 4.4). These changes were seen both in comparison with women with a psychiatric history and those without. As I've said previously about this issue, I have changed my practice to being much more likely to take women who become pregnant off of SSRI antidepressants. Clinically, most women come in and say they have recently discovered that they are pregnant and want to know what to do with the SSRI that they are already on. Other data, not in this study, have demonstrated that staying on the SSRI increases a risk of problems compared with women who stop after they discover that they are pregnant. Therefore, there are increasing reasons for us to not only be careful about this issue, but also to find other ways to treat patients who become pregnant.

J. C. Ballenger, MD

Transcranial direct current stimulation in severe, drug-resistant major depression
Ferrucci R, Bortolomasi M, Vergari M, et al (Centro Clinico per le Neuronanotecnologie e la Neurostimolazione, Fondazione IRCCS Ospedale Maggiore Policlinico, Mangiagalli e Regina Elena, Milan, Italy; Unità Operativa di Psichiatria, Ospedale Villa Santa Chiara, Verona, Italy)
J Affective Disord 118:215-219, 2009

Background.—Though antidepressant drugs are the treatment of choice for severe major depression, a number of patients do not improve with pharmacologic treatment. This study aimed to assess the effects of transcranial direct current stimulation (tDCS) in patients with severe, drug-resistant depression.

Methods.—Fourteen hospitalized patients aged 37–68, with severe major depressive disorder according to DSM-IV.TR criteria, drug resistant, with high risk of suicide and referred for ECT were included. Mood was evaluated using the Beck Depression Inventory (BDI), the Hamilton Depression Rating Scale (HDRS) and the Visual Analogue Scale (VAS). We also administered cognitive tasks to evaluate the possible cognitive effects on memory and attention. tDCS was delivered over the dorsolateral prefrontal cortex (DLPC) (2 mA, 20 min, anode left, cathode right) twice a day.

Results.—After five days of treatment although cognitive performances remained unchanged, the BDI and HDRS scores improved more than 30% (BDI $p = 0.001$; HDRS $p = 0.017$). The mood improvement persisted and even increased at four (T2) weeks after treatment ended. The feeling of sadness and mood as evaluated by VAS improved after tDCS (Sadness $p = 0.007$; Mood $p = 0.036$).

Conclusions.—We conclude that frontal tDCS is a simple, promising technique that can be considered in clinical practice as adjuvant treatment for hospitalized patients with severe, drug-resistant major depression.

▶ These authors did a preliminary study of the effects of a relatively simple brain stimulation technique, transcranial direct current stimulation (tDCS) in severe drug-resistant depression. They treated 14 hospitalized patients who were drug resistant and had a high risk of suicide who had been referred for electroconvulsive therapy (ECT). They delivered tDCS over a dorsal lateral prefrontal cortex (2 mA, 20 min, anode left, cathode right) twice a day. After only 5 days of this experimental treatment, they did see improvement without cognitive impairment. These improvements were over 30% and persisted and even increased over the next 4 weeks. Brain stimulation techniques aimed at the frontal lobes are being explored in multiple different forms. This relatively simple technique is promising given these early results. This technique is potentially simple enough that it might even be an outpatient procedure, and I'll look forward to further studies of it.

J. C. Ballenger, MD

Bipolar Disorder

A brief dyadic group based psychoeducation program improves relapse rates in recently remitted bipolar disorder: A pilot randomised controlled trial

D'Souza R, Piskulic D, Sundram S (Mental Health Res Inst, Melbourne, Australia)
J Affect Disord 120:272-276, 2010

Background.—Various adjunctive psychotherapies assist in decreasing relapse and improving outcomes for people with bipolar disorder (BD). Psychoeducation programs involving patientonly or caregiver-only groups have demonstrated some efficacy. We tested in recently remitted BD if a combined group based psychoeducation program involving patient–companion dyads decreased relapse.

Method.—58 recently remitted BD out-patients were randomised to receive either treatment as usual (TAU, $n = 31$) or 12×90 minute psycho-education sessions delivered weekly in a group program to the patient and companion (SIMSEP, $n = 27$). After 12 weeks SIMSEP patients reverted to TAU and all patients were followed until week 60 or relapse. The primary outcome measure was relapse requiring hospital or intensive community intervention.

Results.—45 patients completed the study. 29 patients remained well at week 60 (SIMSEP $n = 17$, TAU $n = 12$), whilst 16 had relapsed (SIMSEP $n = 3$, TAU $n = 13$). The SIMSEP group were less likely to relapse (Fisher's exact test $p = 0.013$; OR $= 0.16$; 95% CI 0.04–0.70) and had an 11 week longer time to relapse compared to the TAU group (chi-square $(1) = 8.48$, $p < 0.01$). At study completion SIMSEP compared to TAU patients had lower Young Mania Rating Scale scores (Mann–Whitney $U = 255$, $p < 0.01$).

Limitations.—The study was limited by a small sample size.

Conclusion.—A brief group psychoeducation program with recently remitted BD patients and their companions resulted in a decreased relapse rate, longer time to relapse, decreased manic symptoms and improved medication adherence suggesting utility in the adjunctive psychotherapeutic treatment of BD.

▶ This is another study demonstrating that psychoeducation psychotherapy or family-oriented interventions actually seem to be very powerful in bipolar patients, particularly in reducing relapse. These authors tested recently remitted bipolar patients and used a group-based psychoeducational program involving the patients and their companion dyad to demonstrate again a decreased relapse rate. They observed 58 outpatients who received treatment as usual or 12- to 90-minute psychoeducational group sessions of the patient and their companion. After 5 weeks, both groups received treatment as usual until week 60 or relapse (defined as hospitalization or intensive intervention). The intervention group was less likely to relapse and took longer to relapse. Both of these findings were significant. Not surprisingly, they also observed greater medication adherence. This is another study that I use in teaching residents and fellows to try to counter the widespread simplistic idea that all bipolar patients need or can benefit from is medication. This is clearly not the case, and there is now a large body of evidence documenting this.

J. C. Ballenger, MD

The International Society for Bipolar Disorders (ISBD) consensus guidelines for the safety monitoring of bipolar disorder treatments
Ng F, Mammen OK, Wilting I, et al (Univ of Adelaide, South Australia, Australia; Univ of Pittsburgh School of Medicine, PA; Univ Med Ctr Utrecht, Netherlands; et al)
Bipolar Disord 11:559-595, 2009

Objectives.—Safety monitoring is an important aspect of bipolar disorder treatment, as mood-stabilising medications have potentially serious side effects, some of which may also aggravate existing medical comorbidities. This paper sets out the International Society for Bipolar Disorders (ISBD) guidelines for the safety monitoring of widely used agents in the treatment of bipolar disorder. These guidelines aim to provide recommendations that take into consideration the balance between safety and cost-effectiveness, to highlight iatrogenic and preventive clinical issues, and to facilitate the broad implementation of therapeutic safety monitoring as a standard component of treatment for bipolar disorder.

Methods.—These guidelines were developed by an ISBD workgroup, headed by the senior author (MB), through an iterative process of serial consensus-based revisions. After this, feedback from a multidisciplinary group of health professionals on the applicability of these guidelines was sought to develop the final recommendations.

Results.—General safety monitoring recommendations for all bipolar disorder patients receiving treatment and specific monitoring recommendations for individual agents are outlined.

Conclusions.—These guidelines are derived from evolving and often indirect data, with minimal empirical cost-effectiveness data available to provide guidance. These guidelines will therefore need to be modified to adapt to different clinical settings and health resources. Clinical acumen and vigilance remain critical ingredients for safe treatment practice.

▶ These authors provide a very useful article and reference for clinicians. They looked at most of the consensus-based guidelines for bipolar disorder and pulled together a set of recommendations for monitoring of bipolar patients taking mood stabilizers, which included anticonvulsants and atypicals. Their recommendations included (1) waist circumference and body mass index, (2) blood pressure, (3) fasting glucose and lipid levels, (4) blood counts, electrolytes, urea, and creatinine, and (5) liver function tests. They also have individual recommendations for specific medications like lithium and suggest renal function testing at every 2 to 6 months. They stated that this is a good article for us all to have available on our desks.

J. C. Ballenger, MD

Efficacy of ziprasidone in dysphoric mania: Pooled analysis of two double-blind studies

Stahl S, Lombardo I, Loebel A, et al (UCSD, San Diego, CA; Pfizer Inc, NY)
J Affect Disord 122:39-45, 2010

Background.—Dysphoric mania is a common and often difficult to treat subset of bipolar mania that is associated with significant depressive symptoms.

Objective.—This post hoc analysis was designed to evaluate the efficacy of ziprasidone in the treatment of depressive and other symptoms in a cohort of patients with dysphoric mania.

Methods.—Pooled data were examined from two similarly designed, 3-week placebo-controlled trials in acute bipolar mania. Patients scoring ≥ 2 on at least two items of the extracted Hamilton Rating Scale for Depression (HAM-D) met criteria for dysphoric mania and were included in the post hoc analysis. Changes from baseline in symptom scores were evaluated by a mixed-model analysis of covariance.

Results.—179 patients with dysphoric mania were included in the post hoc analysis (ziprasidone, $n = 124$; placebo, $n = 55$). Beginning at day 4, HAM-D scores were significantly lower at all visits in patients treated with ziprasidone compared with those treated with placebo ($p < 0.05$). Ziprasidone-treated patients also demonstrated significant improvements on the Mania Rating Scale and all secondary efficacy measures, and had significantly higher response and remission rates compared with placebo.

Limitations.—The main limitations are the use of a post hoc analysis and the pooling of two studies with slightly different designs.

Conclusion.—In this analysis, ziprasidone significantly improved both depressive and manic mood symptoms in patients with dysphoric mania, suggesting that it might be a useful treatment option in this patient population. Further prospective controlled trials are needed to confirm these findings.

▶ From the beginning, our efforts to study how to treat bipolar illness hit a frequent snag with dysphoric mania. This subtype has traditionally been a great deal more difficult to treat and sometimes responds differentially to medications, often responding better to anticonvulsants in some trials. These authors studied 179 patients with dysphoric mania (124 on ziprasidone and 55 on placebo). By day 4, the Hamilton Rating Scale for Depression scores were significantly lower in the ziprasidone group versus the placebo group. Patients treated with ziprasidone also demonstrated significant improvements in the mania scales. It would appear that ziprasidone did work not only in treating the manic symptoms but also in reducing the depressive symptoms, suggesting that it might be an effective treatment for dysphoric mania.

J. C. Ballenger, MD

Effectiveness of the extended release formulation of quetiapine as monotherapy for the treatment of acute bipolar depression

Suppes T, Datto C, Minkwitz M, et al (Stanford Univ School of Medicine and VA Palo Alto Health Care System, CA; AstraZeneca Pharmaceuticals LP, Wilmington, DE; et al)

J Affect Disord 121:106-115, 2010

Background.—To evaluate the effectiveness of quetiapine extended release once daily in bipolar depression.

Methods.—Double-blind, placebo-controlled study in acutely depressed adults with bipolar I or II disorder, with or without rapid cycling. Patients were randomized to 8 weeks of quetiapine extended release (XR) 300 mg daily monotherapy or placebo. The primary outcome measure was change from baseline to Week 8 in MADRS total score.

Results.—Quetiapine XR 300 mg once daily (N = 133) showed significantly greater improvement in depressive symptoms compared with placebo (N = 137) from Week 1 (p < 0.001) through to Week 8 (p < 0.001). Mean change in MADRS total score at Week 8 was -17.4 in the quetiapine XR group and -11.9 in the placebo group (p < 0.001). Response (≥50 reduction in MADRS total score) and remission (MADRS total score ≤ 12) rates at Week 8 were significantly higher with quetiapine XR (p < 0.001) compared with placebo (p < 0.05). Quetiapine XR improved core symptoms of depression. The most common adverse events associated with quetiapine XR were dry mouth, somnolence, and sedation. Greater weight gain was observed in patients on quetiapine XR relative to placebo.

Limitations.—Fewer patients with bipolar II disorder included, only one fixed dose tested and the lack of an active comparator.

Conclusions.—Quetiapine XR (300 mg) once daily monotherapy was significantly more effective than placebo for treating episodes of depression in bipolar I disorder, throughout the 8-week study, with significance observed as early as Day 7. Adverse events were consistent with the known effects of quetiapine.

▶ This is another study demonstrating that quetiapine is effective in bipolar depression, this time with a once-daily extended release (XR) preparation of quetiapine (300 mg). The quetiapine group (N = 133) showed significantly greater improvements than placebo on most measures beginning at week 1, with higher rates of > 50% reduction in Montgomery-Åsberg Depression Rating Scale total scores and remission. They also observed weight gain in patients on quetiapine XR. This trial demonstrates the efficacy of a once-daily preparation, but perhaps even more importantly, it was a confirmation of previous studies that the difficult-to-treat bipolar-depressed patient does respond to this second-generation antipsychotic (and perhaps others).

J. C. Ballenger, MD

Early stages in the development of bipolar disorder

Duffy A, Alda M, Hajek T, et al (Dalhousie Univ, Canada; et al)
J Affect Disord 121:127-135, 2010

Background.—Numerous studies have observed that offspring of bipolar parents manifest a broad spectrum of psychiatric disorders. We tested the hypothesis that in high risk offspring, bipolar disorder evolves in a predictable clinical sequence from non-specific (non-mood) to specific (mood) psychopathology.

Methods.—Offspring from well-characterized families with one bipolar parent (high risk) or two well parents (controls) were assessed annually or at anytime symptoms developed using KSADS-PL interviews for up to 15 years. DSM-IV diagnoses were made on blind consensus review using all available clinical material. We compared the age-adjusted risks of lifetime psychopathology between high risk and control subjects and assessed the conditional probability of developing a mood disorder given a history of non-mood disorders. In subjects meeting full DSM-IV criteria for bipolar disorder, we assessed the sequence of psychopathology against a clinical staging model.

Results.—High risk offspring manifest higher rates of anxiety and sleep disorders, as well as major mood and substance use disorders compared to controls. Antecedent anxiety increased the age-adjusted risk of mood disorder from 40 to 85% (hazard ratio of 2.6). High risk subjects who developed a mood disorder had an increased risk of a substance use disorder (hazard ratio of 2.4), typically meeting diagnostic criteria during or after the first major mood episode. The evolution of psychopathology leading to bipolar disorder generally followed the proposed sequence, although not all subjects manifest all stages.

Limitations.—Larger numbers of high risk offspring prospectively assessed over the risk period would allow confirmation of these preliminary findings.

Conclusions.—Clinical staging may be a useful approach to refine the early diagnosis and facilitate research into the evolution of bipolar disorder in those at familial risk.

▶ I have been interested in bipolar disorder for a long time, and this study concerns a fascinating subject, that is, the evolution of the illness over time in high-risk offspring of a well-diagnosed bipolar parent. The high-risk offspring in this study had very high rates of anxiety, sleep disorders, mood disorders, and substance abuse disorders compared with controls. Anxiety increased the risk of an ultimate mood disorder 2.65 times and raised it from 40% to 80%. Substance abuse disorder had a hazard ratio of 2.4. There was a fair bit of variability in these subjects, but these findings definitely suggest that there are early stages that could help us diagnose and treat early illness in high-risk individuals.

J. C. Ballenger, MD

Antidepressant Discontinuation in Bipolar Depression: A Systematic Treatment Enhancement Program for Bipolar Disorder (STEP-BD) Randomized Clinical Trial of Long-Term Effectiveness and Safety

Ghaemi SN, Ostacher MM, El-Mallakh RS, et al (Tufts Med Ctr, Boston, MA; Harvard Med School, Boston, MA; Univ of Louisville School of Medicine, KY; et al)
J Clin Psychiatry 71:372-380, 2010

Objective.—To assess long-term effectiveness and safety of randomized antidepressant discontinuation after acute recovery from bipolar depression.

Method.—In the Systematic Treatment Enhancement Program for Bipolar Disorder (STEP-BD) study, conducted between 2000 and 2007, 70 patients with *DSM-IV*–diagnosed bipolar disorder (72.5% non–rapid cycling, 70% type I) with acute major depression, initially responding to treatment with antidepressants plus mood stabilizers, and euthymic for 2 months, were openly randomly assigned to antidepressant continuation versus discontinuation for 1–3 years. Mood stabilizers were continued in both groups.

Results.—The primary outcome was mean change on the depressive subscale of the STEP-BD Clinical Monitoring Form. Antidepressant continuation trended toward less severe depressive symptoms (mean difference in *DSM-IV* depression criteria = −1.84 [95% CI, −0.08 to 3.77]) and mildly delayed depressive episode relapse (HR = 2.13 [1.00–4.56]), without increased manic symptoms (mean difference in *DSM-IV* mania criteria = +0.23 [−0.73 to 1.20]). No benefits in prevalence or severity of new depressive or manic episodes, or overall time in remission, occurred. Type II bipolar disorder did not predict enhanced antidepressant response, but rapid-cycling course predicted 3 times more depressive episodes with antidepressant continuation (rapid cycling = 1.29 vs non–rapid cycling = 0.42 episodes/year, *P* = .04).

Conclusions.—This first randomized discontinuation study with modern antidepressants showed no statistically significant symptomatic benefit with those agents in the long-term treatment of bipolar disorder, along with neither robust depressive episode prevention benefit nor enhanced remission rates. Trends toward mild benefits, however, were found in subjects who continued antidepressants. This study also found, similar to studies of tricyclic antidepressants, that rapid-cycling patients had worsened outcomes with modern antidepressant continuation.

Trial Registration.—clinicaltrials.gov Identifier: NCT00012558.

▶ These authors used data from the Systematic Treatment Enhancement Program for Bipolar Disorder conducted between 2000 and 2007 in bipolar patients with acute depression. After initial response, they were randomly assigned to either continuation or discontinuation of the antidepressants, while mood stabilizers were continued in both groups. Antidepressant continuation did lead to less severe depressive symptoms and mildly delayed depressive relapses, although there were no real benefits in prevalence or severity of new depressive or manic episodes or overall time in remission. Interestingly, patients with a rapid cycling course had 3 times more depressive episodes if the antidepressants were continued. The authors conclude, as have most of the other recent trials, that continued use of antidepressants in bipolar patients did not lead to any major benefits. However, this study did demonstrate a trend toward minor benefits. This is an important study and one of several on this topic that I have reviewed in recent years because it is contrary to how most psychiatrists practice. Even though most studies show little-to-no benefit, and some harm, for continued antidepressant use in bipolar patients, almost all bipolar patients end up on an antidepressant and are chronically treated with them.

J. C. Ballenger, MD

A Double-Blind, Placebo-Controlled Study of Quetiapine and Paroxetine as Monotherapy in Adults With Bipolar Depression (EMBOLDEN II)
McElroy SL, for the EMBOLDEN II (Trial D1447C00134) Investigators (Lindner Ctr of HOPE, Mason, OH; et al)
J Clin Psychiatry 71:163-174, 2010

Objective.—The aim of this study was to evaluate the efficacy and tolerability of quetiapine and paroxetine monotherapy for major depression in bipolar disorder.

Method.—740 patients (478 bipolar I, 262 bipolar II) with major depressive episodes (*DSM-IV*) were randomly assigned to quetiapine 300 mg/d (n = 245), quetiapine 600 mg/d (n = 247), paroxetine 20 mg/d (n = 122), or placebo (n = 126) for 8 weeks. The primary end point was the change from baseline in Montgomery-Asberg Depression Rating Scale (MADRS) total score. The study was conducted from May 2005 to May 2007.

Results.—Mean MADRS score change from baseline at 8 weeks was −16.19 for quetiapine 300 mg, −16.31 for quetiapine 600 mg, −13.76 for paroxetine, and −12.60 for placebo ($P < .001$ for both quetiapine doses, $P = .313$ for paroxetine, vs placebo). Quetiapine-treated (both doses), but not paroxetine-treated, patients showed significantly greater improvements ($P \leq .05$) in most secondary outcomes measures at week 8 versus the placebo group. Paroxetine significantly improved Hamilton Anxiety Rating Scale scores versus placebo ($P < .05$) but not MADRS or Hamilton Depression Rating Scale (HDRS) scores. Both quetiapine doses were associated with greater improvements than paroxetine for MADRS and HDRS scores. The most common adverse events were dry mouth, somnolence, sedation, and dizziness with quetiapine (both doses) and dry mouth, sedation, headache, insomnia, and nausea with paroxetine. The incidence of treatment-emergent mania/hypomania was lower with quetiapine compared with paroxetine and placebo.

Conclusions.—Quetiapine (300 or 600 mg/d), but not paroxetine, was more effective than placebo for treating acute depressive episodes in bipolar I and II disorder. Quetiapine treatment was generally well tolerated.
Trial Registration.—clinicaltrials.gov Identifier: NCT00119652.

► This study compared the new treatment for bipolar depression (quetiapine) with paroxetine in the treatment of major depression in bipolar disorder. In this study (n = 740), bipolar I and bipolar II depressed patients were treated with 300 or 600 mg of quetiapine or 20 mg of paroxetine and compared with placebo in this 8-week trial. Both treatments beat placebo, but some results favored quetiapine, including the Montgomery-Asberg Depression Rating Scale and Hamilton Depression Rating Scale scores and the secondary outcome measures, but anxiety improvements were perhaps better with paroxetine. Emergent mania or hypomania was lower with quetiapine, which was to be expected. On some aspects of analysis, quetiapine worked when paroxetine did not work. This study is primarily consistent with the rest of recent studies' finding that quetiapine is effective in bipolar depression, whereas the antidepressants generally are not. This study sheds further light on the treatment of this very-difficult-to-treat group, that is, the bipolar depressed.

J. C. Ballenger, MD

Olanzapine vs. lithium in management of acute mania
Shafti SS (Univ of Social Welfare and Rehabilitation Sciences [USWR], Tehran, Iran)
J Affect Disord 122:273-276, 2010

Objective.—Among the available mood stabilizers, it appears that lithium may share an important role for treatment of acute mania. In a study from Sep. 2007 to Apr. 2008 at Razi Psychiatric Hospital we evaluated the efficiency of olanzapine vs. lithium.

Methods.—Forty (40) female inpatients meeting DSM-IV-TR criteria for acute mania were entered into a 3-week parallel group, double-blind study for random assignment to olanzapine or lithium carbonate in a 1:1 ratio.

Primary outcome measurements were the changes in Manic State Rating Scale (MSRS) at baseline and weekly intervals up to the third week. Similarly, overall illness severity was rated using the Clinical Global Impression-Severity of illness scale (CGI-S) at baseline and at the end of the third week. Analysis of the data was accomplished by means of split-plot (mixed) and repeated measures analysis of variance (ANOVA) and t test.

Results.—While both olanzapine and lithium were found to be significantly helpful in the improvement of manic symptoms ($p < 0.05$), lithium was considerably more successful by the end of the third week ($p < 0.0002$ and $p < 0.003$, for frequency and intensity of the symptoms). CGI-S also showed important improvements with both olanzapine and lithium ($p < 0.043$ and $p < 0.015$ for olanzapine and lithium).

Conclusion.—Though both olanzapine and lithium were effective in the improvement of manic symptoms, lithium was more beneficial.

▶ Old codgers like me are often fans of lithium in the treatment of bipolar illness. I sometimes have felt like a dinosaur trying to teach residents and psychopharm fellows the value of lithium compared with the new agents that have come out in the last 40 years, even though they know I was involved in the development of the anticonvulsants for bipolar illness. However, recent studies are beginning to document quite clearly that lithium is not only an excellent drug but is probably better than the other treatments available. One large study mentioned elsewhere documents that lithium outperformed Depakote. In this trial, olanzapine (Zyprexa) and lithium were compared head to head in treating consecutive females with acute mania in a 3-week parallel group double-blind study. Strikingly, lithium was found to be "considerably more successful" by the end of the third week. This difference was highly statistically significant, both for frequency and intensity of manic symptoms and overall function. I would like to think that modern psychiatrists would be swayed by these types of studies into being more comfortable with the use of lithium in treating bipolar illness.

J. C. Ballenger, MD

Efficacy and acceptability of mood stabilisers in the treatment of acute bipolar depression: systematic review
Van Lieshout RJ, MacQueen GM (McMaster Univ, Hamilton, Canada)
Br J Psychiatry 196:266-273, 2010

Background.—Although people with bipolar disorder spend more time in a depressed than manic state, little evidence is available to guide the treatment of acute bipolar depression.

Aims.—To compare the efficacy, acceptability and safety of mood stabiliser monotherapy with combination and antidepressant treatment in adults with acute bipolar depression.

Method.—Systematic review and meta-analysis of randomised, double-blind controlled trials.

Results.—Eighteen studies with a total 4105 participants were analysed. Mood stabiliser monotherapy was associated with increased rates of response (relative risk (RR) = 1.30, 95% Cl 1.16–1.44, number needed to treat (NNT) = 10, 95% Cl 7–18) and remission (RR = 1.51, 95% Cl 1.27–1.79, NNT = 8, 95% Cl 5–14) relative to placebo. Combination therapy was not statistically superior to monotherapy. Weight gain, switching and suicide rates did not differ between groups. No differences were found between individual medications or drug classes for any outcome.

Conclusions.—Mood stabilisers are moderately efficacious for acute bipolar depression. Extant studies are few and limited by high rates of discontinuation and short duration. Further study of existing and novel agents is required.

▶ With the increasing evidence that antidepressants are not effective in the treatment of bipolar depression, this is a welcome meta-analysis of what physicians can do. These authors reviewed 18 studies with 44105 participants and compared monotherapy with mood stabilizers to placebo. They were able to certainly demonstrate an increased rate of response and remission. This study is consistent with the extensive but scattered and unsystematic studies in the literature that the mood stabilizers are in fact at least moderately effective or better treatment for bipolar depression even when used in monotherapy.

J. C. Ballenger, MD

A Double-Blind, Placebo-Controlled Study of Quetiapine and Lithium Monotherapy in Adults in the Acute Phase of Bipolar Depression (EMBOLDEN I)

Young AH, for the EMBOLDEN I (Trial 001) Investigators (The Univ of British Columbia, Vancouver, Canada; et al)
J Clin Psychiatry 71:150-162, 2010

Objective.—The aim of this study was to compare the efficacy and tolerability of quetiapine and lithium monotherapy with that of placebo for a major depressive episode in bipolar disorder.

Method.—802 patients with *DSM-IV*–defined bipolar disorder (499 bipolar I, 303 bipolar II) were randomly allocated to quetiapine 300 mg/d (n = 265), quetiapine 600 mg/d (n = 268), lithium 600 to 1800 mg/d (n = 136), or placebo (n = 133) for 8 weeks. Primary endpoint was the change in Montgomery-Asberg Depression Rating Scale (MADRS) total score. The study was conducted from August 2005 to May 2007.

Results.—Mean MADRS total score change from baseline at week 8 was −15.4 for quetiapine 300 mg/d, −16.1 for quetiapine 600 mg/d, −13.6 for lithium, and −11.8 for placebo ($P < .001$ for both quetiapine doses, $P = .123$ for lithium, vs placebo). Quetiapine 600 mg/d was significantly more effective than lithium in improving MADRS total score at week 8 ($P = .013$). Quetiapine-treated (both doses), but not lithium-treated, patients showed significant improvements ($P < .05$) in MADRS response and remission rates, Hamilton Depression Rating Scale (HDRS), Clinical Global Impressions-Bipolar-Severity of Illness and -Change, and Hamilton Anxiety Rating Scale (HARS) scores at week 8 versus placebo. Both quetiapine doses were more effective than lithium at week 8 on the HDRS and HARS. The most common adverse events were somnolence, dry mouth, and dizziness with quetiapine (both doses) and nausea with lithium.

Conclusions.—Quetiapine (300 or 600 mg/d) was more effective than placebo for the treatment of episodes of acute depression in bipolar disorder. Lithium did not significantly differ from placebo on the main measures of efficacy. Both treatments were generally well tolerated.
Trial Registration.—clinicaltrials.gov Identifier: NCT00206141.

▶ This is the large Efficacy of Monotherapy Seroquel in BipOLar DEpressioN I study in which 802 patients with bipolar disorder were studied in a major depressive episode. Two hundred and sixty-five patients were treated with quetiapine (300 mg), 268 with quetiapine (600 mg), 136 with lithium (600-1800 mg), or 133 with placebo for 8 weeks. During this trial, both doses of quetiapine were significantly more effective than placebo. The 600-mg dose group had significantly greater response than lithium in Montgomery-Åsberg Depression Rating Scale total scores. Quetiapine-treated (both doses), but not lithium-treated, patients showed significant improvements in the response and remission rates, Hamilton Depression Rating Scale, the Clinical Global Impressions-Bipolar-Severity of Illness, and the Hamilton Anxiety Scales at 8 weeks versus placebo. In this trial, lithium did not significantly differ from placebo in the main measures of efficacy, and therefore, it is not clear whether this trial can be considered a valid trial. As stated in my review of previous articles, in most recent trials, lithium has done quite well in manic patients. However, this study's results may reflect our long-standing feeling that lithium may have only modest effects in treating bipolar depression and leaves open the clear suggestion that perhaps quetiapine is particularly effective in bipolar depression.

J. C. Ballenger, MD

Association between consistent purchase of anticonvulsants or lithium and suicide risk: A longitudinal cohort study from Denmark, 1995–2001
Smith EG, Søndergård L, Lopez AG, et al (Univ of Massachusetts Med School, Worcester; Univ Hosp Copenhagen, Rigshospitalet, Denmark; Univ of Copenhagen, Denmark)
J Affect Disord 117:162-167, 2009

Background.—Prior studies suggest anticonvulsants purchasers may be at greater risk of suicide than lithium purchasers.
Methods.—Longitudinal, retrospective cohort study of all individuals in Denmark purchasing anticonvulsants (valproic acid, carbamazepine, oxcarbazepine or lamotrigine) ($n = 9952$) or lithium ($n = 6693$) from 1995–2001 who also purchased antipsychotics at least once (to select out nonpsychiatric anticonvulsant use). Poisson regression of suicides by medication purchased (anticonvulsants or lithium) was conducted, controlling for age, sex, and calendar year. Confounding by indication was addressed by restricting the comparison to individuals prescribed the same medication: individuals with minimal medication exposure (e.g., who purchased only a single prescription of anticonvulsants) were

compared to those individuals with more consistent medication exposure (i.e., purchasing ≥ 6 prescriptions of anticonvulsants).

Results.—Demographics and frequency of anticonvulsant, lithium, or antipsychotic use were similar between lithium and anticonvulsant purchasers. Among patients who also purchased antipsychotic at least once during the study period, purchasing anticonvulsants more consistently (≥6 prescriptions) was associated with a substantial reduction in the risk of suicide (RR $= 0.22$, 95% CI $= 0.11$-0.42, $p < 0.0001$), similar to patients consistently purchasing lithium (RR $= 0.27$, 95% CI $= 0.12$-0.62, $p = 0.006$). Absolute suicide risks of consistent anticonvulsant and consistent lithium purchasers were similar.

Limitations.—Lack of information about diagnoses and potential confounders, as well as other covariates that may differ between minimal and consistent medication purchasers, are limitations to this study.

Conclusions.—In this longitudinal study of anticonvulsant purchasers likely to have psychiatric disorders, consistent anticonvulsant treatment was associated with decreased risk of completed suicide.

▶ There have been studies suggesting that both lithium and the anticonvulsants can reduce the risk of suicide. In this large study in Denmark, patients purchasing the anticonvulsants carbamazepine, oxcarbazepine, and lamotrigine ($N = 9952$) or lithium ($N = 6693$) between 1995 and 2001, who also purchased antipsychotics at least once, were studied. The large numbers in this retrospective study allowed for control of various pertinent variables, including patients who were treated consistently versus inconsistently. The authors were able to discern that patients consistently on anticonvulsants did experience a substantial reduction of the risk of suicide. The same was also seen in those who were consistently on lithium. These observations are potentially important. We have thought for some time that lithium reduces the risk of suicide, but had questions about the anticonvulsants. This study would suggest that both reduce suicide if taken consistently.

J. C. Ballenger, MD

A comparison of life events in patients with unipolar disorder or bipolar disorder and controls
Horesh N, Iancu I (Bar Ilan Univ, Ramat Gan, Israel; Rehovot Community Mental Health Clinic, Israel)
Compr Psychiatry 51:157-164, 2010

Objective.—The present study aimed to explore the association between stressful life events (LEs) and the development of affective psychopathology.

Method.—Thirty patients with unipolar disorder and 30 patients with bipolar disorder were compared to 60 matched healthy controls in regard to the rate of stressful LEs. Assessment measures included the Beck

Depression Inventory, the Adult Life Events Questionnaire, and the Childhood Life Events List.

Results.—The entire sample of affective patients had more LEs in general, more negative LEs, and more loss-related LEs in the year preceding their first depressive episode as compared with normal controls. Subjects with unipolar disorder had more positive LEs and more achievement LEs, whereas subjects with bipolar disorder had more uncontrollable LEs in the year preceding the first depressive episode. The relationship between LEs and manic episodes was prominent in the year preceding the first manic episode, with subjects with bipolar disorder reporting more LEs in general and more ambiguous events in that year. Almost no significant differences on LE frequency were observed in the year before the last depressive and manic episodes in the patient groups with unipolar and bipolar disorder. A significant relationship was found between childhood LEs and the development of affective disorders in adulthood, with patients with unipolar disorder exhibiting less positive and achievement LEs.

Conclusions.—In both the unipolar and the bipolar groups, the major impact of LEs on the onset of affective disorders was found in the year before the first depressive or manic episodes. This suggests that the accumulation of stressful LEs at this crucial period contributes to the precipitation of a pathological response mechanism. Once established, this mechanism would be reactivated in the future by even less numerous and less severe stressors, compatible with the kindling hypothesis.

▶ A long time ago, I was involved with Bob Post in theorizing that stressful life events (LEs) were involved in triggering or even causing the worsening of affective disorder, perhaps by a kindling-type mechanism. These authors compared 30 patients with unipolar disorder and 30 more with bipolar disorder with 60 healthy matched controls and compared their rate of stressful LEs. They did show that the entire affectively ill group had more LEs in general as well as more negative ones and more loss-related LEs in the year prior to their first depressive episode when compared with normals. Interestingly, the unipolar patients had more positive achievement-oriented LEs compared with the bipolar patients who had more uncontrollable LEs. The most powerful effect of the LEs appeared to be in the year prior to the first affective episode and those in childhood. LEs seemed to have less effect after the illness was underway. This certainly is consistent with the idea that stressful events in critical periods can seemingly precipitate a pathological affective response. The authors even repeat our original speculation that whatever process was established could be reactivated by future, less severe stressors and even document that this is consistent with the kindling hypothesis. The hypothesis 37 years ago was based on much less evidence, but the evidence continues to build that there is some interaction between stressful LEs changing something in the brain. This process is perhaps akin to kindling that gets established and makes the affectively ill patient much more vulnerable to the stresses and strains of life. It never ceases to amaze me that someone actually reads one's articles and attempts to replicate findings.

J. C. Ballenger, MD

Benzodiazepine Use and Risk of Recurrence in Bipolar Disorder: A STEP-BD Report
Perlis RH, Ostacher MJ, Miklowitz DJ, et al (Massachusetts General Hosp and Harvard Med School, Boston; Univ of California, Los Angeles; et al)
J Clin Psychiatry 71:194-200, 2010

Objective.—Benzodiazepines are widely prescribed to patients with bipolar disorder, but their impact on relapse and recurrence has not been examined.

Method.—We examined prospective data from a cohort of *DSM-IV* bipolar I and II patients who achieved remission during evidence-guided naturalistic treatment in the Systematic Treatment Enhancement Program for Bipolar Disorder (STEP-BD) study (conducted in the United States between 1999 and 2005). Risk for recurrence among individuals who did or did not receive benzodiazepine treatment was examined using survival analysis. Cox regression was used to adjust for clinical and socio-demographic covariates. Propensity score analysis was used in a confirmatory analysis to address the possible impact of confounding variables.

Results.—Of 1,365 subjects, 349 (25.6%) were prescribed a benzodiazepine at time of remission from a mood episode. After adjusting for potential confounding variables, the hazard ratio for mood episode recurrence among benzodiazepine-treated patients was 1.21 (95% CI, 1.01–1.45). The effects of benzodiazepine treatment on relapse remained significant after excluding relapses occurring within 90 days of recovery, or stratifying the sample by propensity score, a summary measure of likelihood of receiving benzodiazepine treatment. In an independent cohort of 721 subjects already in remission at study entry, effects of similar magnitude were observed.

Conclusion.—Benzodiazepine use may be associated with greater risk for recurrence of a mood episode among patients with bipolar I and II disorder. The prescribing of benzodiazepines, at a minimum, appears to be a marker for a more severe course of illness.

▶ I have tried to understand the appropriate use of benzodiazepines and the real risks associated with their use versus alleged risks for quite a while. In this study of 1365 bipolar patients, 349 (25.6%) were prescribed a benzodiazepine sometime during remission of their bipolar illness. They did find in that group that there was a higher risk of recurrence of a mood episode that was statistically significant at 1.21. They again studied in an independent cohort of 721 subjects in remission at study entry and found similar results. This may well indicate that benzodiazepines are associated with a greater risk of a future mood episode in bipolar patients or that they are used in patients with a more severe course of illness, also obviously a reasonable hypothesis.

J. C. Ballenger, MD

Sleep, illness course, and concurrent symptoms in inter-episode bipolar disorder
Eidelman P, Talbot LS, Gruber J, et al (Univ of California, Berkeley)
J Behav Ther Exp Psychiat 41:145-149, 2010

We investigated associations between sleep, illness course, and concurrent symptoms in 21 participants with bipolar disorder who were inter-episode. Sleep was assessed using a week-long diary. Illness course and symptoms were assessed via validated semi-structured interviews. Lower and more variable sleep efficiency and more variable total wake time were associated with more lifetime depressive episodes. Variability in falling asleep time was positively correlated with concurrent depressive symptoms. Sleep efficiency was positively correlated with concurrent manic symptoms. These findings suggest that inter-episode sleep disturbance is associated with illness course and that sleep may be an important intervention target in bipolar disorder.

▶ I have been glad to see the increased study of the daily type symptoms that patients with bipolar disorder have, particularly when they are not in a depressive or manic episode. In this study, symptoms were studied in 21 patients with bipolar disorder who were between episodes. They discovered multiple parameters of poor sleep, including sleep efficiency, total wake time, and difficulty falling asleep, which were correlated with the illness course. These authors then go on to suggest that studying and modifying sleep parameters and sleep disturbances in patients with bipolar disorder should be an important intervention target. I follow the sleep field, and this is actually no surprise. Poor sleep appears to make many illnesses worse. That it does in bipolar illness is not a surprise in that we have known for some time that regular sleep and circadian rhythms are important to the stability of most patients with bipolar disorder.

J. C. Ballenger, MD

Response to ECT in bipolar I, bipolar II and unipolar depression

Medda P, Perugi G, Zanello S, et al (Pharmacology, and Biotecnology, Univ of Pisa, Italy)
J Affective Disord 118:55-59, 2009

Objectives.—A significant body of evidence indicates the efficacy of electroconvulsive therapy (ECT) in unipolar depression but mixed results have been reported in bipolar depression. We explored difference of response to ECT in unipolar (UP), bipolar I (BP I) and bipolar II (BP II) depression, in a sample of patients resistant to pharmacological treatment.

Methods.—One hundred and thirty depressive patients (17 with Major Depression (UP), 67 with bipolar disorder II (BP II) and 46 with bipolar disorder I (BP I) according to DSM-IV criteria) were included in the study and treated with bilateral ECT, on a twice-a-week schedule. The patients were assessed before (baseline) and a week after the ECT course (final score), using the Hamilton Rating Scale for Depression (HAM-D), Young Mania Rating Scale (YMRS), Brief Psychiatric Rating Scale (BPRS) and the Clinical Global Improvement (CGI).

Results.—The three groups (UP, BP II, BP I) showed a significant improvement after the ECT course. Global response rate (CGI < 2) was 94.1% for UP, 79.1% for BP II and 67.4% for BP I. Concerning depressive symptomatology, the remission rate (HAM-D < 8) was respectively 70.5 for UP, 56.7% for BP II and 65.3% for BP I. The best results were achieved by UP patients, while BP I group showed the worst results with a lower remission rate and higher scores in YMRS and BPRS psychotic cluster at the final evaluation.

Conclusion.—ECT turns out to be a viable option for the treatment of both unipolar and bipolar depressive patients resistant to pharmacological treatment. Nevertheless, while the UP group showed the best response and clinical outcomes, the BP I patients tended to exhibit residual manic and psychotic symptomatology.

▶ The literature about whether electroconvulsive therapy (ECT) works as well in bipolar depression as it does in unipolar (UP) depression is unclear. These authors studied 130 depressed patients, 17 with unipolar depression, 67 with bipolar II (BP II), and 46 with bipolar I (BP I) depression. They treated them with bilateral ECT twice a week, and although the UP patients did respond best, the BP I and II did respond well. The global response rates for UP were 94.1%, BP II 79.1%, and BP I 67.4% with similar remission rates (70.5 for UP, 56.7% for BP II, and 65.3% for BP I). They did observe that the bipolar patients tended to have more residual manic and psychotic symptomatology, but the study makes clear that ECT is one of the important options to treat severe bipolar depression.

J. C. Ballenger, MD

Suicide

Suicide Attempts, Gender, and Sexual Abuse: Data From the 2000 British Psychiatric Morbidity Survey

Bebbington PE, Cooper C, Minot S, et al (Dept of Mental Health Sciences, UCL, London; Univ of Leicester, UK; Kings College London; et al)
Am J Psychiatry 166:1135-1140, 2009

Objective.—The purpose of this study was to utilize data from the 2000 British National Survey of Psychiatric Morbidity, a randomized cross-sectional survey of the British population that included questions relating to the phenomena of suicidality and sexual abuse, to test the hypothesis that suicide attempts in women are significantly associated with a history of sexual abuse.

Method.—Participants were male and female volunteers, ages 16 to 74 years old (N = 8,580), interviewed in the 2000 British National Survey of Psychiatric Morbidity.

Results.—Sexual abuse was strongly associated with a history of suicide attempts as well as of suicidal intent and was more common in women. The population attributable risk fraction was considerably greater in female respondents (28%) than in male respondents (7%), which is consistent with more prevalent exposure to sexual abuse among women. The effect of sexual abuse on suicidal attempts and suicidal intent was reduced by controlling for affective symptoms, suggesting that the effect of the former was likely to be mediated by affective changes.

Conclusions.—Sexual abuse is a significant antecedent of suicidal behavior, particularly among women. In identifying suicidal behavior, it is important to consider the possibility of sexual abuse, since it implies a need for focused treatment.

▶ These authors used the large British national survey in psychiatric morbidity and used a sample of 8580 patients. They found that childhood sexual abuse was strongly associated with both a history of suicidal attempts and intent, more commonly in women. This suggests that among suicide attempters we should more directly investigate for a history of sexual abuse so that we can direct treatment efforts at that specifically. The evidence continues to mount that early adversity, and perhaps particularly sexual abuse, leads to lifelong severe psychiatric and physical difficulties.

J. C. Ballenger, MD

Clinical features of patients with treatment-emergent suicidal behavior following initiation of paroxetine therapy

Kraus JE, Horrigan JP, Carpenter DJ, et al (GlaxoSmithKline, Res Triangle Park, NC; et al)
J Affect Disord 120:40-47, 2010

Background.—Understanding suicidal behavior is an important component of assessing suicidality in psychiatric patients. GlaxoSmithKline (GSK) conducted a meta-analysis of randomized, placebo-controlled trials to compare suicidality in adult patients treated with paroxetine vs. placebo. The goal was to identify emergent clinical characteristics of patients with definitive suicidal behavior (DSB: preparatory act, suicide attempt, completed suicide).

Methods.—The dataset comprised 14,911 patients from 57 placebo-controlled paroxetine trials. Possible cases of suicidality were identified and were blindly reviewed by an expert panel, which categorized cases as suicidal or non-suicidal. DSB incidences were compared between paroxetine and placebo. Clinical narratives and case report forms for major depressive disorder (MDD) and anxiety disorder patients with DSB were reviewed. For MDD, rating scale items relating to suicidality, insomnia, agitation, and anxiety were examined.

Results.—Overall (all indications) there were no differences between paroxetine and placebo for DSB (50/8958 [0.56%] vs. 40/5953 [0.67%], respectively; OR = 1.2 [CI 0.8, 1.9]; $p = 0.483$). However, in patients with major depressive disorder (MDD), the incidence of DSB was greater for paroxetine (11/3455 [0.32%] vs. 1/1978 [0.05%], OR = 6.7 [CI 1.1, 149.4]; $p = 0.058$). Review of the 11 paroxetine MDD cases revealed common clinical features: symptomatic improvement; younger age (18–30 years); psychosocial stressors; overdose as method; and absent/mild suicidal ideation at the visit prior to the event. There was no evidence for a consistent adverse event profile or onset of akathisia/agitation or a manic/mixed state. Anxiety disorder patients with DSB had a heterogeneous clinical picture.

Limitations.—Limitations to the study include the relatively small number of cases and the retrospective nature of the study.

Conclusions.—DSB incidence was similar between paroxetine and placebo overall, but a higher frequency of DSB was found for paroxetine in MDD patients, driven by young adults aged ≤30 years. Most MDD patients with DSB improved prior to the attempt and experienced a psychosocial stressor. Patients should receive careful monitoring for suicidality during paroxetine therapy.

▶ GlaxoSmithKline performed a meta-analysis of randomized placebo-controlled trials and suicidality in adult patients treated with paroxetine versus placebo. In a dataset of 14 911 patients in 57 placebo-controlled trials, they identified emergent behavior that they classified as definitive suicidal behaviors, which included preparatory acts, suicide attempts, or completed suicide, which were blindly rated by an expert panel. In the major depressive disorder (MDD) patients, the incidence of definite suicidal behavior was greater for the paroxetine patients (11/3455 or 0.32% vs placebo 1/1978 or 0.05%) and the OR was 6.7. These 11 cases had in common symptomatic improvement, ages between 18 and 30 years, and psychosocial stressors. Overdose was their usual method, and they had absent or mild suicidal ideation at the visit prior to the event. There is no evidence of akathisia/agitation or a manic/mixed state preceding this behavior. Interestingly, the overall rate for all diagnoses demonstrated no differences for paroxetine or placebo for anxious patients who had suicidal behavior or a very mixed state. Many of these MDD patients had improved prior to the suicidal attempt but had experienced a psychosocial stressor. This may provide some clue as to what may be going on.

J. C. Ballenger, MD

Reducing Suicidal Ideation and Depression in Older Primary Care Patients: 24-Month Outcomes of the PROSPECT Study

Alexopoulos GS, Reynolds CF III, Bruce ML, et al (Weill Med College of Cornell Univ, White Plains, NY; Univ of Pittsburgh School of Medicine, PA; Univ of Pennsylvania, Philadelphia; et al)
Am J Psychiatry 166:882-890, 2009

Objective.—The Prevention of Suicide in Primary Care Elderly: Collaborative Trial (PROSPECT) evaluated the impact of a care management intervention on suicidal ideation and depression in older primary care patients. This is the first report of outcomes over a 2-year period.

Method.—Study participants were patients 60 years of age or older (N = 599) with major or minor depression selected after screening 9,072 randomly identified patients of 20 primary care practices randomly assigned to provide either the PROSPECT intervention or usual care. The intervention consisted of services of 15 trained care managers, who offered algorithm-based recommendations to physicians and helped patients with treatment adherence over 24 months.

Results.—Compared with patients receiving usual care, those receiving the intervention had a higher likelihood of receiving antidepressants and/or psychotherapy (84.9%–89% versus 49%–62%) and had a 2.2 times greater decline in suicidal ideation over 24 months. Treatment response occurred earlier on average in the intervention group and increased from months 18 to 24, while no appreciable increase in treatment response occurred in the usual care group during the same period. Among patients with major depression, a greater number achieved remission in the intervention group than in the usual-care group at 4 months (26.6% versus 15.2%), 8 months (36% versus 22.5%), and 24 months (45.4% versus 31.5%). Patients with minor depression had favorable outcomes regardless of treatment assignment.

Conclusions.—Sustained collaborative care maintains high utilization of depression treatment, reduces suicidal ideation, and improves the outcomes of major depression over 2 years.

▶ The large Prevention of Suicide in Primary Care Elderly Collaborative Trial (PROSPECT) involved patients 60 years of age or older ($N = 599$) followed over a 2-year period in 20 primary care practices. They received either the PROSPECT intervention (15 care managers using algorithms to make recommendations to physicians) or usual care. They did in fact find that those who received the intervention had a significantly higher likelihood of receiving antidepressants and/or psychotherapy (84.9%-89% vs 49%-62%) and had a 2.2 times greater reduction of suicidal ideation. The intervention group experienced improvements earlier and these increased from months 18 to 24, while these increases in treatment response did not happen in the usual care. Larger numbers reached remission (26.6% vs 15.2%) at 4 months and 24 months (45.4% vs 31.5%). Interestingly, patients with minor depression had favorable outcomes whichever treatment they received. This study replicates what is almost always found in primary care studies of depression, that is, any algorithm-based additional care over the usual care leads to quite significant increases in treatment of depression and response to these treatments. For this most common illness, it really is worth the effort and expense to add algorithm-based treatments for the depressed patients in primary care.

J. C. Ballenger, MD

Anxiety

Panic disorder as a risk factor for post-partum depression: Results from the Perinatal Depression-Research & Screening Unit (PND-ReScU) study

Rambelli C, Montagnani MS, Oppo A, et al (Univ of Pisa, Italy; et al)
J Affect Disord 122.139-143, 2010

Background.—Although the role of anxiety disorders on the development of Post-partum Depression (PPD) have already been studied in literature, that of individual anxiety disorders has not received specific attention. The aim of this study is to investigate the role of Panic Disorder (PD) and family history for PD as risk factors for PPD.

Methods.—Six hundred women were recruited in a prospective, observational study at the 3rd month of pregnancy and followed up until the 6th month after delivery. At baseline, risk factors for PPD, Axis-I disorders and family history for psychiatric disorders were assessed. We investigated minor and major depression (mMD) occurred at 1st, 3rd and 6th months post-partum. Logistic regression models were used to estimate the association between PD, family history for PD and PPD.

Results.—Forty women had mMD in the post-partum. PD during pregnancy (RR=4.25; 95%CI:1.48–12.19), a history of PD (RR 2.47; 95%CI:1.11–5.49) and family history for PD (RR=2.1; 95%CI:1.06–4.4) predicted PPD after adjusting for lifetime depression and risk factors for PPD.

Limitations.—The response rate is moderately low, but it is similar to other studies. The drop out rate is slightly high, however the 600 women who completed the 6th month follow-up did not differ from the presence of PD at baseline.

Conclusions.—PD is an independent risk factor for PPD, underscoring need to assess PD symptoms during pregnancy. Furthermore, PD represents an important risk factor for the development of PPD and should be routinely screened in order to develop specific preventive interventions.

▶ In previous years I have closely followed the issue of postpartum depression with the hope that we would learn more about it and how to effectively prevent and treat it. These authors studied the role of panic disorder (PD) and a family history of PD as risk factors for postpartum depression. They recruited 600 women in a prospective study at the third month of pregnancy and observed them 6 months after delivery. They were able to demonstrate that both PD and a family history of PD were predictive of postpartum depression. This is one of the clear historical factors that we can assess during pregnancy to help us more intelligently follow up those women who are at risk for postpartum depression.

J. C. Ballenger, MD

Dimensional predictors of response to SRI pharmacotherapy in obsessive–compulsive disorder
Landeros-Weisenberger A, Bloch MH, Kelmendi B, et al (Yale Univ School of Medicine, New Haven, CT; et al)
J Affect Disord 121:175-179, 2010

Background.—Obsessive–compulsive disorder (OCD) is clinically heterogeneous. Previous studies have reported different patterns of treatment response to serotonin reuptake inhibitors (SRI) based on symptom dimension. Our objective was to replicate these results in OCD patients who participated in one of four randomized, placebo-controlled, clinical trials (RCT).

Methods.—A total of 165 adult OCD subjects participated in one or more eight-week RCT with clomipramine, fluvoxamine, or fluoxetine. All subjects were classified as having major or minor symptoms in four specific OC symptom dimensions that were derived in a previous factor analytic study involving many of these same patients. Ordinal logistic regression was used to test the association between OC symptom dimensions and SRI response.

Results.—We found a significant association between the symptom dimension involving sexual, religious and harm-related obsessions as well as checking compulsions (AGG/SR) and improved SRI response.

This increased rate of SRI response was experienced primarily by individuals with harm-related obsessions. Over 60% of patients with AGG/SR OCD symptoms were rated as very much improved after SRI treatment.

Limitations.—As some of the RCTs included were conducted prior to the development of the Yale–Brown Obsessive–Compulsive Scale (Y–BOCS), improvement in OCD severity was assessed using the Clinical Global Improvement (CGI) Scale. Data from the double-blind and open-label continuation phases of these trials was collapsed together to increase statistical power.

Conclusions.—Patients with OCD vary in their response to SRIs. The presence of AGG/SR symptoms is associated with an initial positive response to SRIs. These data add to the growing body of work linking central serotonin systems with aggressive behavior.

▶ It is difficult for us to predict which obsessive-compulsive disorder (OCD) patient will respond to serotonin reuptake inhibitors (SRI) pharmacotherapy. This trial of 165 OCD patients compared clomipramine, fluvoxamine, and fluoxetine in 4 randomized placebo-controlled trials. Interestingly, they did observe significant association between the symptom clusters involving sexual, religious, or harm-related obsessions and checking compulsions and improvement to an SRI. This was particularly noted in those with harm-related obsessions. However, it is striking that more than 60% of the patients with aggressive and sexual or religious obsessions were rated as very much improved after a selective serotonin reuptake inhibitor treatment.

J. C. Ballenger, MD

Early Temperament Prospectively Predicts Anxiety in Later Childhood
Grant VV, Bagnell AL, Chambers CT, et al (Dalhousie Univ, Halifax, Nova Scotia)
Can J Psychiatry 54:320-330, 2009

Objective.—To investigate the contribution of early childhood temperamental constructs corresponding to 2 subtypes of general negative emotionality—fearful distress (unadaptable temperament) and irritable distress (fussy–difficult temperament)—to later anxiety in a nationally representative sample.

Method.—Using multiple linear regression analyses, we tested the hypothesis that caregiver-reported child unadaptable temperament and fussy–difficult temperament scales of children aged 2 to 3 years (in 1995) would prospectively predict caregiver-reported child anxiety symptoms at ages 4 to 5, 6 to 7, 8 to 9, and 10 to 11 years, and child-reported anxiety at 10 to 11 years (controlling for sex, age, and socioeconomic status) in a nationally representative sample from Statistics Canada's National Longitudinal Survey of Children and Youth (initial weighted $n = 768\ 600$).

Results.—Only fussy–difficult temperament predicted anxiety in children aged 6 to 7 years. In separate regressions, unadaptable temperament and fussy–difficult temperament each predicted anxiety at 8 to 9 years, but when both were entered simultaneously, only unadaptable temperament remained a marginal predictor. Temperament did not significantly predict caregiver- or child-reported anxiety at 10 to 11 years, suggesting that as children age, environmental factors may become more important contributors to anxiety than early temperament.

Conclusion.—Our results provide the first demonstration that early temperament is related to later childhood anxiety in a nationally representative sample.

▶ These authors looked at whether fearful distress or irritable distress (2 recognized types of early childhood temperament) were predictive of later anxiety in a nationally representative sample. Reports were from caregivers (initially) of whether the child had an unadaptable temperament or a fussy difficult temperament at ages 2 to 3, and caregiver reported anxiety symptoms at 4 to 5, 6 to 7, 8 to 9, and 10 to 11 years, and child reported anxiety at 10 to 11 years. This sample involved a Canadian sample of 768 600. The fussy difficult temperament did predict anxiety at age 6 to 7, but at 8 to 9 only an unadaptable temperament was marginally predictive, and neither significantly predicted caregiver or child reported anxiety at 10 to 11 years. This suggests that as children age, environmental factors become more important than early temperament. This article and its results enter a complex literature that in general does suggest that early temperament is predictive for anxiety as children age into adulthood. There are excellent studies stemming from Jerome Kagan's early work at Harvard that demonstrate that early characteristics (behavioral inhibition) are predictive of development of social anxiety of a problematic nature in 7- to 10-year olds and certainly increased rates of social anxiety disorder and other anxiety disorders in the teenage years. In this area, it is clear that genetics play a large role, but this study, which is certainly based on a large sample, suggests that environment has increasing importance as children age.

J. C. Ballenger, MD

Diagnosis of multiple anxiety disorders predicts the concurrent comorbidity of major depressive disorder
Miyazaki M, Yoshino A, Nomura S (Natl Defense Med College, Saitama, Japan)
Compr Psychiatry 51:15-18, 2010

Purpose.—It has been established that a single anxiety disorder (AD) is more likely to be comorbid with other ADs as well as major depressive disorder (MDD). However, little is known about the comorbidity risks of MDD in patients with double or multiple ADs in comparison with those with a single AD. In this study, we estimated the comorbidity risks of MDD in patients with multiple ADs.

Method.—The subjects were 217 consecutive outpatients with any ADs who were comprehensively diagnosed using the Mini International Neuropsychiatric Interview. The comorbidity rates of MDD in subjects with 2 or more ADs were compared with those in subjects with a single AD.

Results.—The comorbidity rates of MDD in subjects with a single AD (n = 119), 2 ADs (n = 75), and 3 or more ADs (n = 23) were 20.1%, 45.3%, and 87.0%, respectively. The relative risks of the comorbidity of MDD in subjects with 2 and with 3 or more ADs compared with those with a single AD were 3.3 (95% confidence interval, 1.7-6.3) and 26.4 (95% confidence interval, 8.2-118.7), respectively. Generalized anxiety disorder was associated with a higher comorbidity rate of MDD in subjects with a single AD but not in subjects with 2 or more ADs.

Conclusion.—The results showed that the presence of multiple ADs strongly predicts comorbidity with MDD in an exponential manner, suggesting that we should pay attention to the fact that patients with multiple ADs are more likely to be comorbid with MDD.

▶ It has become clear that anxiety disorders (ADs) often come comorbid with other ADs as well as major depressive disorder (MDD). We don't know much about what the risk is of multiple ADs in terms of depression. I end up seeing a lot of patients with multiple ADs these days and was intrigued by this study of 217 outpatients. The rate of MDD in patients with 2 or more ADs was markedly higher, the more ADs that were present the more likely the patients had MDD. With a single AD, the comorbidity rate with MDD was 20.1%, but with 2, it rose to 45.3% and with 3, to 87.0%. Generalized AD had the highest comorbidity rate if it was a single AD but not with 2 or more. This documents the intuitive and clinical experience that multiple ADs are not good for a patient's prognosis, particularly for depression.

J. C. Ballenger, MD

Deep Brain Stimulation for Intractable Obsessive Compulsive Disorder: Pilot Study Using a Blinded, Staggered-Onset Design

Goodman WK, Foote KD, Greenberg BD, et al (Mount Sinai School of Medicine, NY; Univ of Florida, Gainesville; Brown Univ, Providence, RI)
Biol Psychiatry 67:535-542, 2010

Background.—Prior promising results have been reported with deep brain stimulation (DBS) of the anterior limb of the internal capsule in cases with severe obsessive compulsive disorder (OCD) who had exhausted conventional therapies.

Methods.—In this pilot study, six adult patients (2 male; 4 female) meeting stringent criteria for severe (minimum Yale-Brown Obsessive Compulsive Scale [Y-BOCS] of 28) and treatment-refractory OCD had

DBS electrode arrays placed bilaterally in an area spanning the ventral anterior limb of the internal capsule and adjacent ventral striatum referred to as the ventral capsule/ventral striatum. Using a randomized, staggered-onset design, patients were stimulated at either 30 or 60 days following surgery under blinded conditions.

Results.—After 12 months of stimulation, four (66.7%) of six patients met a stringent criterion as "responders" (≥35% improvement in the Y-BOCS and end point Y-BOCS severity ≤16). Patients did not improve during sham stimulation. Depressive symptoms improved significantly in the group as a whole; global functioning improved in the four responders. Adverse events associated with chronic DBS were generally mild and modifiable with setting changes. Stimulation interruption led to rapid but reversible induction of depressive symptoms in two cases.

Conclusions.—This pilot study suggests that DBS of the ventral capsule/ventral striatum region is a promising therapy of last resort for carefully selected cases of severe and intractable OCD. Future research should attend to subject selection, lead location, DBS programming, and mechanisms underpinning therapeutic benefits.

▶ I continue to review articles about various brain manipulations with severe obsessive-compulsive disorder (OCD) patients who have not responded to conventional therapies. I do this because the number of OCD patients remaining severely ill is a distressingly common occurrence, and these types of studies are continuing to prove to be helpful in this severe patient group. This is a pilot study of 6 adult patients who had electrode arrays bilaterally placed deep in their brain in an area of the ventral anterior limb of the internal capsule and adjacent ventral striatum. In a randomized staggered-onset design, they were stimulated either 30 or 60 days under blind conditions. After 12 months of stimulation, 4 of the 6 patients met stringent criteria as responders (≥35% improvement in the Yale-Brown Obsessive Compulsive Scale [Y-BOCS] and end point Y-BOCS severity ≤16). In contrast, they did not improve during sham stimulation. Depressive symptoms improved in the group as a whole. Global functioning did improve in the 4 responders. Adverse events were generally mild and could be reduced by changing the setting of the stimulation. This particular technique is less invasive than the neurosurgical approaches that have been applied previously and appears to be at least as effective in this small pilot study. I look forward to the follow-up of this particular methodology.

J. C. Ballenger, MD

Association of Poor Childhood Fear Conditioning and Adult Crime

Gao Y, Raine A, Venables PH, et al (Univ of Pennsylvania, Philadelphia; Univ of York, England, UK; Univ of Southern California, Los Angeles, CA)
Am J Psychiatry 167:56-60, 2010

Objective.—Amygdala dysfunction is theorized to give rise to poor fear conditioning, which in turn predisposes to crime, but it is not known whether poor conditioning precedes criminal offending. This study prospectively assessed whether poor fear conditioning early in life predisposes to adult crime in a large cohort.

Method.—Electrodermal fear conditioning was assessed in a cohort of 1,795 children at age 3, and registration for criminal offending was ascertained at age 23. In a case-control design, 137 cohort members with a criminal record were matched on gender, ethnicity, and social adversity with 274 noncriminal comparison members. Statistical analyses compared childhood fear conditioning for the two groups.

Results.—Criminal offenders showed significantly reduced electrodermal fear conditioning at age 3 compared to matched comparison subjects.

Conclusions.—Poor fear conditioning at age 3 predisposes to crime at age 23. Poor fear conditioning early in life implicates amygdala and ventral prefrontal cortex dysfunction and a lack of fear of socializing punishments in children who grow up to become criminals. These findings are consistent with a neurodevelopmental contribution to crime causation.

► This is an interesting study suggesting that amygdala dysfunction that is thought to result in poor fear conditioning could in fact lead to adult crime through a lack of fear of the kind of punishments, which shapes behavior in socialized versus criminal directions. They studied 1795 children at age 3 with electrodermal fear conditioning and ascertained 137 individuals who at age 23 had criminal records and compared them to 294 noncriminal comparison individuals. Interestingly, they did find significantly reduced electrodermal fear conditioning at age 3 in the criminal offenders supporting their hypothesis. Poor fear conditioning in early life, perhaps implicating amygdala and ventral prefrontal cortex dysfunction, appears to lead to an increase in future criminal behavior. This reminds me of when I presented an article at the American Psychological Association more than 30 years ago demonstrating low cerebrospinal fluid 5HIAA associated with increased aggression, only to find when I left the presentation hall that there were picketers outside outraged by such a finding. I hope this does not happen to these authors, but also it does underscore the complexity of neurobiological findings in larger sociological contexts like crime or violence.

J. C. Ballenger, MD

An Increased Risk of Stroke Among Panic Disorder Patients: A 3–Year Follow–up Study

Chen Y-H, Hu C-J, Lee H-C, et al (Taipei Med Univ, Taiwan)
Can J Psychiatry 55:43-49, 2010

Objective.—To explore whether panic disorder (PD) increases the risk for stroke, using a nationwide, population-based dataset.

Methods.—Our study used data from Taiwan's National Health Insurance Research Database. The study cohort included patients who received ambulatory psychiatric care for PD between 2002 and 2003, inclusive ($n = 3891$). We selected our comparison cohort by randomly recruiting enrollees ($n = 19\,455$) matched with the study group by sex and age. Each patient was tracked for 3 years, from their index ambulatory care visit until the end of 2006, to identify whether or not a patient had a stroke during the follow-up period. Cox proportional hazard regressions were performed as a means of computing the 3-year survival rate, adjusting for potential confounding factors.

Results.—Among the total sample, 2029 patients (8.7%) experienced a stroke during the 3-year follow-up period, including 647 from the study cohort (16.6% of the PD patients) and 1382 (7.1%) from the comparison cohort. After adjusting for the patients' sex, age, monthly income, level of urbanization, and comorbid medical disorders, the hazard of stroke occurring during the 3-year follow-up period was 2.37 ($P < 0.001$) times greater for patients with PD than for patients in the comparison cohort. In further analyses, stratified by medical diseases and age, the significant risk of PD on subsequent stroke persisted.

Conclusions.—We conclude that PD is an independent risk factor for stroke. For patients with PD, aggressive treatment of PD may be considered as part of stroke prevention.

▶ I have followed panic disorder for a very long time and seen it go from being a rare, poorly recognized, harmless condition to our more appropriate modern understanding that it is a common and very serious psychiatric condition with considerable morbidity. These Taiwanese researchers used a large database ($n = 3891$) of panic patients receiving outpatient psychiatric care and compared them with a random-matched sample of 19 455. They followed them over a 3-year period for whether they suffered a stroke during that time. In the total sample of 2029 patients, 8.7% experienced a stroke during that period, but the percentage was 16.6% of the panic disorder patients, compared with 7.1% in the comparison cohort, which was a 2.37 times increase in the panic disorder patients. Previous studies have found increases in various cardiovascular outcomes in the panic disorder patients, and this study again documented that this is hardly a harmless illness, either psychiatrically or medically.

J. C. Ballenger, MD

Schizophrenia

11-year follow-up of mortality in patients with schizophrenia: a population-based cohort study (FIN11 study)
Tiihonen J, Lönnqvist J, Wahlbeck K, et al (Helsinki Univ Central Hosp, Finland; Vaasa Central Hosp, Finland; et al)
Lancet 374:620-627, 2009

Background.—The introduction of second-generation antipsychotic drugs during the 1990s is widely believed to have adversely affected mortality of patients with schizophrenia. Our aim was to establish the long-term contribution of antipsychotic drugs to mortality in such patients.

Methods.—Nationwide registers in Finland were used to compare the cause-specific mortality in 66 881 patients versus the total population (5·2 million) between 1996, and 2006, and to link these data with the use of antipsychotic drugs. We measured the all-cause mortality of patients with schizophrenia in outpatient care during current and cumulative exposure to any antipsychotic drug versus no use of these drugs, and exposure to the six most frequently used antipsychotic drugs compared with perphenazine use.

Findings.—Although the proportional use of second-generation antipsychotic drugs rose from 13% to 64% during follow-up, the gap in life expectancy between patients with schizophrenia and the general population did not widen between 1996 (25 years), and 2006 (22·5 years). Compared with current use of perphenazine, the highest risk for overall mortality was recorded for quetiapine (adjusted hazard ratio [HR] 1·41, 95% CI 1·09–1·82), and the lowest risk for clozapine (0·74, 0·60–0·91; p=0·0045 for the difference between clozapine vs perphenazine, and p<0·0001 for all other antipsychotic drugs). Long-term cumulative exposure (7–11 years) to any antipsychotic treatment was associated with lower mortality than was no drug use (0·81, 0·77–0·84). In patients with one or more filled prescription for an antipsychotic drug, an inverse relation between mortality and duration of cumulative use was noted (HR for trend per exposure year 0·991; 0·985–0·997).

Interpretation.—Long-term treatment with antipsychotic drugs is associated with lower mortality compared with no antipsychotic use. Second-generation drugs are a highly heterogeneous group, and clozapine seems to be associated with a substantially lower mortality than any other antipsychotics. Restrictions on the use of clozapine should be reassessed.

▶ Because of the metabolic changes discussed with the second-generation antipsychotic drugs (SGAs), there has been considerable concern that population studies might show greater mortality in patients with schizophrenia treated with these medications. These authors used the nationwide registers available in Finland to compare mortality in 66 881 patients versus the total population of 5.2 million between 1996 and 2006 when there was a marked increase in the use of SGAs. During that period, their use rose from 13% to 64% of antipsychotic use. However, reassuringly, the life expectancy gap between patients with schizophrenia and the population did not widen and actually slightly decreased from 1996 in which it was 25 years to 2006 where it was 22.5 years. The highest risk was with quetiapine with a hazard ratio of 1.41, and the lowest risk was seen with clozapine (HR 0.74). In contrast to the worry that the long-term use of these SGAs (7-11 years) would be associated with greater mortality, this was not seen. In fact, they found lower mortality with SGA use versus no drugs at all. In fact, there was an inverse relationship between mortality and duration of use. The data of lowest risk with clozapine (even compared with a first generation antipsychotics perphenazine) are interesting. Certainly, clozapine has been demonstrated to have decreased deaths from suicide, but this study and others would suggest that it also reduces the death rate through other largely unknown mechanisms. Given how clozapine is often considered a dangerous drug, these data should lead us to rethink and reassess that issue.

J. C. Ballenger, MD

Association Between *HTR2C* and *HTR2A* Polymorphisms and Metabolic Abnormalities in Patients Treated With Olanzapine or Clozapine

Gunes A, Melkersson KI, Scordo MG, et al (Uppsala Univ, Sweden; Karolinska Institutet, Stockholm, Sweden)
J Clin Psychopharmacol 29:65-68, 2009

Serotonin 2C and 2A receptor (5-HT$_{2C}$ and 5-HT$_{2A}$) antagonisms are hypothesized to play a role in the metabolic adverse effects induced by olanzapine and clozapine. Associations between polymorphisms in 5-HT$_{2C}$ and 5-HT$_{2A}$ receptor coding genes, *HTR2C* and *HTR2A*, with antipsychotic-induced weight gain have been reported. The impact of *HTR2C* and *HTR2A* polymorphisms on body mass index (BMI), glucose-insulin homeostasis, and blood lipid levels was evaluated in 46 patients with schizophrenia or schizoaffective disorder and treated with olanzapine (n = 28) or clozapine (n = 18) for at least 6 months. Olanzapine-treated patients with *HTR2C* haplotype C (−759C, −697C, and 23Ser) had higher BMI ($P = 0.029$) and C peptide levels ($P = 0.029$) compared with patients with haplotype B (−759 T, −697C, and 23Cys). The frequency of patients homozygous for the *HTR2C* haplotype A (−759C, −697 G, and 23Cys) was significantly higher among clozapine-treated patients with obesity (BMI $\geq$ 30 kg/m^2) compared with nonobese patients ($P = 0.015$; odds ratio, 28; 95% confidence interval, 2–380). Patients carrying the *HTR2A* haplotype 2 (−1438A, 102T, and 452His) had significantly higher C peptide levels compared with haplotype 3 (−1438A, 102T, and 452Tyr) carriers in the olanzapine group ($P = 0.034$) and in the overall study population ($P = 0.019$). None of the haplotypes were associated with serum levels of insulin, triglycerides, and cholesterol or with homeostasis model assessment index for insulin resistance. In conclusion, both *HTR2C* and *HTR2A* gene polymorphisms seem to be associated with the occurrence of metabolic abnormalities in patients treated with olanzapine or clozapine.

▶ The use of both olanzapine and clozapine has been associated with metabolic abnormalities, the most common of which are weight gain, insulin resistance changes, and increased lipid levels. This study in 46 patients with schizophrenia or schizoaffective disorder treated with olanzapine or clozapine for at least 6 months were genotyped. As predicted, the polymorphisms for *HTR2C* and *HTR2A* were significantly associated with some of the metabolic abnormalities in patients treated with these 2 drugs. These abnormalities are to varying degrees seen with all of the second-generation antipsychotics. They are most associated certainly with olanzapine and clozapine, and this study and others like it will perhaps provide us a handle on how to manage the patients in whom we need to use these medications. This is a good example of the treatment model of the future in which genetic subtyping of patients before treatment will be predictive of side effects, and in some cases, of treatment response.

J. C. Ballenger, MD

Does Adherence to Medications for Type 2 Diabetes Differ Between Individuals With Vs Without Schizophrenia?
Kreyenbuhl J, Dixon LB, McCarthy JF, et al (Univ of Maryland School of Medicine, Baltimore; VA Serious Mental Illness Treatment Res and Evaluation Ctr [SMITREC], Ann Arbor, MI; et al)
Schizophr Bull 36:428-435, 2010

Individuals with schizophrenia are at increased risk for poor health outcomes and mortality. This may be due to inadequate self-management of co-occurring conditions, such as type 2 diabetes. We compared adherence to oral hypoglycemic medications for diabetes patients with vs without comorbid schizophrenia. Using Veterans Affairs (VA) health system administrative data, we identified all patients with both schizophrenia and type 2 diabetes and with at least one oral hypoglycemic prescription fill in fiscal year 2002 (N = 11 454) and a comparison group of patients with diabetes who were not diagnosed with schizophrenia (N = 10 560). Nonadherence was operationalized as having a medication possession ratio indicating receipt of less than 80% of needed hypoglycemic medications. Poor adherence was less prevalent among diabetes patients with (43%) than without schizophrenia (52%, $P < .001$). In multivariable analyses, having schizophrenia was associated with a 25% lower likelihood of poor adherence compared with not having schizophrenia (adjusted odds ratio: 0.75, 95% confidence interval: 0.70–0.80).

Poorer adherence was associated with black race, homelessness, depression, substance use disorder, and medical comorbidity. Having more outpatient visits, a higher proportion of prescriptions delivered by mail, lower prescription copayments, and more complex medication regimens were each associated with increased adherence. Among veterans with diabetes receiving ongoing VA care, overall hypoglycemic medication adherence was low, but individuals with comorbid schizophrenia were more likely to be adherent to these medications. Future studies should investigate whether factors such as comanagement of a chronic psychiatric illness or regular contact with mental health providers bestow benefits for diabetes self-management in persons with schizophrenia.

▶ In evaluating the risk of chronic medical conditions in people with schizophrenia, we are often tempted to assume that they take care of their illnesses like diabetes less well than those without schizophrenia. These authors used a huge Veterans Affairs (VA) database to document that poor adherence (receiving less than 80% of hypoglycemic medications) was in fact less prevalent among the diabetes patients with schizophrenia (43%) than those without schizophrenia (52%). It is unclear why there was 25% better adherence in the schizophrenic diabetics, but the authors suggest that maybe the regular visits to the mental health providers in the VA setting led to better care of their diabetes.

J. C. Ballenger, MD

A Comparison Study of Multiple Measures of Adherence to Antipsychotic Medication in First-Episode Psychosis
Cassidy CM, Rabinovitch M, Schmitz N, et al (McGill Univ, Montreal, Quebec, Canada)
J Clin Psychopharmacol 30:64-67, 2010

This study evaluates how much agreement there is between subjective reports of adherence to antipsychotic medication and objective or derived measures of adherence in first-episode psychosis (FEP) and asks if any adherence measure could approximate a gold standard based on correlation to symptom improvement in the early phase of treatment. Adherence was assessed in 81 FEP subjects on a monthly basis by reports from patients, clinicians, family, and pill counting. A consensus measure of adherence was derived from all available sources of adherence data. Symptoms were measured using the Positive and Negative Syndrome Scale at study entry and 3 months subsequently. Adherence as measured by patient report, pill count, and clinician report were in good agreement with each other (intraclass correlation coefficient $= 0.84$), and all of these measures were highly correlated to consensus adherence (r values between 0.86 and 0.98). Mean adherence was slightly higher as rated by patients (83% full doses taken per month) and family members (91%) than by clinicians (76%), pill counting (73%), or consensus value (74%). Early in treatment, each measure of adherence (except family report) was significantly associated with positive symptom reduction, although the order of magnitude of this correlation was greater for pill count and consensus adherence ($P < 0.01$) compared with patient- or clinician-reported adherence ($P < 0.05$). Patient or clinician reports provide a reasonable estimate of medication adherence in FEP, but introducing pill counting or a derived measure of adherence may allow more accurate measurement.

▶ This is an interesting study in which they studied 81 first-episode psychosis patients with multiple measures of adherence to see if they could develop a standard that would correlate actually to symptom improvement in the early phases of treatment. In fact, patient report, pill count, and clinician report actually agreed well with each other and were highly correlated with consensus adherence. Adherence was rated as higher by patients and family members than by clinicians, pill counting, or consensus value. Most of these measures actually did significantly correlate with positive symptom reduction, although the magnitude of this correlation was greater for pill count and consensus adherence than patient or clinician reports. Not surprisingly, the external measure of pill counting was more highly associated with response than the others.

J. C. Ballenger, MD

A Double-Blind, Randomized Study of Minocycline for the Treatment of Negative and Cognitive Symptoms in Early-Phase Schizophrenia

Levkovitz Y, Mendlovich S, Riwkes S, et al (Shalvata Mental Health Care Ctr, Hod-Hasharon, Israel; et al)
J Clin Psychiatry 71:138-149, 2010

Background.—Current antipsychotics have only a limited effect on 2 core aspects of schizophrenia: negative symptoms and cognitive deficits. Minocycline is a second-generation tetracycline that has a beneficial effect in various neurologic disorders. Recent findings in animal models and human case reports suggest its potential for the treatment of schizophrenia. These findings may be linked to the effect of minocycline on the glutamatergic system, through inhibition of nitric oxide synthase and blocking of nitric oxide-induced neurotoxicity. Other proposed mechanisms of action include effects of minocycline on the dopaminergic system and its inhibition of microglial activation.

Objective.—To examine the efficacy of minocycline as an add-on treatment for alleviating negative and cognitive symptoms in early-phase schizophrenia.

Method.—A longitudinal double-blind, randomized, placebo-controlled design was used, and patients were followed for 6 months from August 2003 to March 2007. Seventy early-phase schizophrenia patients (according to *DSM-IV*) were recruited and 54 were randomly allocated in a 2:1 ratio to minocycline 200 mg/d. All patients had been initiated on treatment with an atypical antipsychotic ≤ 14 days prior to study entry (risperidone, olanzapine, quetiapine, or clozapine; 200–600 mg/d chlorpromazine-equivalent doses). Clinical, cognitive, and functional assessments were conducted, with the Scale for the Assessment of Negative Symptoms (SANS) as the primary outcome measure.

Results.—Minocycline was well tolerated, with few adverse events. It showed a beneficial effect on negative symptoms and general outcome (evident in SANS, Clinical Global Impressions scale). A similar pattern was found for cognitive functioning, mainly in executive functions (working memory, cognitive shifting, and cognitive planning).

Conclusions.—Minocycline treatment was associated with improvement in negative symptoms and executive functioning, both related to frontal-lobe activity. Overall, the findings support the beneficial effect of minocycline add-on therapy in early-phase schizophrenia.

Trial Registration.—clinicaltrials.gov Identifier: NCT00733057.

▶ Most current antipsychotics have limited efficacy against 2 of the most important aspects of schizophrenia: negative symptoms and cognitive deficits. Minocycline is a second-generation tetracycline that has been shown to have beneficial effects in various neurological disorders, and it was the hope that it would have these types of effects in schizophrenia. In this trial, 54 patients were treated initially with an atypical antipsychotic and then had minocycline added as an adjunctive treatment. In fact, it did show beneficial effects on negative symptoms and general outcome and in many ways for cognitive function, particularly in executive functions, including memory, cognitive shift, and cognitive planning. It is certainly an exciting trial, and I look forward to replications and further exploration of this interesting agent with actions on the glutamate system.

J. C. Ballenger, MD

Cognitive Effects of Antipsychotic Drugs in First-Episode Schizophrenia and Schizophreniform Disorder: A Randomized, Open-Label Clinical Trial (EUFEST)

Davidson M, Galderisi S, Weiser M, et al (Sheba Med Ctr, Tel-Hashomer, Israel; Univ of Naples SUN, Italy; Med Univ of Innsbruck, Austria; et al)
Am J Psychiatry 166:675-682, 2009

Objective.—Cognitive impairment, manifested as mild to moderate deviations from psychometric norms, is present in many but not all schizophrenia patients. The purpose of the present study was to compare the effect of haloperidol with that of second-generation antipsychotic drugs on the cognitive performance of patients with schizophreniform disorder or first-episode schizophrenia.

Methods.—Subjects were 498 patients with schizophreniform disorder or first-episode schizophrenia who were randomly assigned to open-label haloperidol (1 to 4 mg/day [N = 103]), amisulpride (200 to 800 mg/day [N = 104]), olanzapine (5 to 20 mg/day [N = 105]), quetiapine (200 to 750 mg/day [N = 104]), or ziprasidone (40 to 160 mg/day [N = 82]). The Rey Auditory Verbal Learning Test, Trail Making Test Part A and Part B, WAIS Digit Symbol Test, and Purdue Pegboard Test were administered at baseline and the 6-month follow-up evaluation.

Results.—Compared with scores at baseline, composite cognitive test scores improved for all five treatment groups at the 6-month follow-up evaluation. However, there were no overall differences among the treatment groups. In addition, there was a weak correlation between the degree of cognitive improvement and changes in Positive and Negative Syndrome Scale scores.

Conclusion.—Treatment with antipsychotic medication is associated with moderate improvement in the cognitive test performance of patients who have schizophreniform disorder or who are in their first episode of schizophrenia. The magnitude of improvement does not differ between treatment with haloperidol and treatment with second-generation antipsychotics. Moreover, cognitive improvement is weakly related to symptom change.

▶ Studies now tell us that much of the disability in schizophrenia and schizophreniform disorders is secondary to the cognitive dysfunction caused by these illnesses. One promise of the second-generation antipsychotics is that many studies have demonstrated greater improvement in cognitive performance in people with schizophrenia with the second-generation antipsychotics versus the first generation. This study had 498 patients randomly assigned to the first-generation haloperidol (1-4 mg a day), amisulpride (200-800 mg a day), olanzapine (5-0 mg a day), quetiapine (200-750 mg a day), or ziprasidone (40-160 mg a day). This is the largest number of second-generation antipsychotics to be compared with a first generation antipsychotic. Surprisingly, the cognitive test scores improved in all 5 treatment groups at the 6 months evaluation. However, there were no overall differences among the treatment groups. Interestingly, the cognitive improvement was somewhat related to symptom improvement. This particularly well-done study would not support the suggestions from other trials that second-generation antipsychotics have greater ability to improve cognition in schizophrenia. This question remains an open one.

Cuesta et al[1] compared olanzapine and risperidone in first-episode psychosis (schizophrenia). These authors were able to estimate how significant the cognitive improvement was with olanzapine and risperidone. In contrast to Davidson et al's article where improvement with the various medications was described as moderate, in this trial, improvement ranged from 17% to 54%. Most improvement appeared related to greater difficulties at baseline and poorer academic performance and IQ.

J. C. Ballenger, MD

Reference

1. Cuesta MJ, Jalon EG, Campos MS, Peralta V. Cognitive effectiveness of olanzapine and risperidone in first-episode psychosis. *B J Psychiatry.* 2009;194:439-445.

Efficacy and effectiveness of individual family intervention on social and clinical functioning and family burden in severe schizophrenia: a 2-year randomized controlled study

Girón M, Fernández-Yañez A, Mañá-Alvarenga S, et al (Univ Miguel Hernández, Alacant, Spain; Florida-Babel Mental Health Centre, Alacant, Spain; Petrer Mental Health Centre, Spain; et al)
Psychol Med 40:73-84, 2010

Background.—Empirical evidence of the efficacy and effectiveness of psychosocial family intervention and of the specificity of its effects on the course of schizophrenia is limited. The aim was to study the efficacy and effectiveness of psychosocial family intervention with regard to clinical and social functioning and family burden after controlling for compliance and several prognostic factors.

Method.—A 2-year randomized controlled trial with blind assessments. Fifty patients with DSM-IV schizophrenia and persistent positive symptoms and/or previous clinical relapse were allocated to psychosocial family intervention, individual counselling and standard treatment *versus* individual counselling and standard treatment.

Results.—Family intervention was associated with fewer clinical relapses, hospitalizations and major incidents, and an improvement in positive and negative symptoms, social role performance, social relations, employment and family burden. The reduction in hospitalizations in the family intervention group was significantly greater than that observed in the group of patients who refused to participate but this was not the case for the control group. The effects of family intervention were independent of compliance and prognostic factors.

Conclusions.—Family intervention is effective in severe schizophrenia independently of compliance and prognostic factors.

▶ This is a striking study of 50 patients with schizophrenia with persistent positive symptoms who were randomly allocated to a psychosocial family intervention with individual counseling and standard treatment versus just individual counseling and standard treatment. The results were striking in that the family intervention group had fewer clinical relapses, hospitalizations, improvement in positive and negative symptoms, social relations, employment, and family burden. The effects in this study would suggest that a cost-effectiveness study would probably demonstrate that this is cost effective and ought to be more widely applied.

J. C. Ballenger, MD

A 24-Week, Multicenter, Open-Label, Randomized Study to Compare Changes in Glucose Metabolism in Patients With Schizophrenia Receiving Treatment With Olanzapine, Quetiapine, or Risperidone

Newcomer JW, Ratner RE, Eriksson JW, et al (Washington Univ School of Medicine, St Louis, MO; MedStar Res Inst, Hyattsville, MD; Sahlgrenska Univ Hosp, Gothenburg, Sweden; et al)
J Clin Psychiatry 70:487-499, 2009

Objective.—This randomized, 24-week, flexible-dose study compared changes in glucose metabolism in patients with DSM-IV schizophrenia receiving initial exposure to olanzapine, quetiapine, or risperidone.

Method.—The hypothesized primary endpoint was change (baseline to week 24) in area under the curve (AUC) 0- to 2-hour plasma glucose values during an oral glucose tolerance test (OGTT); primary analysis: olanzapine versus quetiapine. Secondary endpoints included mean change in AUC 0- to 2-hour plasma insulin values, insulin sensitivity index, and fasting lipids. The first patient enrolled on April 29, 2004, and the last patient completed the study on October 24, 2005.

Results.—Mean weight change (kg) over 24 weeks was +3.7 (quetiapine), +4.6 (olanzapine), and +3.6 (risperidone). Based on data from 395 patients (quetiapine, N − 115 [mean dose = 607.0 mg/day], olanzapine, N = 146 [mean dose = 15.2 mg/day], and risperidone, N = 134 [mean dose = 5.2 mg/day]), mean change in AUC 0- to 2-hour glucose value (mg/dL × h) at week 24 was significantly lower for quetiapine versus olanzapine (t = 1.98, df = 377, p = .048). Increases in AUC 0- to 2-hour glucose values were statistically significant with olanzapine (+21.9 mg/dL × h, 95% CI = 11.5 to 32.4 mg/dL × h) and risperidone (+18.8 mg/dL × h, 95% CI = 8.1 to 29.4 mg/dL × h), but not quetiapine (+9.1 mg/dL × h, 95% CI = −2.3 to 20.5 mg/dL × h). AUC 0- to 2-hour insulin values increased statistically significantly with olanzapine (+24.5%, 95% CI = 11.5% to 39.0%), but not with quetiapine or risperidone. Reductions in insulin sensitivity index were statistically significant with olanzapine (−19.1%, 95% CI = −27.9% to −9.3%) and risperidone (-15.8%, 95% CI = −25.1% to −5.4%), but not quetiapine. Total cholesterol and low-density lipoprotein levels increased statistically significantly with olanzapine (+21.1 mg/dL, 95% CI = 13.0 to 29.2 mg/dL, and +20.5 mg/dL, 95% CI = 13.8 to 27.1 mg/dL, respectively) and quetiapine (+13.1 mg/dL, 95% CI = 4.3 to 21.9 mg/dL, and +13.3 mg/dL, 95% CI = 6.1 to 20.5 mg/dL, respectively), but not risperidone. Statistically significant increases in triglycerides (+30.9 mg/dL, 95% CI = 10.9 to 51.0 mg/dL), total cholesterol/high-density lipoprotein (HDL) ratio (0.5, 95% CI = 0.2 to 0.8), and triglyceride/HDL ratio (0.3, 95% CI = 0.0 to 0.6) were observed with olanzapine only.

Conclusion.—The results indicate a significant difference in the change in glucose tolerance during 6 months' treatment with olanzapine versus quetiapine, with significant reductions on olanzapine and risperidone, but not quetiapine; these differential changes were largely explained by changes in insulin sensitivity.

Trial Registration.—clinicaltrials.gov Identifier: NCT00214578.

▶ The arrival of the second-generation antipsychotics (called atypicals initially) was suggested to be revolutionary by many authors and clinicians. In many studies, they do show greater promise in schizophrenia with greater efficacy in certain areas (eg, negative symptoms, depression, cognition) and are certainly better tolerated by patients. This has made them more widely used in the outpatient setting, and in particular in other conditions than the original labeled conditions of schizophrenia and bipolar illness. They are now widely used in treatment resistant depression, and treatment resistant anxiety, as well as in some insomnia difficulties in patients with psychiatric disorders, and in substance abuse, aggression, etc. However, their biggest drawback (beyond cost) has been the worry of increased weight gain and metabolic changes in insulin sensitivity and poor glucose control and lipid metabolism. The literature continues to evolve, but clearly finds the greatest difficulties in these areas with clozapine and olanzapine. There remain questions about the risks and liabilities with the other SGAs, particularly quetiapine, risperidone, and aripiprazole. This study is a large study ($N = 395$ patients) on quetiapine, olanzapine, and risperidone. The mean changes in glucose measured by a 2-hour glucose tolerance test (GTT) was significantly lower for quetiapine versus olanzapine with significant increases seen in 2-hour GTT with olanzapine and risperidone but not quetiapine. The 2-hour insulin values also increased with olanzapine but not quetiapine or risperidone, and the insulin sensitivity index was significantly different for olanzapine and risperidone but not quetiapine. The total cholesterol also increased with olanzapine and quetiapine but not risperidone. There were significant increases in triglycerides, total cholesterol/high-density lipoprotein (HDL) changes only with olanzapine. These studies are consistent with the literature as a whole suggesting that these problematic side effects are primarily observed with olanzapine and clozapine. Unfortunately, these 2 medications also appear to be the most effective against psychosis. Clozapine and olanzapine trials use has mutated over time to a second line use in many practices because of these metabolic changes.

J. C. Ballenger, MD

General Psychiatry

Does Clozapine Promote Employability and Reduce Offending Among Mentally Disordered Offenders?

Balbuena L, Mela M, Wong S, et al (Carleton Univ, Ottawa, Ontario; Univ of Saskatchewan, Saskatoon; Inst of Mental Health, Nottingham, UK; et al)
Can J Psychiatry 55:50-56, 2010

Objective.—To compare employment pay, count of infractions, and clinical symptoms in psychiatric inmates treated with clozapine or other antipsychotics after 6 months of treatment.

Methods.—Clinical charts and institutional offence records of psychiatric inmates ($n = 98$), comprised of those on clozapine ($n = 65$) and on other antipsychotics ($n = 33$), were reviewed at baseline and after 6 months of treatment. The outcome measures used were Brief Psychiatric Rating Scale (BPRS) scores, employment pay, medication compliance, and the frequency of institutional offences. A binary logistic regression model was used to analyze a categorical change in pay variable, while a negative binomial model was used to analyze the frequency of infractions.

Results.—Treatment with clozapine was associated with greater odds of a pay increase (OR = 3.13; 95% CI 1.3 to 7.53, $P = 0.01$). However, patients on other antipsychotics had a more favourable improvement in BPRS ($F = 5.44$, $df = 1,57$, $P = 0.02$). Patients on other antipsychotics also had a higher count of posttreatment offences (Incidence Rate Ratio = 2.22; 95% CI 1.11 to 4.41, $P = 0.02$).

Conclusion.—Clozapine probably has a favourable effect on inmate behaviour and institutional adjustment. This effect can last up to 36 months after the initial dose.

▶ The use of clozapine in psychotic patients has been suggested to have several remarkable benefits, including a 30% response rate in the treatment of nonresponsive patients and reduction of suicide. These authors demonstrated that treatment with clozapine was also associated with better chances of having pay increases or reduced incidence of criminal offenses when compared with other antipsychotics. There is increasing evidence that we should be using clozapine more frequently than we have because it has largely been relegated to a last-resort antipsychotic.

J. C. Ballenger, MD

Early outcomes and predictors in 260 patients with psychogenic nonepileptic attacks

McKenzie P, Oto M, Russell A, et al (Southern General Hosp, Glasgow, Scotland; et al)
Neurology 74:64-69, 2010

Objective.—To determine short-term outcome and its predictors in patients with psychogenic nonepileptic attacks (PNEA).

Methods.—Retrospective cohort study of outcomes relating to attendance at follow-up, spells, use of emergency services, employment, and social security payments recorded at 6 and 12 months post diagnosis in 260 consecutive patients.

Results.—A total of 187 patients (71.9%) attended at least 1 follow-up visit, and 105 patients (40.4%) attended 2. A total of 71/187 patients (38.0%) were spell-free at last follow-up. In contrast, 35/187 patients (18.7%) had marked increase in spell frequency postdiagnosis. Delay to diagnosis had no relationship to outcome. Patients with anxiety or depression were 2.32 times less likely to become spell-free ($p = 0.012$), and patients drawing social security payments at baseline were 2.34 times less likely to become spell-free ($p = 0.014$), than patients without those factors. Men were 2.46 times more likely to become spell-free than women ($p = 0.016$). While 93/187 patients (49.7%) were using emergency medical services at baseline, only 29/187 (15.5%) were using them at follow-up ($p < 0.001$). This was independent of whether or not the patient became spell-free.

Conclusion.—A substantial minority of our patients became spell-free with communication of the diagnosis the only intervention. Previous psychiatric diagnoses, social security payments, and gender were important predictors of outcome. Most patients stopped using emergency services, irrespective of whether or not spells continued. Outcomes other than spell frequency may be important in patients with psychogenic nonepileptic attacks.

▶ These authors followed what has always been a fascinating group to me, that is, patients who have psychogenic nonepileptic attacks. They followed 187 patients for whom the only intervention was making the diagnosis. This single intervention lead to improvement in a large number of these patients. At follow-up in 12 months after diagnosis, 38% were spell free, while 18.7% had marked increases in their spell frequency. Those with anxiety and depression were less likely to improve, and those receiving social security payments were 2.34 times less likely to become spell free. Interestingly, while almost half were using emergency medical services before diagnosis, this fell to 15.5% whether they became spell free or not. It is a little surprising to me that just making the diagnosis would be so helpful, but it is an encouraging result nonetheless.

J. C. Ballenger, MD

Effects of Olanzapine and Haloperidol on the Metabolic Status of Healthy Men
Vidarsdottir S, de Leeuw van Weenen JE, Frölich M, et al (Leiden Univ Med Ctr, The Netherlands)
J Clin Endocrinol Metab 95:118-125, 2010

Background.—A large body of evidence suggests that antipsychotic drugs cause body weight gain and type 2 diabetes mellitus, and atypical (new generation) drugs appear to be most harmful. The aim of this study was to determine the effect of short-term olanzapine (atypical antipsychotic drug) and haloperidol (conventional antipsychotic drug) treatment on glucose and lipid metabolism.

Research Design and Methods.—Healthy normal-weight men were treated with olanzapine (10 mg/d; n = 7) or haloperidol (3 mg/d, n = 7) for 8 d. Endogenous glucose production, whole body glucose disposal (by [6,6-^{2}H$_2$]glucose dilution), lipolysis (by [^{2}H$_5$]glycerol dilution), and substrate oxidation rates (by indirect calorimetry) were measured before and after intervention in basal and hyperinsulinemic condition.

Results.—Olanzapine hampered insulin-mediated glucose disposal (by 1.3 mg·kg^{-1}·min^{-1}), whereas haloperidol did not have a significant effect. Endogenous glucose production was not affected by either drug. Also, the glycerol rate of appearance (a measure of lipolysis rate) was not affected by either drug. Olanzapine, but not haloperidol, blunted the insulin-induced decline of plasma free fatty acid and triglyceride concentrations. Fasting free fatty acid concentrations declined during olanzapine treatment, whereas they did not during treatment with haloperidol.

Conclusions.—Short-term treatment with olanzapine reduces fasting plasma free fatty acid concentrations and hampers insulin action on glucose disposal in healthy men, whereas haloperidol has less clear effects. Moreover, olanzapine, but not haloperidol, blunts the insulin-induced decline of plasma free fatty acids and triglyceride concentrations. Notably, these effects come about without a measurable change of body fat mass.

▶ One of the important and controversial areas that we have followed in our reviews is the metabolic issues with the second-generation antipsychotics. These authors studied a small group of healthy normal weight men who were treated with olanzapine or haloperidol, and insulin measures were closely followed. Olanzapine did change and hamper insulin-mediated glucose disposal, but haloperidol did not. Olanzapine, but not haloperidol, blunted the insulin-induced decline of plasma free acid and triglyceride concentrations. The fasting free fatty acids were reduced during olanzapine treatment but not during haloperidol treatment. These effects occurred without a measurable change in body fat and mass. This is one more piece of evidence further clarifying the effects on glucose insulin and triglycerides with olanzapine.

J. C. Ballenger, MD

Which Physician and Practice Characteristics are Associated With Adherence to Evidence-Based Guidelines for Depressive and Anxiety Disorders?
Smolders M, Laurant M, Verhaak P, et al (Radboud Univ Nijmegen Med Centre [RUNMC], The Netherlands; Netherlands Inst for Health Services Res, Utrecht; et al)
Med Care 48:240-248, 2010

Background.—Research on quality of care for depressive and anxiety disorders has reported low rates of adherence to evidence-based depression and anxiety guidelines. To improve this care, we need a better understanding of the factors determining guideline adherence.

Objective.—To investigate how practice- and professional-related factors are associated with adherence to these guidelines.

Design.—Cross-sectional cohort study.

Participants.—A total of 665 patients with a composite interview diagnostic instrument diagnosis of depressive or anxiety disorders, and 62 general practitioners from 21 practices participated.

Measures.—Actual care data were derived from electronic medical record data. The measurement of guideline adherence was based on performance indicators derived from evidence-based guidelines. Practice-, professional-, and patient-related characteristics were measured with questionnaires. The characteristics associated with guideline adherence were assessed by multivariate multilevel regression analysis.

Results.—A number of practice and professional characteristics showed a significant univariate association with guideline adherence. The multivariate multilevel analyses revealed that, after controlling for patient characteristics, higher rates of guideline adherence were associated with stronger confidence in depression identification, less perceived time limitations, and less perceived barriers for guideline implementation. These professional-related determinants differed among the overall concept of guideline adherence and the various treatment options.

Conclusions.—This study showed that rates of adherence to guidelines on depressive and anxiety disorders were not associated with practice characteristics, but to some extent with physician characteristics. Although most of the identified professional-related determinants are very difficult to change, our results give some directions for improving depression and anxiety care.

▶ One of the most distressing things in the field of developing guidelines for treatment is that no matter how good they are, they are frequently not followed by most practitioners. It is unclear why this occurs, but issues about practice characteristics and physician characteristics have been shown to influence adherence and nonadherence. In this study, the authors studied 655 patients and 62 general practitioners from 21 practices. They were in fact able to show higher rates of adherence to the guidelines in the physicians with stronger confidence in their ability to identify depression, fewer perceived time limitations, and fewer perceived barriers for implementation of guidelines. It does provide some of the areas where we might work to change these issues, albeit changing some characteristics will be difficult.

J. C. Ballenger, MD

Efficacy and safety of quetiapine in critically ill patients with delirium: A prospective, multicenter, randomized, double-blind, placebo-controlled pilot study
Devlin JW, Roberts RJ, Fong JJ, et al (Northeastern Univ School of Pharmacy, Boston, MA; Massachusetts College of Pharmacy, Worcestor; et al)
Crit Care Med 38:419-427, 2010

Objective.—To compare the efficacy and safety of scheduled quetiapine to placebo for the treatment of delirium in critically ill patients requiring as-needed haloperidol.

Design.—Prospective, randomized, double-blind, placebo-controlled study.

Setting.—Three academic medical centers.

Patients.—Thirty-six adult intensive care unit patients with delirium (Intensive Care Delirium Screening Checklist score ≥4), tolerating enteral nutrition, and without a complicating neurologic condition.

Interventions.—Patients were randomized to receive quetiapine 50 mg every 12 hrs or placebo. Quetiapine was increased every 24 hrs (50 to 100 to 150 to 200 mg every 12 hrs) if more than one dose of haloperidol was given in the previous 24 hrs. Study drug was continued until the intensive care unit team discontinued it because of delirium resolution, therapy ≥10 days, or intensive care unit discharge.

Measurements and Main Results.—Baseline characteristics were similar between the quetiapine (n = 18) and placebo (n = 18) groups. Quetiapine was associated with a shorter time to first resolution of delirium [1.0 (interquartile range [IQR], 0.5–3.0) vs. 4.5 days (IQR, 2.0–7.0; $p = .001$)], a reduced duration of delirium [36 (IQR, 12–87) vs. 120 hrs (IQR, 60–195; $p = .006$)], and less agitation (Sedation-Agitation Scale score ≥5) [6 (IQR, 0–38) vs. 36 hrs (IQR, 11–66; $p = .02$)]. Whereas mortality (11% quetiapine vs. 17%) and intensive care unit length of stay (16 quetiapine vs. 16 days) were similar, subjects treated with quetiapine were more likely to be discharged home or to rehabilitation (89% quetiapine vs. 56%; $p = .06$). Subjects treated with quetiapine required fewer days of as-needed haloperidol [3 [(IQR, 2–4)] vs. 4 days (IQR, 3–8; $p = .05$)]. Whereas the incidence of QTc prolongation and extrapyramidal symptoms was similar between groups, more somnolence was observed with quetiapine (22% vs. 11%; $p = .66$).

Conclusions.—Quetiapine added to as-needed haloperidol results in faster delirium resolution, less agitation, and a greater rate of transfer to home or rehabilitation. Future studies should evaluate the effect of quetiapine on mortality, resource utilization, post-intensive care unit cognition, and dependency after discharge in a broader group of patients.

▶ This study compares the previous standard of care, haloperidol, with the new second-generation antipsychotic quetiapine in treating delirium in critically ill patients in 3 academic medical centers. Patients received either quetiapine or placebo, with intensive care unit (ICU) patients in each group.

Quetiapine was initiated at 50 mg every 12 hours and was increased every 24 hours to 200 mg in 12 hour intervals. Those on quetiapine had shorter time to resolution of delirium and less agitation, mortality was similar (11% on quetiapine vs 17%) as was ICU length of stay (both 16 days), but the quetiapine subjects were more likely to be discharged home or to rehab (89% vs 56%) and had fewer days of the as-needed haloperidol rescue medication. While some results with the second-generation antipsychotics in dementia patients have been worrisome, this study documents that quetiapine given to seriously ill delirious patients actually reduced delirium and other complications and led to more rapid rehabilitation of these patients. To me, this was a surprisingly positive result.

J. C. Ballenger, MD

Cognitive behavioral therapy versus paroxetine in the treatment of hypochondriasis: An 18-month naturalistic follow-up

Greeven A, van Balkom AJLM, van der Leeden R, et al (Leiden Univ, The Netherlands; VU-Univ Med Centre, Amsterdam, The Netherlands; et al)
J Behav Ther Exp Psychiatry 40:487-496, 2009

Background.—The present maintenance study investigated whether the reduction in hypochondriacal complaints after initial treatment with CBT or paroxetine sustained during a follow-up period and whether psychiatric severity at pretest predicted the course of hypochondriacal symptoms.

Method.—A naturalistic follow-up period of 18 months after a 16-week RCT consisting of 33 patients initially allocated to a CBT condition and 29 patients to a paroxetine condition. The main outcome measure was the Whiteley Index.

Results.—The initial treatment effect of CBT and paroxetine sustained during the follow-up period. No significant differences between CBT and paroxetine were found. Treatment course could not be predicted by psychiatric comorbidity.

Conclusion.—CBT and paroxetine are both effective treatments for hypochondriasis in the long term.

▶ Hypochondriasis is certainly a difficult condition to treat, and good scientific study of its treatments have been slow in evolving. This article reviewed a maintenance study with a naturalistic follow-up study after a 16-week randomized controlled trial of 33 patients treated with Cognitive Behavior Therapy (CBT) versus 29 patients with paroxetine. Interestingly, the significantly positive treatment effects of both treatments were sustained throughout the follow-up period without significant differences between them. Both treatments were effective. This trial is somewhat different from most in that treatment results were sustained in the paroxetine cell equally well as in the CBT cell. This study and the original one gives us considerable guidance that this condition can and should be treated rather than just considered a problematic personality type.

J. C. Ballenger, MD

Adult Outcomes of Youth Irritability: A 20-year Prospective Community-Based Study
Stringaris A, Cohen P, Pine DS, et al (Mood and Anxiety Program, NIMH, Bethesda, MD; New York State Psychiatric Inst)
Am J Psychiatry 166:1048-1054, 2009

Objective.—Irritability is a widely occurring DSM-IV symptom in youths. However, little is known about the relationship between irritability in early life and its outcomes in mid-adulthood. This study examines the extent to which youth irritability is related to adult psychiatric outcomes by testing the hypothesis that it predicts depressive and generalized anxiety disorders.

Method.—The authors conducted a longitudinal community-based study of 631 participants whose parents were interviewed when participants were in early adolescence (mean age = 13.8 years [SD = 2.6]) and who were themselves interviewed 20 years later (mean age = 33.2 years [SD = 2.9]). Parent-reported irritability in adolescence was used to predict self-reported psychopathology, assessed by standardized diagnostic interview at 20-year follow-up.

Results.—Cross-sectionally, irritability in adolescence was widely associated with other psychiatric disorders. After adjustment for baseline emotional and behavioral disorders, irritability in adolescence predicted major depressive disorder (odds ratio = 1.33, 95% confidence interval [CI] – 1.00–1.78]), generalized anxiety disorder (odds ratio = 1.72, 95% CI = 1.04–2.87), and dysthymia (odds ratio = 1.81, 95% CI = 1.06–3.12) at 20-year follow-up. Youth irritability did not predict bipolar disorder or axis II disorders at follow-up.

Conclusions.—Youth irritability as reported by parents is a specific predictor of self-reported depressive and anxiety disorders 20 years later. The role of irritability in developmental psychiatry, and in the pathophysiology of mood and anxiety disorders specifically, should receive further study.

▶ These authors conducted a longitudinal community-based study of 631 children whose parents were interviewed when the children were in early adolescence. These individuals were interviewed themselves 20 years later (mean age 33.2 years). Those individuals whose parents reported irritability in them in adolescence had more psychiatric disorders, including major depressive disorder and generalized anxiety disorder and dysthymia, but not bipolar disorder. To my knowledge, this type of work with irritability in childhood is underdeveloped in our field, particularly given that this study strongly suggests it may be a major predictor of adult difficulties.

J. C. Ballenger, MD

Did Medicare Part D Improve Access to Medications?
Domino ME, Farley JF (Univ of North Carolina at Chapel Hill)
Psychiatr Serv 61:118-120, 2010

This study examined medication use among Medicare beneficiaries and dually eligible beneficiaries before and after the implementation of Medicare Part D on January 1, 2006. Nationally representative 2004–2006 data from the Medical Expenditure Panel Survey were used. Two large classes of psychotropic medications (antidepressant and antipsychotic medications) and two large classes of nonpsychotropic medications (lipid-lowering and antihypertensive agents) were examined to determine whether changes in prescription patterns occurred as a result of the implementation of Part D. There was no strong evidence that Part D was associated with large changes in access to medications in the four classes of medications examined here.

▶ After implementation of Medicare Part D in January 1, 2006, I certainly hoped that there would be improvement in the availability of treatment with psychotropic and other medications. However, this article documents that there has been little evidence that Part D has been associated with any large increase in access in psychiatric medicines, lipid-lowering agents, or any antihypertensive medications. This is a disappointing result (and an expensive one), and one would have to wonder whether the recently approved Obama-Care will correct this.

J. C. Ballenger, MD

Does the judicious use of safety behaviors improve the efficacy and acceptability of exposure therapy for claustrophic fear?
Deacon BJ, Sy JT, Lickel JJ, et al (Univ of Wyoming, Laramie)
J Behav Ther Exp Psychiatry 41:71-80, 2010

Exposure therapy is traditionally conducted with an emphasis on the elimination of safety behaviors. However, theorists have recently suggested that the judicious use of safety behaviors may improve the tolerability of this treatment without reducing its efficacy. The present study tested this notion by randomly assigning participants with high claustrophobic fear to receive a single-session intervention with or without access to safety aids during early exposure trials. Improvement was generally equivalent between the treatment conditions, and no reliable benefits or drawbacks were associated with the judicious use of safety behaviors. The theoretical and clinical implications of these findings are discussed.

▶ It has been a raging debate in the field whether exposure therapy is somehow interfered with if we allow patients to use safety behaviors. Recently, therapists have suggested that careful use of some safety behaviors may help with tolerability of this treatment without reducing its effectiveness, and this certainly seems clinically rational. Although this study was only in a group with high claustrophobic fears and in a single session intervention, these authors did not demonstrate any negative or positive difference by judicious use of safety behaviors. This is an important debate because the consistent 25% refusal rates for exposure therapy greatly reduces the effectiveness of this excellent treatment.

J. C. Ballenger, MD

Low early-life social class leaves a biological residue manifested by decreased glucocorticoid and increased proinflammatory signaling
Miller GE, Chen E, Fok AK, et al (Univ of British Columbia, Vancouver, Canada; et al)
Proc Natl Acad Sci U S A 106:14716-14721, 2009

Children reared in unfavorable socioeconomic circumstances show increased susceptibility to the chronic diseases of aging when they reach the fifth and sixth decades of life. One mechanistic hypothesis for this phenomenon suggests that social adversity in early life programs biological systems in a manner that persists across decades and thereby accentuates vulnerability to disease. Here we examine the basic tenets of this hypothesis by performing genome-wide transcriptional profiling in healthy adults who were either low or high in socioeconomic status (SES) in early life. Among subjects with low early-life SES, there was significant up-regulation of genes bearing response elements for the CREB/ATF family of transcription factors that conveys adrenergic signals to leukocytes, and significant down-regulation of genes with response elements for the glucocorticoid receptor, which regulates the secretion of cortisol and transduces its antiinflammatory actions in the immune system. Subjects from low-SES backgrounds also showed increased output of cortisol in daily life, heightened expression of transcripts bearing response elements for NF-κB, and greater stimulated production of the proinflammatory cytokine interleukin 6. These disparities were independent of subjects' current SES, lifestyle practices, and perceived stress. Collectively, these data suggest that low early-life SES programs a defensive phenotype characterized by resistance to glucocorticoid signaling, which in turn facilitates exaggerated adrenocortical and inflammatory responses. Although these response patterns could serve adaptive functions during acute threats to well-being, over the long term they might exact an allostatic toll on the body that ultimately contributes to the chronic diseases of aging.

▶ We have repeatedly observed that early adversity leads to long lasting vulnerability. This study observes a distressing finding that patients who, as children, were in low socioeconomic situations (SES) experienced long lasting significant upregulations of the genes leading to CREB/ATF transcription factors. These convey adrenergic input to leukocytes, as well as significant down regulation of the genes controlling the glucocorticoid receptor regulating cortisol. These differences were independent of their current socioeconomic status or lifestyle or even their perceived stress. The authors suggest that these data indicate that low early life SES leaves an individual with a defensive phenotype characterized by resistance to glucocorticoid negative feedback which then leads to increased cortisol secretion and increased inflammatory responses. The suggestion is that these changes are helpful when they were in an adverse early experience, but are definitely damaging over the entire life and that one does not outgrow this early difficulty. As I stated in response to another article, it seems very clear that in early life we are vulnerable to adversity of all types, and this often leads to lifelong difficulties psychiatrically and physically.

J. C. Ballenger, MD

Effectiveness of second-generation antipsychotics: a naturalistic, randomized comparison of olanzapine, quetiapine, risperidone, and ziprasidone
Johnsen E, Kroken RA, Wentzel-Larsen T, et al (Haukeland Univ Hosp, Sandviken, Bergen, Norway)
BMC Psychiatry 10:26, 2010

Background.—No clear recommendations exist regarding which antipsychotic drug should be prescribed first for a patient suffering from psychosis. The primary aims of this naturalistic study were to assess the head-to-head effectiveness of first-line second-generation antipsychotics with regards to time until drug discontinuation, duration of index admission, time until readmission, change of psychopathology scores and tolerability outcomes.

Methods.—Patients $\geq$ 18 years of age admitted to the emergency ward for symptoms of psychosis were consecutively randomized to risperidone (n = 53), olanzapine (n = 52), quetiapine (n = 50), or ziprasidone (n = 58), and followed for up to 2 years.

Results.—A total of 213 patients were included, of which 68% were males. The sample represented a diverse population suffering from psychosis. At admittance the mean Positive and Negative Syndrome Scale (PANSS) total score was 74 points and 44% were antipsychotic drug naïve. The primary intention-to-treat analyses revealed no substantial differences between the drugs regarding the times until discontinuation of initial drug, until discharge from index admission, or until readmission.

Quetiapine was superior to risperidone and olanzapine in reducing the PANSS total score and the positive subscore. Quetiapine was superior to the other drugs in decreasing the PANSS general psychopathology subscore; in decreasing the Clinical Global Impression - Severity of Illness scale score (CGI-S); and in increasing the Global Assessment of Functioning - Split version, Functions scale score (GAF-F). Ziprasidone was superior to risperidone in decreasing the PANSS positive symptoms subscore and the CGI-S score, and in increasing the GAF-F score. The drugs performed equally with regards to most tolerability outcomes except a higher increase of hip-circumference per day for olanzapine compared to risperidone, and more galactorrhoea for risperidone compared to the other groups.

Conclusions.—Quetiapine appears to be a good starting drug candidate in this sample of patients admitted to hospital for symptoms of psychosis.

Trial Registration.—ClinicalTrials.gov ID; URL: http://www.clinicaltrials. gov/: NCT00932529.

▶ In this naturalistic 24-month effectiveness trial, the second-generation antipsychotics were compared (without industry funding). The patients (n = 213) were randomly assigned to olanzapine, quetiapine, risperidone, or ziprasidone. Patients were followed for 2 years. Assignment was not entirely random. Quetiapine was consistently superior to the other agents in terms of the Positive and Negative Syndrome Scale total score, positive symptoms, general psychopathology subscore, Clinical Global Impression - Severity of Illness scale score, and Global Assessment of Functioning - Split version, Functions scale scores. It was not superior in the negative symptoms or depressive symptoms. There were few differences in tolerability, although risperidone patients had greater weight gain and required more anticholinergics (27% vs 0%-13%). Most studies and meta-analyses find little effectiveness differences in these second-generation antipsychotics. This study did. This may be because they had more antipsychotic naïve patients (44%) than other studies. Also, it was a relatively small study, and that may have prevented smaller differences from being discerned.

J. C. Ballenger, MD

Cost-effectiveness of a stepped care intervention to prevent depression and anxiety in late life: randomised trial
van't Veer-Tazelaar P, Smit F, van Hout H, et al (Vrije Universiteit [VU] Medical Centre, Amsterdam, The Netherlands; VU Med Centre, Amsterdam, The Netherlands)
Br J Psychiatry 196:319-325, 2010

Background.—There is an urgent need for the development of cost-effective preventive strategies to reduce the onset of mental disorders.

Aims.—To establish the cost-effectiveness of a stepped care preventive intervention for depression and anxiety disorders in older people at high risk of these conditions, compared with routine primary care.

Method.—An economic evaluation was conducted alongside a pragmatic randomised controlled trial (ISRCTN26474556). Consenting individuals presenting with subthreshold levels of depressive or anxiety symptoms were randomly assigned to a preventive stepped care programme ($n = 86$) or to routine primary care ($n = 84$).

Results.—The intervention was successful in halving the incidence rate of depression and anxiety at €563 (£412) per recipient and €4367 (£3196) per disorder-free year gained, compared with routine primary care. The latter would represent good value for money if the willingness to pay for a disorder-free year is at least €5000.

Conclusions.—The prevention programme generated depression- and anxiety-free survival years in the older population at affordable cost.

▶ These investigators studied a pragmatic randomized controlled trial of adults with subthreshold levels of anxiety and depression, who were either randomly followed or put into a preventive stepped care program. Interestingly, they were able to clearly reduce the incident rate of depression and anxiety by half. They were also able to demonstrate decreased cost of €563 per recipient and cost of €4367 per disorder-free year gained compared with routine primary care. This area is open to individual values about whether preventing a year of depression or anxiety is worth this amount of money, but it is good data to demonstrate that it is possible and sharpens the questions involved in this type of policy decision.

J. C. Ballenger, MD

Consequences of Receipt of a Psychiatric Diagnosis for Completion of College
Hunt J, Eisenberg D, Kilbourne AM (Univ of Arkansas for Med Sciences, Little Rock; Univ of Michigan School of Public Health, Ann Arbor; Univ of Michigan Med School, Ann Arbor)
Psychiatr Serv 61:399-404, 2010

Objective.—The purpose of this study was to evaluate the independent associations between *DSM-IV* psychiatric disorders and the failure to complete college among college entrants.

Methods.—Data were from the 2001–2002 National Epidemiologic Survey on Alcohol and Related Conditions (NESARC). The sample included 15,800 adults, aged 22 years and older, who at least entered college. Diagnoses were made with the NESARC survey instrument, the Alcohol Use Disorder and Associated Disability Interview Schedule—DSM-IV Version. The large sample permitted analysis of multiple psychiatric disorders in the same multivariable logistic regression models. Given the frequent comorbidity of these disorders, this approach is an important step toward disentangling the independent roles of disorders in postsecondary educational outcomes.

Results.—Evaluation of the independent associations between specific psychiatric disorders and postsecondary educational attainment showed that five diagnoses were positively and significantly associated with the failure to graduate from college. Four were axis I diagnoses: bipolar I disorder, marijuana use disorder, amphetamine use disorder, and cocaine use disorder. One was an axis II diagnosis: antisocial personality disorder.

Conclusions.—This study provides new data on *DSM-IV* diagnoses associated with the failure to complete postsecondary education. The findings suggest that psychiatric factors play a significant role in college academic performance, and the benefits of prevention, detection, and treatment of psychiatric illness may therefore include higher college graduation rates.

▶ These authors used a large epidemiologic sample of 15 800 adults age 22 years and older who had entered college in 2001/2002. Not surprisingly, they found that bipolar I disorder, marijuana use disorder, amphetamine use disorder, cocaine use disorder, and antisocial personality disorder were all associated with a higher graduation failure rate. In my experience, these 5 disorders are certainly obviously associated with poor performance in college, but in fact, I am surprised that anxiety disorders and depression don't figure more prominently in this dataset. They are certainly more common and are frequent reasons in my experience for serious difficulty in completing college work.

J. C. Ballenger, MD

Association of Western and Traditional Diets With Depression and Anxiety in Women
Jacka FN, Pasco JA, Mykletun A, et al (Univ of Melbourne, Geelong, Australia)
Am J Psychiatry 167:305-311, 2010

Objective.—Key biological factors that influence the development of depression are modified by diet. This study examined the extent to which the high-prevalence mental disorders are related to habitual diet in 1,046 women ages 20–93 years randomly selected from the population.

Method.—A diet quality score was derived from answers to a food frequency questionnaire, and a factor analysis identified habitual dietary patterns. The 12-item General Health Questionnaire (GHQ-12) was used to measure psychological symptoms, and a structured clinical interview was used to assess current depressive and anxiety disorders.

Results.—After adjustments for age, socioeconomic status, education, and health behaviors, a "traditional" dietary pattern characterized by vegetables, fruit, meat, fish, and whole grains was associated with lower odds for major depression or dysthymia and for anxiety disorders.

A "western" diet of processed or fried foods, refined grains, sugary products, and beer was associated with a higher GHQ-12 score. There was also an inverse association between diet quality score and GHQ-12 score that was not confounded by age, socioeconomic status, education, or other health behaviors.

Conclusions.—These results demonstrate an association between habitual diet quality and the high-prevalence mental disorders, although reverse causality and confounding cannot be ruled out as explanations. Further prospective studies are warranted.

▶ These authors present an intriguing idea. They studied the diet in 1046 women and compared them with the 12-item General Health Questionnaire measure of current depression and anxiety symptoms. Interestingly, they found that people on a Western diet of processed or fried foods, high sugar intake, and beer and refined grains had higher symptom scores compared with those on a more Eastern traditional diet of vegetables, fruits, meats, and whole grains. It is obviously hard to know whether people with these disorders eat poorer foods or whether the poorer dietary habits lead to these symptoms, but it certainly poses an interesting question.

J. C. Ballenger, MD

Dizziness, migrainous vertigo and psychiatric disorders
Teggi R, Caldirola D, Colombo B, et al (Vita-Salute Univ, Milan, Italy)
J Laryngol Otol 124:285-290, 2010

Objectives.—This study sought to establish the prevalence of vestibular disorders, migraine and definite migrainous vertigo in patients with psychiatric disorders who were referred for treatment of dizziness, without a lifetime history of vertigo.

Study Design.—Retrospective study.

Setting.—Out-patients in a university hospital.

Materials and Methods.—Fifty-two dizzy patients with panic disorders and agoraphobia, 30 with panic disorders without agoraphobia, and 20 with depressive disorders underwent otoneurological screening with bithermal caloric stimulation. The prevalence of migraine and migrainous vertigo was assessed. The level of dizziness was evaluated using the Dizziness Handicap Inventory.

Results.—Dizzy patients with panic disorders and agoraphobia had a significantly $p = 0.05$ regarding the prevalence of peripheral vestibular abnormalities in the group of subjects with PD and agoraphobia and in those with depressive disorders. Migraine was equally represented in the three groups, but panic disorder patients had a higher prevalence of migrainous vertigo definite migrainous vertigo. Almost all patients with a peripheral vestibular disorder had a final diagnosis of definite migrainous vertigo according to Neuhauser criteria. These patients had higher

Dizziness Handicap Inventory scores. The Dizziness Handicap Inventory total score was higher in the subgroup of patients with panic disorders with agoraphobia also presenting unilateral reduced caloric responses or definite migrainous vertigo, compared with the subgroup of remaining subjects with panic disorders with agoraphobia ($p < 0.001$).

Conclusions.—Our data support the hypothesis that, in patients with panic disorders (and especially those with additional agoraphobia), dizziness may be linked to malfunction of the vestibular system. However, the data are not inconsistent with the hypothesis that migrainous vertigo is the most common pathophysiological mechanism for vestibular disorders.

▶ One of the most common symptoms that take patients to see doctors is dizziness. It is also an especially complex symptom to understand in patients with panic disorder and even with depression. In dizziness clinics, perhaps the largest group of patients are in fact those with panic disorder. In this study, the panic disorder patients had a higher prevalence of migrainous vertigo-type dizziness. It was particularly higher in the group with agoraphobia. It was these patients who had the greatest demonstrated abnormalities in caloric responses of the vestibular system. This study adds some light to this extremely murky clinical area of whether patients need ear, nose, and throat evaluation.

J. C. Ballenger, MD

State anxiety and subjective well-being responses to acute bouts of aerobic exercise in patients with depressive and anxiety disorders
Knapen J, Sommerijns E, Vancampfort D, et al (Katholieke Universiteit Leuven, Belgium; et al)
Br J Sports Med 43:756-759, 2009

Objective.—Acute aerobic exercise is associated with a reduction in state anxiety and an improvement in subjective well-being. The objective of the present study was to contrast the effects of aerobic exercise at self-selected intensity versus prescribed intensity on state anxiety and subjective well-being (negative affect, positive well-being and fatigue) in patients with depressive and/or anxiety disorders. In addition, the potential impact of heart rate feedback was assessed.

Methods.—Nineteen men and 29 women performed three test conditions on a bicycle ergometer during 20 minutes: two tests at self-selected intensity; one with and another without heart rate feedback, and a third test at the prescribed intensity of 50% of the maximal heart rate reserve according to Karvonen. Tests were executed in random order. State anxiety and subjective well-being were evaluated using the state anxiety inventory and the subjective exercise experiences scale.

Results.—After 20 minutes cycling, patients showed significantly decreased state anxiety and negative affect in the three conditions. The magnitude of the reduction did not differ significantly between the three conditions. Only cycling at self-selected intensity enhanced positive well-being. Cycling at 50% of the maximal heart rate reserve decreased fatigue, whereas cycling at self-selected intensity increased fatigue.

Conclusions.—The response in state anxiety and negative affect was unaffected by the type of aerobic exercise. Self-selected intensity influenced exercise-induced changes in positive well-being and fatigue in a positive and negative way, respectively.

▶ While I was in medical school, I spent a summer working with a very busy practitioner faculty member who treated a lot of depressed, largely middle aged people. The very successful program he implemented had liberal amounts of exercise for these largely sedentary patients. Since that time, we've learned that exercise has antidepressant activity, both on the current episode of depression and at a population level retarding the development of depression. In this trial, the authors studied 19 men and 29 women who they had perform 3 different types of aerobic exercise. The 3 conditions included 2 tests where the patients selected the intensity of the bicycle exercise, one with and one without heart rate feedback. The third condition prescribed the intensity of the workout at 50% of maximal heart rate. These were done in random order and state anxiety and subjective wellbeing were evaluated after 20 minutes of cycling. Patients did in fact have decreased state anxiety and negative affect in all 3 conditions, with improvements not differing between the conditions. However, only cycling at a self selected intensity enhanced positive wellbeing. Cycling at the 50% maximal heart rate did decrease fatigue but at the self selected intensity actually increased fatigue. It seems odd to juxtapose in these reviews a study directly stimulating the brain electrically with another showing exercise on a bicycle both being antidepressants, but that is the state of the current science in psychiatry.

J. C. Ballenger, MD

A Randomized, Double-Blind, Placebo-Controlled Trial of St John's Wort for Treating Irritable Bowel Syndrome
Saito YA, Rey E, Almazar-Elder AE, et al (Mayo Clinic, Rochester, MN; et al)
Am J Gastroenterol 105:170-177, 2010

Objectives.—St John's wort (SJW) is known to effectively treat patients with mild-to-moderate depression. Antidepressants are frequently used to treat irritable bowel syndrome (IBS). To date, no study that examines the efficacy of SJW in IBS has been carried out. The aim of this study was to evaluate the efficacy of SJW in IBS after 12 weeks.

Methods.—In this randomized, double-blind, placebo-controlled trial, 70 participants with an established diagnosis of IBS were randomized and assigned by concealed allocation to either SJW or placebo. Both treatment arms were balanced on symptom subtype. The primary end point was self-reported overall bowel symptom score (BSS) at 12 weeks.

Secondary end points were individual BSS for diarrhea (D-BSS), constipation (C-BSS), pain or discomfort, and bloating; adequate relief (AR) of IBS on at least 50% of the last 4 weeks of therapy; and IBS quality-of-life score at 12 weeks.

Results.—In all, 86% of the participants were women, and the median age was 42 years. Overall, 29% had C-IBS, 37% D-IBS, and 31% had mixed IBS. Both groups reported decreases in overall BSS from baseline, with the placebo arm having significantly lower scores at 12 weeks ($P = 0.03$) compared with SJW. These patterns of improvement were mirrored in the secondary end points with the placebo group faring better than the SJW-treated group, with significant differences observed at week 12 for D-BSS ($P = 0.03$) and percent with AR ($P = 0.02$). A similar proportion of subjects in each treatment group (SJW: 51% vs. placebo: 54%) believed that the study drug they received decreased IBS life interferences ($P = 0.79$).

Conclusions.—SJW was a less effective treatment for IBS than placebo.

▶ This is apparently the first controlled trial of St John's wort in irritable bowel syndrome where many antidepressants have been shown to be effective. The authors randomized 70 patients to St John's wort or placebo and followed them for 12 weeks. The placebo group actually did better at 12 weeks compared with those on St John's wort. This better response on placebo was mirrored on both the primary outcome measures and the secondary ones. I report this study because it is good science actually informing an area that is often plagued by beliefs and wishes that natural treatments will work better for chronic problems that have poor response to traditional treatments. However, as was the case with St John's in depression, rigorous National Institute of Health-sponsored trials failed to show that it was more effective than placebo, and this is the case again in this particular study as well.

J. C. Ballenger, MD

Miscellaneous

Cardiometabolic Risk of Second-Generation Antipsychotic Medications During First-Time Use in Children and Adolescents

Correll CU, Manu P, Olshanskiy V, et al (Zucker Hillside Hosp, Glen Oaks, NY)
JAMA 302:1765-1773, 2009

Context.—Cardiometabolic effects of second-generation antipsychotic medications are concerning but have not been sufficiently studied in pediatric and adolescent patients naive to antipsychotic medication.

Objective.—To study the association of second-generation antipsychotic medications with body composition and metabolic parameters in patients without prior antipsychotic medication exposure.

Design, Setting, and Patients.—Nonrandomized Second-Generation Antipsychotic Treatment Indications, Effectiveness and Tolerability in Youth (SATIETY) cohort study, conducted between December 2001 and

September 2007 at semi-urban, tertiary care, academic inpatient and outpatient clinics in Queens, New York, with a catchment area of 4.5-million individuals. Of 505 youth aged 4 to 19 years with 1 week or less of antipsychotic medication exposure, 338 were enrolled (66.9%). Of these patients, 272 had at least 1 postbaseline assessment (80.5%), and 205 patients who completed the study (60.7%). Patients had mood spectrum (n = 130; 47.8%), schizophrenia spectrum (n = 82; 30.1%), and disruptive or aggressive behavior spectrum (n = 60; 22.1%) disorders. Fifteen patients who refused participation or were nonadherent served as a comparison group.

Intervention.—Treatment with aripiprazole, olanzapine, quetiapine, or risperidone for 12 weeks.

Main Outcome Measures.—Weight gain and changes in lipid and metabolic parameters.

Results.—After a median of 10.8 weeks (interquartile range, 10.5-11.2 weeks) of treatment, weight increased by 8.5 kg (95% confidence interval [CI], 7.4 to 9.7 kg) with olanzapine (n = 45), by 6.1 kg (95% CI, 4.9 to 7.2 kg) with quetiapine (n = 36), by 5.3 kg (95% CI, 4.8 to 5.9 kg) with risperidone (n = 135), and by 4.4 kg (95% CI, 3.7 to 5.2 kg) with aripiprazole (n = 41) compared with the minimal weight change of 0.2 kg (95% CI, −1.0 to 1.4 kg) in the untreated comparison group (n = 15). With olanzapine and quetiapine, respectively, mean levels increased significantly for total cholesterol (15.6 mg/dL [95% CI, 6.9 to 24.3 mg/dL] $P < .001$ and 9.1 mg/dL [95% CI, 0.4 to 17.7 mg/dL] $P = .046$), triglycerides (24.3 mg/dL [95% CI, 9.8 to 38.9 mg/dL] $P = .002$ and 37.0 mg/dL [95% CI, 10.1 to 63.8 mg/dL] $P = .01$), non–high-density lipoprotein (HDL) cholesterol (16.8 mg/dL [95% CI, 9.3 to 24.3 mg/dL] $P < .001$ and 9.9 mg/dL [95% CI, 1.4 to 18.4 mg/dL] $P = .03$), and ratio of triglycerides to HDL cholesterol (0.6 [95% CI, 0.2 to 0.9] $P = .002$ and (1.2 [95% CI, 0.4 to 2.0] $P = .004$). With risperidone, triglycerides increased significantly (mean level, 9.7 mg/dL [95% CI, 0.5 to 19.0 mg/dL]; $P = .04$). Metabolic baseline-to-end-point changes were not significant with aripiprazole or in the untreated comparison group.

Conclusions.—First-time second-generation antipsychotic medication use was associated with significant weight gain with each medication. Metabolic changes varied among the 4 antipsychotic medications.

▶ This *JAMA* article analyzes an important issue, that is, the uses of second-generation antipsychotic (SGA) medications in children where we have seen indications of greater risk of weight gain and metabolic abnormalities. Over the years 2001 and 2007, these authors studied 505 youths aged 4 to 19 years in Queens, NY. Of the 338 enrolled, 205 patients completed the study. These patients had a mixture of mood disorders, schizophrenia, and disruptive aggressive behavior. They were treated for a mean of 10.8 weeks and over that time, weight increased on olanzapine by 8.5 kg, quetiapine 6.1 kg, risperidone 5.3 kg, and aripiprazole 4.4 kg, compared with only 0.2 kg in the small untreated comparison group (N = 15). More than 50% gained more than their 7% total body weight. On olanzapine and quetiapine, choles- terol and tricyclics increased, and triglycerides increased significantly with ris- peridone. It is clear that treatment with these agents in young people is associated with greater risks of weight gain and metabolic changes than with adults. This should give even greater pause to us in using SGAs in young people for the broad range of indications that have evolved in clinical practice.[1]

J. C. Ballenger, MD

Reference

1. Varley CK, McClellan J. Implications of marked weight gain associated with atyp- ical antipsychotic medications in children and adolescents. *JAMA.* 2009;302: 1811-1812.

Comparison of Pharmacokinetic Profiles of Brand-Name and Generic Formulations of Citalopram and Venlafaxine: A Crossover Study

Chenu F, Batten LA, Zernig G, et al (Univ of Ottawa, Canada; Med Univ Innsbruck, Austria)
J Clin Psychiatry 70:958-966, 2009

Background.—Generic drugs are lower-cost versions of patent-expired brand-name medications. Bioequivalence is decreed when the 90% confi- dence intervals for the ratios of the generic to the reference compound for the area under the curve and maximum plasma concentration (C_{max}) fall within a 0.80 to 1.25 range. The aim of the present pilot study was to compare the pharmacokinetic profiles of brand-name and generic formu- lations of citalopram and extended-release venlafaxine.

Method.—Effexor XR/Novo-venlafaxine XR 75 mg and Celexa/Gen- citalopram 40 mg were studied in a randomized crossover design. Healthy male volunteers took either Effexor XR or Novovenlafaxine XR for 4 days, a 4-day washout was allowed, and then participants took the other venlafaxine formulation for 4 days. This was followed by a washout of at least 7 days. The participants then took Celexa or Gen-citalopram for 8 days, a 14-day washout was allowed, and then participants took the other citalopram formulation for 8 days. In each of the study phases, the sequence of treatment (brand-name × generic) was randomly assigned. Plasma levels of drugs were measured at fixed intervals after participants took the drugs and at steady state. The study was conducted from November 2007 through July 2008.

Results.—Twelve participants completed the venlafaxine study. Nine of the participants, plus 3 new participants, were then enrolled in the citalo- pram study, to maintain a total of 12. The plasma levels of citalopram were similar after ingestion of the brand-name and generic drugs. After ingestion of venlafaxine, the C_{max} values were 36 ± 6 ng/mL and 52 ± 8 ng/mL in the brand-name and generic groups, respectively. The ratio of the log-transformed values of C_{max} was 150% and, therefore, not within the acceptable 80% to 125% range. The concentration of the active metabolite of venlafaxine (O-desmethyl-venlafaxine [ODV]) was also significantly increased in the generic group (+43% higher in the generic group at 3 h; +48% higher at 5 h; p < .05). No differences were seen at steady state for either ODV or venlafaxine. Participants taking Novo-venlafaxine reported 3 times more side effects than those taking Effexor XR. Pill contents were identical in the 2 groups, but extraction of venlafaxine occurred more readily with the generic formulation than with the brand-name formulation, which required an additional sonication.

Conclusion.—Gen-citalopram appeared to be bioequivalent to Celexa, whereas Novo-venlafaxine XR was not bioequivalent to Effexor XR. Consequently, the Novo-venlafaxine formulation released its active ingredient more rapidly and outside the acceptable norm.

Trial Registration.—clinicaltrials.gov Identifier: NCT00676039.

▶ My patients and I frequently discuss the use of generic versus brand-name medications because of the often striking savings possible. We have known for some time that the generics are only required to fall within the range of 80% to 125% of the reference compound. Since generics can be changed as frequently as monthly by the pharmacy without knowledge of the physician or patient, this can introduce a great deal of variance if a formulation one month is 80% of the reference compound and the next month, it is 125%. This study actually compared brand-name and generic formulations of citalopram and venlafaxine ER using a randomized crossover design comparing plasma levels. Interestingly, the plasma levels of citalopram were similar for the brand and generic drugs. However, the values for venlafaxine were strikingly different, 36 ± 6 ng/dL (brand) versus 52 ± 8 ng/dL (generic) in the generic groups. This 150% difference is clearly outside the acceptable 125% range. Also, the active metabolite of venlafaxine was also significantly increased by 43% to 48% in the generic group. These differences in the venlafaxine group were reflected in increased side effects. There were 3 times as many side effects with the generic versus the brand Effexor XR. This difference appeared to be related to the fact that the generic (Novo-venlafaxine) released its active drug more rapidly. In my experience, the difference between brand and generic is generally not worth the price. However, I think we should all be alert to the fact that if a patient notices a difference, either in side effects or even clinically, they may very well be accurately noticing the differences in the plasma levels of the medicines that they are receiving.

J. C. Ballenger, MD

Americans' Attitudes Toward Psychiatric Medications: 1998–2006
Mojtabai R (Johns Hopkins Bloomberg School of Public Health, Baltimore, MD)
Psychiatr Serv 60:1015-1023, 2009

Objectives.—This study examined recent changes in attitudes toward psychiatric medications in the U.S. general population.

Methods.—Samples of adult participants in the U.S. General Social Surveys of 1998 (N = 1,387) and 2006 (N = 1,437) were compared for opinions on the benefits and risks of psychiatric medications as well as willingness to take them in hypothetical situations, including experiencing symptoms of panic attacks or major depression and difficulty in coping with stress or having trouble in personal life.

Results.—Public opinions regarding benefits of psychiatric medications became more favorable between 1998 and 2006. More participants in 2006 than in 1998 thought that medications help people to deal with day-to-day stresses (83.4% versus 77.8%), make things easier in relation with family and friends (75.9% versus 68.4%), and help people feel better about themselves (68.0% versus 60.1%). The public expressed a greater willingness to take medications in 2006 compared with 1998 for trouble in personal life (29.1% versus 23.3%), to cope with stresses of life (46.6% versus 35.5%), for depression (49.1% versus 41.2%), and for panic attacks (63.7% versus 55.6%). Opinions regarding the risks of medications did not change between 1998 and 2006.

Conclusions.—Americans' opinions toward psychiatric medications became more favorable over the past decade, and people became more willing to take these medications. These changes have likely contributed to the increased use of psychiatric medications in recent years and will continue to do so in the coming years.

▶ One of the issues I have followed in previous reviews are the slow changes in attitudes toward psychiatric medications in the public. Antidepressants and other psychiatric medications remain woefully underused, largely because of negative attitudes. In this particular study, they compared a large sample of United States adults in 1998 (*N* = 1387) and again from a similar group in 2006 (*N* = 1437) about their opinions of the risks and benefits of these psychiatric medications and their willingness to take them. Interestingly, attitudes in fact did become more favorable between 1998 and 2006. People became significantly more willing to take them to help deal with everyday stress, for improvement in their relationships with family or friends, and to feel better about themselves, as well as for depression and panic attacks. Interestingly, opinions about the risks about these medications did not change. This change in attitude does mirror the increase in use of psychiatric medications that we have observed in recent years and does bode well for future improvements in this area. Still, most people with these illnesses and conditions fail to take these medications, which could be helpful to them. Unlike many situations in our field, this situation does seem to be improving.

J. C. Ballenger, MD

Nortriptyline and gabapentin, alone and in combination for neuropathic pain: a double-blind, randomised controlled crossover trial
Gilron I, Bailey JM, Tu D, et al (Queen's Univ, Kingston, Ontario, Canada; et al)
Lancet 374:1252-1261, 2009

Background.—Drugs for neuropathic pain have incomplete efficacy and dose-limiting side-effects when given as monotherapy. We assessed the efficacy and tolerability of combined nortriptyline and gabapentin compared with each drug given alone.

Methods.—In this double-blind, double-dummy, crossover trial, patients with diabetic polyneuropathy or postherpetic neuralgia, and who had a daily pain score of at least 4 (scale 0–10), were enrolled and treated at one study site in Canada between Nov 5, 2004, and Dec 13, 2007. 56 patients were randomised in a 1:1:1 ratio with a balanced Latin square design to receive one of three sequences of daily oral gabapentin, nortriptyline, and their combination. In sequence, a different drug was given to each randomised group in three treatment periods. During each 6-week treatment period, drug doses were titrated towards maximum tolerated dose. The primary outcome was mean daily pain at maximum tolerated dose. Analysis was by intention to treat. This trial is registered, number ISRCTN73178636.

Findings.—45 patients completed all three treatment periods; 47 patients completed at least two treatment periods and were analysed for the primary outcome. Mean daily pain (0–10; numerical rating scale) was $5 \cdot 4$ (95% CI $5 \cdot 0$ to $5 \cdot 8$) at baseline, and at maximum tolerated dose, pain was $3 \cdot 2$ ($2 \cdot 5$ to $3 \cdot 8$) for gabapentin, $2 \cdot 9$ ($2 \cdot 4$ to $3 \cdot 4$) for nortriptyline, and $2 \cdot 3$ ($1 \cdot 8$ to $2 \cdot 8$) for combination treatment. Pain with combination treatment was significantly lower than with gabapentin ($-0 \cdot 9$, 95% CI $-1 \cdot 4$ to $-0 \cdot 3$, p=$0 \cdot 001$) or nortriptyline alone ($-0 \cdot 6$, 95% CI $-1 \cdot 1$ to $-0 \cdot 1$, p=$0 \cdot 02$). At maximum tolerated dose, the most common adverse event was dry mouth, which was significantly less frequent in patients on gabapentin than on nortriptyline (p<$0 \cdot 0001$) or combination treatment (p<$0 \cdot 0001$). No serious adverse events were recorded for any patients during the trial.

Interpretation.—Combined gabapentin and nortriptyline seems to be more efficacious than either drug given alone for neuropathic pain, therefore we recommend use of this combination in patients who show a partial response to either drug given alone and seek additional pain relief. Future

trials should compare other combinations to their respective monotherapies for treatment of such pain.

▶ The use of nortriptyline has become very widespread in chronic pain patients,
and more recently, gabapentin has as well. These authors did an excellent
double-blind, double-dummy crossover trial in patients with diabetic neuropathy
or postherpetic neuralgia with significant pain. They studied 56 patients who
received all 3 treatments in random order. They were treated with nortriptyline
alone, gabapentin alone, or the combination. They found very clear results. The
combination treatment led to significantly lower pain when compared with gabapentin or nortriptyline alone. Side effects were minor. This is an important study
because almost everyone treated for chronic pain with either of these 2 drugs, or
other modalities, generally has only a partial response. This study argues strongly
that we should be using the combination of these drugs on a routine basis, particularly in those patients who did not respond completely to either one of these
commonly used treatments.

J. C. Ballenger, MD

**Comparison of Topiramate and Risperidone for the Treatment of Behavioral
Disturbances of Patients With Alzheimer Disease: A Double-Blind,
Randomized Clinical Trial**
Mowla A, Pani A (Bushehr Univ of Med Sciences, Iran)
J Clin Psychopharmacol 30:40-43, 2010

Introduction.—Behavioral disturbances are determining factors in
handling patients with Alzheimer dementia. The current pharmacotherapy
for behavioral symptoms associated with dementia is not satisfactory. Our
goal was to compare a new anticonvulsant, topiramate, with a usually
used medication, risperidone, for controlling behavioral disturbances of
patients with Alzheimer dementia.

Method.—Elderly patients with a *Diagnostic and Statistical Manual of
Mental Disorders, Fourth Edition* diagnosis of Alzheimer disease and
significant behavioral disturbances were randomized to receive, for
a period of 8 weeks, a flexible dose of either topiramate (25–50 mg/d) or
risperidone (0.5–2 mg/d). Outcome measures were the Cohen-Mansfield
Agitation Inventory, Neuropsychiatry Inventory parts 1 and 2, and the
Clinical Global Impression.

Result.—Forty-eight patients were randomized to treatment with either
topiramate or risperidone, and 41 patients (21 of 25 in topiramate group
and 20 of 23 in risperidone group) completed the trial. Both groups
showed significant improvement in all outcome measures without important difference (Neuropsychiatry Inventory total score $P < 0.531$,
$Z = 0.62$; Cohen-Mansfield Agitation Inventory $P < 0.927$, $Z = 0.09$; Clinical Global Impression, $P < 0.654$, $Z = 0.48$). There were no significant

changes in the cognitive status of patients (assessed by Mini-Mental Status Examination) taking topiramate or risperidone during the trial.

Conclusion.—Treatment with a low dose of topiramate (25–50 mg/d) demonstrated a comparable efficacy with risperidone in controlling behavioral disturbances of patients with Alzheimer dementia.

▶ The psychiatric and behavioral difficulties in Alzheimer patients usually end up being one of the issues (if not the most important) we have to wrestle with clinically. This has been complicated recently by observations of increased mortality with certain antipsychotics, including the second generation or atypicals. This study compared the relatively new anticonvulsant, topiramate, and a frequently used second-generation antipsychotic, risperidone, in this population. Doses in this 8-week trial in 48 patients with topiramate were relatively low (25 to 50 mg per day), and they had the same positive improvements as did risperidone (0.1 to 2 mg using a blinded staggered-onset design per day). Often there are complications with topiramate, especially cognitive changes; but there were none observed in this particular study.

J. C. Ballenger, MD

Case Reports of Postmarketing Adverse Event Experiences With Olanzapine Intramuscular Treatment in Patients With Agitation

Marder SR, Sorsaburu S, Dunayevich E, et al (Univ of California, Los Angeles [UCLA]; Lilly Corporate Ctr, Indianapolis, IN; Orexigen Therapeutics, La Jolla, CA; et al)
J Clin Psychiatry 71:433-441, 2010

Objective.—Agitation is a medical emergency with increased risk for poor outcome. Successful treatment often requires intramuscular (IM) psychotropics. Safety data from the first 21 months of olanzapine IM, approved in the United States for the treatment of agitation associated with schizophrenia and bipolar disorder, are presented.

Method.—A Lilly-maintained safety database was searched for all spontaneous adverse events (AEs) reported in temporal association with olanzapine IM treatment.

Results.—The estimated worldwide patient exposure to olanzapine IM from January 1, 2004, through September 30, 2005, was 539,000; 160 cases containing AEs were reported from patients with schizophrenia (30%), bipolar disorder (21%), unspecified psychosis (10%), dementia (8%), and depression (5%). Many reported concomitant treatment with benzodiazepines (39%) or other antipsychotics (54%). The most frequently reported events involved the following organ systems: central nervous (21%), cardiac (12%), respiratory (6%), vascular (6%), and psychiatric (5%). Eighty-three cases were considered serious, including 29 fatalities. In these fatalities, concomitant benzodiazepines or other antipsychotics were reported in 66% and 76% of cases, respectively. The most frequently reported events in the fatal cases involved the following organ systems: cardiovascular (41%), respiratory (21%), general (17%), and central nervous (10%). The majority of fatal cases (76%) included comorbid conditions and potentially clinically significant risk factors for AEs.

Conclusions.—Clinicians should use care when treating agitated patients, especially when they present with concurrent medical conditions and are treated with multiple medications, which may increase the risk of poor or even fatal outcomes. Clinicians should use caution when using olanzapine IM and parenteral benzodiazepines simultaneously.

▶ Severe agitation can be an emergency, and intramuscular treatments are often used in emergency settings. These authors report safety data from the first 21 months after the approval of the intramuscular form of olanzapine for treatment of agitation in patients with schizophrenia and bipolar disorder. The database included a worldwide patient exposure from January 1, 2004 to September 30, 2005 of 539 000 cases. In this dataset, the most commonly reported events in decreasing order occurred in the central nervous system (CNS), cardiac, respiratory, vascular, and psychiatric areas. Eighty-three of the 160 cases were considered serious, including 29 fatalities. In these fatalities, the patients were also being treated with benzodiazepines or other antipsychotics in 66% and 76% of cases, respectively. The most common fatal cases involved the cardiovascular, respiratory, general, or CNS, and most (76%) patients had comorbid conditions and potentially clinically significant risk factors. Whether this particular medication caused or contributed to these fatalities is obviously unclear, given the illness level of the patients being treated. However, it is clear that great caution is called for in using intramuscular olanzapine (and others), especially if benzodiazepines are used at the same time.

J. C. Ballenger, MD

Novelty seeking among adult women is lower for the winter borns compared to the summer borns: replication in a large Finnish birth cohort
Chotai J, Joukamaa M, Taanila A, et al (Univ of Umeå, Sweden; Tampere Univ Hosp, Finland; Univ of Oulu, Finland; et al)
Compr Psychiatry 50:562-566, 2009

Objective.—Earlier general population studies have shown that novelty seeking (NS) of the Temperament and Character Inventory (TCI) of personality is lower for persons born in winter compared to those born in summer, particularly for women. Here, we investigate if this result can be replicated in another population.

Method.—The Northern Finland 1966 Birth Cohort, comprising 4968 subjects (2725 women, 2243 men), was investigated with regard to the temperament dimensions of the TCI and the season of birth.

Results.—Novelty seeking and reward dependence (RD) showed significant variations according to the month of birth. We found that women born during winter have significantly lower levels of NS compared to women born during summer, with a minimum for the birth month November and maximum for May. These results are similar to those found in a previous Swedish study. Furthermore, our study showed that men born during spring had significantly lower mean scores of RD compared to men born during autumn, with a minimum for birth month March. This was in contrast to the Swedish study, where the minimum of RD was obtained for the birth month December.

Conclusion.—Women born in winter have lower NS as adults compared to women born in summer. Because NS is modulated by dopamine, this study gives further support to the studies in the literature that show that dopamine turnover for those born in winter is higher than for those born in summer.

▶ This study is an attempt at replication of the finding that people born in the winter have lower novelty seeking personalities than those in the summer. They studied the Finnish cohort of 4968 subjects, both men and women, and in fact, found significant variations in novelty seeking and reward dependence depending on the month of birth. Women born in the winter had significantly lower levels of novelty seeking versus those born in the summer, similar to results found in a previous Swedish study. Men born in the spring had lower reward dependence compared with those born in the autumn. The authors postulate that because novelty seeking is presumably modulated by dopamine, the supportive evidence in the literature is that dopamine turnover is higher for those born in the winter than those born in the summer, perhaps thereby conferring a protected benefit against novelty seeking. For those not familiar with the novelty seeking idea, it appears to underlie multiple high-risk activities, particularly drug abuse. Although I don't know exactly what to do with this type of finding, I do find it very interesting.

J. C. Ballenger, MD

Acute Psychological Stress Reduces Working Memory-Related Activity in the Dorsolateral Prefrontal Cortex
Qin S, Hermans EJ, van Marle HJF, et al (Radboud Univ Nijmegen Med Ctr, The Netherlands; et al)
Biol Psychiatry 66:25-32, 2009

Background.—Acute psychological stress impairs higher-order cognitive function such as working memory (WM). Similar impairments are seen in various psychiatric disorders that are associated with higher susceptibility to stress and with prefrontal cortical dysfunctions, suggesting that acute stress may play a potential role in such dysfunctions. However, it remains unknown whether acute stress has immediate effects on WM-related prefrontal activity.

Methods.—Using functional magnetic resonance imaging (fMRI), we investigated neural activity of 27 healthy female participants during a blocked WM task (numerical N-back) while moderate psychological stress was induced by viewing strongly aversive (vs. neutral) movie material together with a self-referencing instruction. To assess stress manipulation, autonomic and endocrine, as well as subjective, measurements were acquired throughout the experiment.

Results.—Successfully induced acute stress resulted in significantly reduced WM-related activity in the dorsolateral prefrontal cortex (DLPFC), and was accompanied by less deactivation in brain regions that are jointly referred to as the default mode network.

Conclusions.—This study demonstrates that experimentally induced acute stress in healthy volunteers results in a reduction of WM-related DLPFC activity and reallocation of neural resources away from executive function networks. These effects may be explained by supraoptimal levels of catecholamines potentially in conjunction with elevated levels of cortisol. A similar mechanism involving acute stress as a mediating factor may play an important role in higher-order cognitive deficits and hypofrontality observed in various psychiatric disorders.

▶ We have documented impairment in higher order cognitive functioning (like working memory) in multiple psychiatric disorders. These authors argued that stress may mediate that by interfering with prefrontal cortical function. These authors studied functional magnetic resonance imaging (fMRI) in 27 healthy females who were subjected to moderate psychological stress by viewing strongly aversive movie material. They were able to induce stress, which led to significant reductions in memory related activity in the dorsal lateral prefrontal cortex. This accompanied deactivation in related networks. This certainly suggests a logical brain mechanism for the interference of stress in patients with varied psychiatric disorders or simply stress in general.

J. C. Ballenger, MD

Psychiatry in General Medicine

Distinctiveness of psychological obstacles to recovery in low back pain patients in primary care

Foster NE, Thomas E, Bishop A, et al (Keele Univ, Staffordshire, UK)
Pain 148:398-406, 2010

Many psychological factors have been suggested to be important obstacles to recovery from low back pain, yet most studies focus on a limited number of factors. We compared a more comprehensive range of 20 factors in predicting outcome in primary care. Consecutive patients consulting 8 general practices were eligible to take part in a prospective cohort study; 1591 provided data at baseline and 810 at 6 months. Clinical outcome was defined using the Roland and Morris Disability Questionnaire (RMDQ). The relative strength of the baseline psychological measures to predict outcome was investigated using adjusted multiple linear regression techniques. The sample was similar to other primary care cohorts (mean age 44 years, 59% women, mean baseline RMDQ 8.6). The 20 factors each accounted for between 0.04% and 33.3% of the variance in baseline RMDQ score. A multivariate model including all 11 scales that were associated with outcome in the univariate analysis accounted for 47.7% of the variance in 6 months RMDQ score; rising to 55.8% following adjustment. Four scales remained significantly associated with outcome in the multivariate model explaining 56.6% of the variance: perceptions of personal control, acute/chronic timeline, illness identify and pain self-efficacy. When all independent factors were included, depression, catastrophising and fear avoidance were no longer significant. Thus, a small number of psychological factors are strongly predictive of outcome in primary care low back pain patients. There is clear redundancy in the measurement of psychological factors. These findings should help to focus targeted interventions for back pain in the future.

▶ These authors observed 1591 consecutive patients in 8 general practices. One of the most common problems presenting in clinical medicine is low back pain. Foster et al used psychological tests to try to predict who would recover and found that 56.6% of the variance was determined by 4 factors, including chronic time line illness, identified pain, self-efficacy, and perceptions of personal control. When all factors were included, depression, catastrophising, and fear avoidance stopped having any significance. Hopefully, this type of knowledge would allow us to approach more intelligently this very common and costly problem because of the disability it causes.

J. C. Ballenger, MD

Prevalence and comorbidity of common mental disorders in primary care
Roca M, Gili M, Garcia-Garcia M, et al (Univ of Balearic Islands, Spain; Biométrica Institut, Barcelona, Spain; et al)
J Affective Disord 119:52-58, 2009

Objective.—To estimate the prevalence and comorbidity of the most common mental disorders in primary care practice in Spain, using the Primary Care Evaluation of Mental Disorders (PRIME-MD) questionnaire.

Design.—A systematic sample of 7936 adult primary care patients was recruited by 1925 general practitioners in a large cross-sectional national epidemiological study. The PRIME-MD was used to diagnose psychiatric disorders.

Setting.—1356 primary care units proportionally distributed throughout the country.

Results.—53.6% of the sample presented one or more psychiatric disorder. The most prevalent were affective (35.8%), anxiety (25.6%), and somatoform (28.8%) disorders. 30.3% of the patients had more than one current mental disorder. 11.5% presented comorbidity between affective, anxiety, and somatoform disorders.

Conclusions.—The study provides further evidence of the high prevalence and high comorbidity of mental disorders in primary care. Given the large overlap between affective, anxiety and somatoform disorders, future diagnostic classifications should reconsider the current separation between these entities.

▶ Previous readers of my reviews know that a topic I follow closely is the care of psychiatric patients in primary care. It is clear that much of the care of our patients occurs there, such that Darrel Regier years ago called it the de facto mental health system in the United States. This has recently found widespread media attention in that, with the exception of the antipsychotics, lithium and the anticonvulsants, all the rest of the psychotropics are prescribed 3 or 4 times more frequently by nonpsychiatric physicians than by psychiatrists. This particular trial was a very systematic study of 7936 adult primary care patients seen by 1925 general practitioners (GPs). Not surprisingly, 53.6% of the sample had one or more psychiatric disorders, the most prevalent being affective (35.8%), anxiety (25.6%), and somatoform (28.8%) disorders. Again, not surprisingly, almost a third had more than one mental disorder. There are not really any surprises in this study, although it underscores again the remarkable importance of these issues.

J. C. Ballenger, MD

7 Biological Psychiatry

Introduction

I am delighted to share with you a selection of provocative and interesting articles, a virtual "potpourri" of scientific endeavors over this past year. I have included a wide sample of articles that reflect advances in the neurobiology of mental illness as well as how biology interacts with environment. The articles span some key aspects of current importance—imaging advances, neurotrophins, pathways to addiction, neurobiological expression of common experiences like memory, cognitive performance, and craving. These articles are exciting individually, and I hope that you will find the aggregate and synthesis all the more exciting.
Science marches forward.
Thank you for your interest.

Peter F. Buckley, MD

Schizophrenia

Cardiovascular Disease Mortality in Patients With Chronic Schizophrenia Treated With Clozapine: A Retrospective Cohort Study

Kelly DL, McMahon RP, Liu F, et al (Univ of Maryland School of Medicine, Baltimore; et al)
J Clin Psychiatry 71:304-311, 2010

Background.—Cardiovascular disease (CVD) mortality in schizophrenia is more frequent than in the general population. Whether second-generation antipsychotics (SGAs) increase risk of CVD morbidity and mortality has yet to be determined.

Method.—We conducted a retrospective cohort study using an administrative database to identify patients with *DSM-III–* or *DSM-IV–*diagnosed schizophrenia, treated in Maryland, who started clozapine treatment (n = 1,084) or were never treated with clozapine (initiated on risperidone; n = 602) between 1994 and 2000. Deaths between 1994 and 2004 were identified by the Social Security Death Index, and death records were obtained.

Results.—During the 6- to 10-year follow-up period, there were 136 deaths, of which 43 were attributed to CVD. Cardiovascular disease mortality in patients aged younger than 55 years at medication start was approximately 1.1% (clozapine, 1.1%; risperidone, 1.0%) in both groups at 5 years and 2.7% (clozapine) and 2.8% (risperidone) at 10 years ($\chi_1^2 = 0.12$, $P = .73$). Patients who started treatment at ages ≥ 55 years had CVD mortality of 8.5% (clozapine) and 3.6% (risperidone) at 5 years and 16.0% (clozapine) and 5.7% (risperidone) at 10 years ($\chi_1^2 = 2.13$, $P = .144$). In a Cox regression model, patients aged ≥ 55 years were at greater risk of mortality than younger patients (hazard ratio = 4.6, $P < .001$); whites were at greater risk than nonwhites (HR = 2.1, $P = .046$); however, SGA treatment (HR = 1.2; 95% CI, 0.6–2.4; $P = .61$) and sex (HR = 0.9, $P = .69$) were not statistically significant predictors of CVD, nor was there a significant age × clozapine interaction ($\chi_1^2 = 1.52$, $P = .22$). Age-, race-, and gender-adjusted standardized mortality ratios were significantly elevated (clozapine, 4.70; 95% CI, 3.19–6.67; risperidone, 2.88; 95% CI, 1.38–5.30) compared to year 2000 rates for the Maryland general population but did not differ by antipsychotic group ($\chi_1^2 = 1.42$, $P = .23$).

Conclusions.—The risk of CVD mortality in schizophrenia does not differ between clozapine and risperidone in adults despite known differences in risk profiles for weight gain and metabolic side effects. However, we cannot rule out an increased risk of CVD mortality among those starting treatment at ages 55 years or older (Table 2).

▶ This is a complex but important retrospective pharmacovigilance study of mortality in patients receiving second-generation antipsychotics. It does not address another contentious and unevoked issue as to whether mortality in schizophrenia is higher in patients being treated with first-generation antipsychotic medications or second-generation antipsychotics. The study takes its lead from the earlier, and now confirmed, studies of high rates of weight gain, diabetes, and cardiovascular ill-health in people who stay long term on clozapine. It is perhaps surprising then that the authors did not find any significant differences overall in the rate of deaths from cardiovascular disease between patients who received clozapine and those who were being treated

TABLE 2.—Cardiovascular Disease Mortality in Maryland Persons With Schizophrenia: Age-, Race-, and Sex-Adjusted Standardized Mortality Ratios (SMRs) Compared to the Maryland General Population in 2000[a]

	Overall (n = 1,549)		Clozapine (n = 1,078)		Risperidone (n = 471)		Test for Clozapine-Risperidone Difference	
	SMR	95% CI	SMR	95% CI	SMR	95% CI	χ_1^2	P Value
Male	3.20	2.03–4.81	3.82	2.26–6.03	2.03	0.65–4.74	1.11	.293
Female	6.25	3.70–9.88	6.92	3.68–11.84	4.98	1.61–11.63	0.14	.704
White	6.45	4.38–9.15	7.06	4.52–10.50	4.98	2.00–10.26	0.38	.537
Nonwhite	1.90	0.91–3.50	2.19	0.88–4.52	1.46	0.29–4.25	0.08	.783
All patients	4.08	2.92–5.53	4.70	3.19–6.67	2.88	1.38–5.30	1.42	.233

[a]Test for male-female difference in SMR (pooling across drug): $\chi_1^2 = 3.96$, $P = .047$; test for white-nonwhite difference (pooling across drug): $\chi_1^2 = 11.63$, $P = .001$.

with risperidone. The reason may be that the study, while elegant and important, simply did not have enough power (ie, not enough deaths recorded) to find a difference (Fig 1 in the original article, Table 2). So just because they did not find one, this study is not of robust-enough methodology to entirely refute that a difference (which one might anticipate based on all the literature) actually exists. Age is the strongest predictor (see Fig 1 in the original article). The study does caution the use of clozapine in the elderly. There is also Food and Drug Administration-required black box labeling for the use of any antipsychosis in the elderly.

P. F. Buckley, MD

Dizziness, migrainous vertigo and psychiatric disorders
Teggi R, Caldirola D, Colombo B, et al (Vita-Salute Univ, Milan, Italy)
J Laryngol Otol 124:285-290, 2010

Objectives.—This study sought to establish the prevalence of vestibular disorders, migraine and definite migrainous vertigo in patients with psychiatric disorders who were referred for treatment of dizziness, without a lifetime history of vertigo.

Study Design.—Retrospective study.

Setting.—Out-patients in a university hospital.

Materials and Methods.—Fifty-two dizzy patients with panic disorders and agoraphobia, 30 with panic disorders without agoraphobia, and 20 with depressive disorders underwent otoneurological screening with bithermal caloric stimulation. The prevalence of migraine and migrainous vertigo was assessed. The level of dizziness was evaluated using the Dizziness Handicap Inventory.

Results.—Dizzy patients with panic disorders and agoraphobia had a significantly $p = 0.05$ regarding the prevalence of peripheral vestibular abnormalities in the group of subjects with PD and agoraphobia and in those with depressive disorders. Migraine was equally represented in the three groups, but panic disorder patients had a higher prevalence of migrainous vertigo definite migrainous vertigo. Almost all patients with a peripheral vestibular disorder had a final diagnosis of definite migrainous vertigo according to Neuhauser criteria. These patients had higher Dizziness Handicap Inventory scores. The Dizziness Handicap Inventory total score was higher in the subgroup of patients with panic disorders with agoraphobia also presenting unilateral reduced caloric responses or definite migrainous vertigo, compared with the subgroup of remaining subjects with panic disorders with agoraphobia ($p < 0.001$).

Conclusions.—Our data support the hypothesis that, in patients with panic disorders (and especially those with additional agoraphobia), dizziness may be linked to malfunction of the vestibular system. However, the data are not inconsistent with the hypothesis that migrainous vertigo is the most common pathophysiological mechanism for vestibular disorders.

▶ This is an interesting study from an Italian group comparing migraines and vestibular function among dizzy patients who have either anxiety (panic attacks with/without agoraphobia) or depression. They postulate a relationship between vestibular dysfunction and psychiatric disorders. The finding of a lack of association with vestibular disturbance and depression is surprising. However, this study was retrospective and so symptom constellation and diagnosis may be less clear. Additionally, it is well known that there is substantial overlap and comorbidity between anxiety and depression—these issues could not have been teased out in this retrospective design.

P. F. Buckley, MD

Olanzapine vs. lithium in management of acute mania
Shafti SS (Univ of Social Welfare and Rehabilitation Sciences [USWR], Tehran, Italy)
J Affective Disord 122:273-276, 2010

Objective.—Among the available mood stabilizers, it appears that lithium may share an important role for treatment of acute mania. In a study from Sep. 2007 to Apr. 2008 at Razi Psychiatric Hospital we evaluated the efficiency of olanzapine vs. lithium.

Methods.—Forty (40) female inpatients meeting DSM-IV-TR criteria for acute mania were entered into a 3-week parallel group, double-blind study for random assignment to olanzapine or lithium carbonate in a 1:1 ratio.

Primary outcome measurements were the changes in Manic State Rating Scale (MSRS) at baseline and weekly intervals up to the third week. Similarly, overall illness severity was rated using the Clinical Global Impression-Severity of illness scale (CGI-S) at baseline and at the end of the third week. Analysis of the data was accomplished by means of split-plot (mixed) and repeated measures analysis of variance (ANOVA) and t test.

Results.—While both olanzapine and lithium were found to be significantly helpful in the improvement of manic symptoms ($p < 0.05$), lithium was considerably more successful by the end of the third week ($p < 0.0002$ and $p < 0.003$, for frequency and intensity of the symptoms). CGI-S also showed important improvements with both olanzapine and lithium ($p < 0.043$ and $p < 0.015$ for olanzapine and lithium).

Conclusion.—Though both olanzapine and lithium were effective in the improvement of manic symptoms, lithium was more beneficial.

▶ This is an interesting and provocative study of lithium versus olanzapine, especially given that the total sample size of this study ($n = 40$) is conspicuously smaller than the large comparative trials of putative antimania drugs. Lithium is certainly a robust antimanic agent, and it has stood the test of time. In the United States, its use has declined with the growing availability and use of anticonvulsant agents (most notably valproic acid) and several new antipsychotic medications. The effect of lithium in reducing manic symptoms was most robust at the third week of treatment in this study. Both olanzapine and lithium were pretty well tolerated, with a low study dropout rate (15% and 10%, respectively). Clearly, this is too small a study to pronounce lithium as superior to olanzapine and as an antimanic drug. Moreover, there are variable findings from previous studies—some of which are also quite small.

P. F. Buckley, MD

Transient Estradiol Exposure during Middle Age in Ovariectomized Rats Exerts Lasting Effects on Cognitive Function and the Hippocampus
Rodgers SP, Bohacek J, Daniel JM (Tulane Univ, New Orleans, LA)
Endocrinology 151:1194-1203, 2010

We determined whether transient exposure to estradiol during middle age in ovariectomized rats would exert lasting effects on cognition and the brain beyond the period of exposure. Two experiments were conducted. Rats 10–11 months of age were ovariectomized and received vehicle control treatment throughout the experiment, continuous estradiol treatment throughout the experiment, or 40 d of transient exposure to estradiol that ended 3 d before behavioral training. In the first experiment, rats were trained on a radial-maze working memory task and killed 2 months after the termination of transient exposure to estradiol. The hippocampus was immunostained for choline acetyltransferase and estrogen receptors α (ERα) and β (ERβ) by Western blotting. In a second experiment to determine the durability of treatment effects, rats were behaviorally tested every other month until brains were collected for Western blotting 8 months after the termination of transient exposure to estradiol. Maze testing included delay trials and scopolamine trials, in which dose-effect curves for the muscarinic receptor antagonist were determined. Transient exposure to estradiol enhanced working memory and attenuated amnestic effects of scopolamine as effectively as continuous estradiol exposure. Enhancements persisted for up to 7 months. Transient exposure to estradiol increased hippocampal levels of ERα and choline acetyltransferase 2 months and ERα 8 months after termination of the exposure. Neither estradiol treatment altered estrogen receptor β levels. Results demonstrate that short-term treatment with estradiol during middle age enhances working memory well beyond the duration of treatment and suggest ERα as a potential mechanism for this effect.

▶ This is a complicated series of experiments showing the effects of estrogen exposure and estrogen receptor levels over time in an already well-validated rat model. Estrogen exposure enhances memory. Estrogen-exposed rats also had higher receptor levels over time. This work is important and contributes to a major and ongoing public debate about the risks and benefits of hormone replacement in middle-aged women. Some studies have shown a potentially lower progression to cognitive impairment as well as less cardiovascular disease and osteoporosis. These, if true, are substantial benefits and are consistent with the proposed hypothesis of neuroprotective effects of estrogen therapy. However, these results are not conclusive and must be balanced with an apparently higher risk of breast and uterine cancer in middle-aged females who take estrogens for a long time.

P. F. Buckley, MD

Subjective Experience of Cognitive Failures as Possible Risk Factor for Negative Symptoms of Psychosis in the General Population
Pfeifer S, van Os J, Hanssen M, et al (Maastricht Univ, The Netherlands)
Schizophr Bull 35:766-774, 2009

Objective.—The aim of this study was to examine whether proneness to subjective cognitive failure (cognitive based mistakes) increases the risk for the development of symptoms of psychosis and to what degree any association was familial.

Methods.—At baseline, the Cognitive Failure Questionnaire (CFQ) and the Community Assessment of Psychic Experiences (CAPE) questionnaire were administered in a general population sample of genetically related individuals ($n = 755$). Individuals scoring high (>75th percentile) or average on the CAPE (between 40th and 60th percentile) ($n = 488$) were reinterviewed with the CAPE and Structured Interview for Schizotypy—Revised (SIS-R) at follow-up (mean interval = 7.7 months, SD = 4.8 months).

Results.—Cross-trait, *within*-relative analysis showed a significant association between the CFQ and the negative dimension, assessed with both the CAPE and SIS-R, whereas no association was found between the CFQ and the positive dimension. Cross-trait, *between*-relative analyses showed no association between the CFQ in one relative and any of the dimensions of the subclinical psychosis phenotype in the other relative.

Conclusion.—Proneness to subjective cognitive failure possibly contributes to the development or persistence of negative symptoms and can be seen as potential risk factor for negative symptoms of psychosis. This overlap is due to individual effects rather than familial liability.

▶ A senior author of this article, Professor Jim van Os from the Netherlands, has produced very interesting evidence from several community-based studies of psychopathology that suggest a baseline role of hallucinations of about 8% to 10% in the population (when randomly observed). Their studies then examine factors that might explain these observations, chief among these being the use of illicit drugs (especially marijuana) and genetic risk for psychosis. In this study, the Netherlands group looks at the relationship between cognitive performance and schizotypy—focusing here on negative symptoms. However, although the data are well collected, it is hard to pick up mild negative symptoms in nonschizophrenic patients, even if they have schizotypy. This is an interesting and provocative work because it suggests and reminds us that psychopathology is not static and that there is a constant interplay between (abnormal) mental life and our environment.

P. F. Buckley, MD

Superior temporal gyrus volume in antipsychotic-naive people at risk of psychosis
Takahashi T, Wood SJ, Yung AR, et al (Univ of Melbourne, Australia; et al)
Br J Psychiatry 196:206-211, 2010

Background.—Morphological abnormalities of the superior temporal gyrus have been consistently reported in schizophrenia, but the timing of their occurrence remains unclear.

Aims.—To determine whether individuals exhibit superior temporal gyral changes before the onset of psychosis.

Method.—We used magnetic resonance imaging to examine grey matter volumes of the superior temporal gyrus and its subregions (planum polare, Heschl's gyrus, planum temporale, and rostral and caudal regions) in 97 antipsychotic-naive individuals at ultra-high risk of psychosis, of whom 31 subsequently developed psychosis and 66 did not, and 42 controls.

Results.—Those at risk of psychosis had significantly smaller superior temporal gyri at baseline compared with controls bilaterally, without any prominent subregional effect; however, there was no difference between those who did and did not subsequently develop psychosis.

Conclusions.—Our findings indicate that grey matter reductions of the superior temporal gyrus are present before psychosis onset, and are not due to medication, but these baseline changes are not predictive of transition to psychosis.

▶ These Australian investigators are the world leaders in research on the prodrome in schizophrenia. They published a major article in the *Lancet* in 2003 showing that among those individuals who were at risk to develop psychosis, individuals who went on to have a psychotic episode had a previous MRI showing (as a group) smaller hippocampal and superior temporal gyrus volumes. This study essentially enlarges this sample and approach, now examining 66 patients at risk for psychosis who did not become psychotic, 31 patients who did become psychotic, and 42 normal subjects. The authors replicate the earlier findings of superior temporal gyrus volume reductions in people at risk of psychosis. Because none of these individuals received antipsycotic medication, this effect can be attributed likely to the disease process. However, the authors failed to replicate in this expanded sample their earlier finding of difference between individuals who do and do not go on to become psychotic. Nonetheless, the powerful message of their original article stands and will overshadow the nonreplication of this report. Additionally, other groups have now also found similar neurobiological changes at the conversion point to psychosis.

P. F. Buckley, MD

Prevalence of Negative Symptoms in Outpatients With Schizophrenia Spectrum Disorders Treated With Antipsychotics in Routine Clinical Practice: Findings From the CLAMORS Study
Bobes J, for the CLAMORS Study Collaborative Group (Univ of Oviedo, Asturias, Spain; et al)
J Clin Psychiatry 71:280-286, 2010

Objective.—To analyze the prevalence of negative symptoms in antipsychotic-treated outpatients with schizophrenia spectrum disorders.

Method.—A cross-sectional, retrospective multicenter study was carried out between May 2004 and April 2005 in 1,704 adult psychiatric outpatients meeting *DSM-IV* criteria for schizophrenia, schizophreniform, or schizoaffective disorder. We used 5 items of the Positive and Negative Syndrome Scale (PANSS) negative symptoms subscale to individually determine the presence of a negative symptom when the score on the item was > 3. Primary negative symptoms were considered present when patients fulfilled all of the following: > 3 score on the corresponding item; < 3 score on any positive item; no extrapyramidal symptoms; ≤ 3 score on anxiety and depression items; dose of haloperidol, when applicable, ≤ 15 mg/d; and no antiparkinsonian treatment.

Results.—A total of 1,452 evaluable patients (863 men, 60.9%), 40.7 ± 12.2 (mean ± SD) years of age, were included. One or more negative symptoms were present in 57.6% of patients, with primary negative symptoms in 12.9% of subjects. The most frequent negative symptom items were social withdrawal (45.8%), emotional withdrawal (39.1%), poor rapport (35.8%), and blunted affect (33.1%). Negative symptoms (1-blunted affect, 2-emotional withdrawal, 3-poor rapport, 4-social withdrawal, 5-verbal fluency) were most associated with maleness (symptom 4); age > 40/45 years (men/women; symptoms 1,2,4); single/unmarried status (symptoms 2–4); unemployment (symptoms 3,4); higher score on the Clinical Global Impressions (CGI) scale and PANSS total score (symptoms 1–5); lower score on the PANSS positive symptoms subscale (symptoms 1,3); more than 52 weeks of treatment (symptoms 1–3,5); and high antipsychotic dose (symptom 2).

Conclusions.—The prevalence of negative symptoms in patients with schizophrenia spectrum disorders treated with antipsychotics in routine clinical practice not only is still considerably high but also seems to be related to poorer functioning, unemployment, greater severity, and less positive symptomatology and higher antipsychotic dose (Table 3).

▶ This is a large observational Spanish study that was conducted several years ago to assess the metabolic adverse effects of antipsychotic therapy. Although

TABLE 3.—Factors Associated With the Presence of Negative Symptoms, Symptom-by-Symptom and Overall[a]

	1. Blunted Affect	2. Emotional Withdrawal	3. Poor Rapport	4. Social Withdrawal	5. Verbal Fluency	At Least 1 Negative Symptom	All Negative Symptoms
Sex							
Female (protective factor)				0.697 (0.523–0.931)		0.726 (0.537–0.982)	
Age, y							
≥40 (men)/ ≥45 years (women)	1.574 (1.172–2.115)	1.659 (1.215–2.267)		1.656 (1.237–2.219)		1.732 (1.288–2.330)	
Marital status							
Not married		1.756 (1.211–2.546)	1.547 (1.091–2.194)	1.756 (1.211–2.546)			
Work status							
Unemployed/inactive			1.889 (1.214–2.940)	1.526 (1.040–2.237)			3.815 (1.862–7.816)
CGI severity							
3–4	4.848 (2.050–11.460)	2.819 (1.462–5.433)	6.490 (2.553–16.499)	4.144 (2.287–7.510)	5.251 (2.228–12.376)	5.431 (3.237–9.111)	
5–7	20.896 (8.151–53.571)	8.905 (4.161–19.056)	26.051 (9.418–72.058)	14.626 (7.061–30.295)	10.160 (4.074–25.340)	29.759 (12.492–70.893)	
PANSS total							
> median (68)	7.884 (5.601–11.099)	10.210 (7.347–14.188)	8.275 (5.923–11.561)	5.644 (4.980–8.863)	8.252 (5.873–11.595)	12.773 (9.285–17.572)	22.428 (12.533–40.132)
PANSS positive							
≥ 26 (protective factor)	0.441 (0.232–0.838)		0.373 (0.196–0.709)				
Treatment time, wk							
> 52 weeks	1.501 (1.111–2.038)	1.409 (1.039–1.910)	1.551 (1.151–2.090)		1.512 (1.136–2.014)		2.040 (1.448–2.875)

Abbreviations: CGI = Clinical Global Impressions scale, OR = odds ratio, PANSS = Positive and Negative Syndrome Scale.
[a] All factors are measured as OR (95% CI).

this group clearly has a keen interest in negative symptoms of schizophrenia (indeed Dr Arango, a coauthor, spent many years studying negative symptoms with Drs Carpenter, Buchanan, and Kirkpatrick at the University of Maryland), this particular study was neither conceived nor designed for this purpose. Accordingly, there are shortcomings with this study, particularly the closure of interrater reliability measurements of negative symptoms (which are rated notoriously variable among evaluators) across the investigators. Also, as the data attest to (Table 3) it is not clear about the associations described in the study—eg, are high doses of antipsychotics contributing to the negative symptoms or are clinicians prescribing high doses of medications to counteract severe negative symptoms? Notwithstanding these caveats, the study still highlights the common extent of negative symptoms in people with schizophrenia.

P. F. Buckley, MD

Auditory Hallucinations in Dissociative Identity Disorder and Schizophrenia With and Without a Childhood Trauma History: Similarities and Differences
Dorahy MJ, Shannon C, Seagar L, et al (Univ of Canterbury, Christchurch, New Zealand; Holywell Hosp, Antrim, Northern Ireland; Belmont Private Hosp, Brisbane, Australia; et al)
J Nerv Ment Dis 197:892-898, 2009

Little is known about similarities and differences in voice hearing in schizophrenia and dissociative identity disorder (DID) and the role of child maltreatment and dissociation. This study examined various aspects of voice hearing, along with childhood maltreatment and pathological dissociation in 3 samples: schizophrenia without child maltreatment (n = 18), schizophrenia with child maltreatment (n = 16), and DID (n = 29). Compared with the schizophrenia groups, the DID sample was more likely to have voices starting before 18, hear more than 2 voices, have both child and adult voices and experience tactile and visual hallucinations. The 3 groups were similar in that voice content was incongruent with mood and the location was more likely internal than external. Pathological dissociation predicted several aspects of voice hearing and appears an important variable in voice hearing, at least where maltreatment is present (Table 3).

▶ This is an often-neglected topic of hearing voices. It's difficult to study because hearing voices is an entirely subjective experience. This is a clever study, comparing adults with schizophrenia (with and without a history of childhood trauma) and people with dissociative identity disorder. Although the data are interesting and suggest at least some qualitative (and timing) differences in the experience of hearing voices between schizophrenia and dissociative identity disorder, the number of patients in each group is relatively small. Unfortunately, this is a key methodological issue because it does not really allow for strong statistical inferences. Nevertheless, these data do

TABLE 3.—Frequency of Complex Phenomenological Aspects of Voice Hearing Experience Across Groups

	SwithoutM; N = 18		SwithM; N = 16		DID; N = 29	
	n	%	n	%	n	%
Voice in relation to person						
Voice/s talk about themselves in relation to you (eg "We are normal, YOU are mad")	5	28	4	25	18	62
Voices *often* comment to each other about you	4	24	3	19	18	62
Voices *sometime* or *often* talk among themselves without reference to you	2	12	3	19	23	79
Voice/s often make a running commentary on your behavior/thoughts	5	31	4	28	16	55
Voices *sometime* or *often* address you	10	59	8	50	23	79
The voice/s *often* told you what to do	8	44	13	81	21	72
Yes, I am able to resist the voice/s[c]	11	61	14	88	24	83
Sometimes or often feel controlled by the voices	9	50	13	81	24	83
Would miss voice if/when stopped	3	16	2	13	20	69
Content of voices and identifiability						
The content reflects thoughts I have	8	44	4	25	17	59
Content related to someone influential in your life	4	22	6	38	22	76
Voices were replays of memories of previous things said to you	4	22	7	44	22	76
Mood congruency						
Mood of voice/s is *different* from your mood at the time	11	61	10	63	22	76
Mood of voice/s is *different* from your general mood throughout day/wk	13	72	11	69	20	69
Accompanying sensation and other types of hallucinations						
Had sign voice/s were coming	3	17	4	25	22	76
Experienced accompanying physical sensation with voices	9	50	8	50	28	97
Headaches	2	11	3	19	14	48
Experienced visual hallucinations	8	44	7	44	24	83
Experienced tactile hallucinations	6	33	3	19	26	90
Experienced olfactory hallucinations	4	22	6	38	22	76
Experienced gustatory hallucinations	1	6	4	25	16	55
Other hallucinations happen around same time as auditory hallucinations	5	28	9	56	23	79

[c]Five schizophrenia without maltreatment and 1 Schizophrenia with maltreatment reported "NO" command hallucinations.

highlight the real experience of voices occurring in a nonpsychotic state where trauma is the underlying etiological factor.

P. F. Buckley, MD

Misattributions of agency in schizophrenia are based on imprecise predictions about the sensory consequences of one's actions

Synofzik M, Thier P, Leube DT, et al (Univ of Tübingen, Germany; Univ Hosp Marburg, Germany; et al)

Brain 133:262-271, 2010

The experience of being the initiator of one's own actions seems to be infallible at first glance. Misattributions of agency of one's actions in certain neurological or psychiatric patients reveal, however, that the central mechanisms underlying this experience can go astray. In

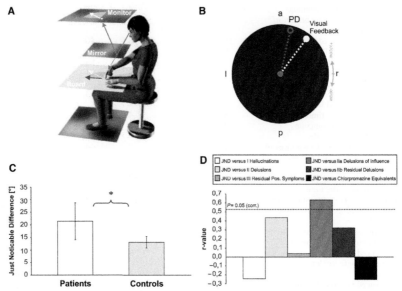

FIGURE 1.—Thresholds for the detection of experimental distortion of visual feedback about pointing and their relation to delusions of control. (**A**) Setup: Subjects viewed a virtual image of their finger (white disc) on the feedback monitor via a mirror (solid orange line) while performing pointing movements. This setup allowed subjects to perceive the virtual image in the same plane as their actual finger while the direction of movement could be manipulated (red arrow: movement vector; solid/broken white arrow: actual/perceived visual feedback). (**B**) Experiment 1: On-line visual feedback (white disc) about pointing (red circle) was either rotated in a counter-clockwise (ccw) or—as in this example—in a clockwise direction (cw) and the size of the rotation angle (x) was varied across trials. Dotted lines indicate the pointing movement (red) and the respective visual feedback trajectory (white). PD denotes the actual pointing direction, a, p, l, r denote anterior, posterior, left and right, respectively. The subject's task was to indicate the direction of perceived visual feedback rotation in a two-alternative forced-choice manner (clockwise versus counterclockwise). (**C**) Just noticeable difference: On average, schizophrenia patients showed a significantly larger just noticeable difference (JND) between the actual and the perceived pointing direction, indicating an impaired ability to detect visual feedback manipulations (means ± 95% confidence intervals, uncorrected). (**D**) Correlation between psychopathology and the just noticeable difference: The bar plot shows correlation coefficients (r-values) for the linear correlations between the just noticeable difference and (i) the SAPS sub-scores as well as (ii) patients' medication (chlorpromazine equivalents). The corrected P-threshold of P < .05 is indicated by the dotted line. For further explanation please refer to the main text. For interpretation of the references to color in this figure legend, the reader is referred to web version of this article. (Reprinted from Synofzik M, Thier P, Leube DT, et al. Misattributions of agency in schizophrenia are based on imprecise predictions about the sensory consequences of one's actions. *Brain.* 2010;133:262-271, with permission from Oxford University.)

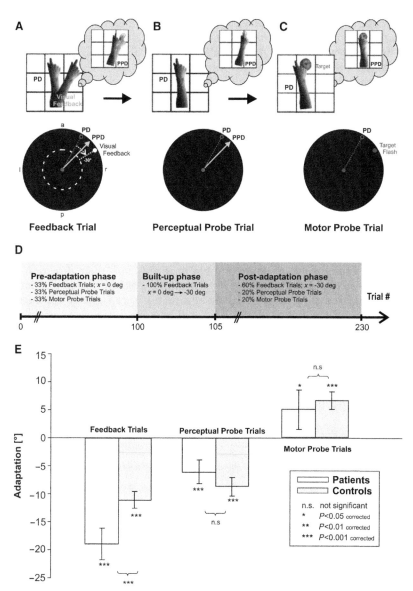

FIGURE 2.—Adaptation of self-action estimates and motor performance to a constant visual feedback rotation. (A–C) Paradigm Experiment 2: The top row provides a graphical illustration of each of our three experimental conditions as well as the expected perceptual and motor effects of feedback adaptation on both controls [*cf.* Synofzik *et al.* (2006); skin coloured arms] and schizophrenia patients [*cf.* Lindner *et al.* (2005) green arms]: (**A**) if subjects were constantly provided rotated visual feedback with respect to their actual pointing direction (PD, grey arm), controls would tend to perceive their arm as pointing into the direction of visual feedback. This perceived pointing direction of controls (PPD) is indicated by the skin coloured arm. (**B**) Even without visual feedback, they would continue to perceive their arm as pointing into the same visual direction (as in **A**) since they would have 'internalized' the new visual consequences associated with this action. (**C**) Finally, if asked to reach for a specific visual target (apple) without visual feedback, controls would reach in a direction opposite to the feedback rotation in order to account for the

particular, delusions of influence in schizophrenia might result from deficits in an inferential mechanism that allows distinguishing whether or not a sensory event has been self-produced. This distinction is made by comparing the actual sensory information with the consequences of one's action as predicted on the basis of internal action-related signals such as efference copies. If this internal prediction matches the actual sensory event, an action is registered as self-caused; in case of a mismatch, the difference is interpreted as externally produced. We tested the hypothesis that delusions of influence are based on deficits in this comparator mechanism. In particular, we tested whether patients' impairments in action attribution tasks are caused by imprecise predictions about the sensory consequences of self-action. Schizophrenia patients and matched controls performed pointing movements in a virtual-reality setup in which the visual consequences of movements could be rotated with respect to the actual movement. Experiment 1 revealed higher thresholds for detecting experimental feedback rotations in the patient group. The size of these thresholds correlated positively with patients' delusions of influence. Experiment 2 required subjects to estimate their direction of pointing visually in the presence of constantly rotated visual feedback. When compared to controls, patients' estimates were significantly better adapted to the feedback rotation and exhibited an increased variability. In interleaved trials without visual feedback, i.e. when pointing estimates relied solely on internal action-related signals, this variability was likewise increased and correlated with both delusions of influence and the size of patients' detection thresholds as assessed in the first experiment. These findings support the notion that delusions of influence are based on imprecise internal predictions about the sensory consequences of one's actions.

---

altered visual consequences of their movement. In the case of schizophrenia patients we hypothesized that—due to imprecise internal predictions—these patients would over-rely on visual feedback about self-action and thus perceive their arm as even further rotated into the direction of the visual feedback manipulation (**A**, green arm). In addition, imprecise internal predictions should cause a higher variability of the visual selfaction estimates (**A** and **B**, green dots indicate variably perceived movement directions). Finally, we did not expect any alteration in patients' motor performance (**C**). The bottom row of panels A–C depicts the three different experimental conditions that we used to obtain the aforementioned measures. For a complete description of these conditions please refer to the methods section. Exemplary pointing and a rotated feedback trajectory are shown by the dotted red lines and the dotted white line, respectively. Exemplary perceived pointing directions are indicated by the solid grey arrows. The dashed circle in (**A**) indicates that the first half of subjects' visual movement trajectory was occluded to avoid any online-corrections of pointing. An explicit pointing target (red circle) was only flashed in motor probe trials (**C**), while in the remaining conditions (**A** and **B**) subjects where free to point in any freely chosen direction between subjective 0° (r) and 90° (a, anterior). No visual feedback was provided in probe trials (**B** and **C**). (**D**) Time-line of Experiment 2: This illustration indicates the share of each experimental condition and also specifies x, namely the angle of visual feedback rotation, for each of the different stages of adaptation. (**E**) Group results: Both groups showed a significant, adaptation-induced shift of their perceived pointing direction into the direction of feedback rotation. Schizophrenia patients thereby expressed significantly higher levels of adaptation as long as visual feedback was present (feedback trials). In the absence of visual feedback, the adaptation of the perceived pointing direction was significant in both groups and of a comparable amount (perceptual probe trials). Moreover, both groups significantly adjusted their motor behaviour by a comparable amount (motor probe trials; figure-conventions as in Fig. 1). For interpretation of the references to color in this figure legend, the reader is referred to web version of this article. (Reprinted from Synofzik M, Thier P, Leube DT, et al. Misattributions of agency in schizophrenia are based on imprecise predictions about the sensory consequences of one's actions. *Brain*. 2010;133:262-271, with permission from Oxford University.)

Moreover, we suggest that such imprecise predictions prompt patients to rely more strongly on (and thus adapt to) external agency cues, in this case vision. Such context-dependent weighted integration of imprecise internal predictions and alternative agency cues might thus reflect the common basis for the various misattributions of agency in schizophrenia patients.

▶ The reasons and interactions between external and internal perceptions and the symptoms of schizophrenia remain an intriguing question. Venables, Mehl, and others proposed an external stimuli filtering failure that resulted in a "flooding" or bombardment of stimuli, which the patient cannot manage, thereby resulting in hyperarousal to the external environment and misattribution of experiences as paranoid delusions, etc. This is a more modern-day explication of this notion—this time focusing more on the internal experiences between perceptions and thoughts (Figs 1 and 2). The relationships of their process to psychopathology are surprisingly weak. These are detailed and complicated studies. However, the findings are certainly interesting.

P. F. Buckley, MD

Brain-Derived Neurotrophic Factor and Initial Antidepressant Response to an *N*-Methyl-ᴅ-Aspartate Antagonist

Machado-Vieira R, Yuan P, Brutsche N, et al (Natl Insts of Health [NIH], Bethesda, MD)
J Clin Psychiatry 70:1662-1666, 2009

Objective.—A model has been proposed to explain the pathophysiology of mood disorders based on decreased neurotrophin levels during mood episodes; treatment with antidepressants and mood stabilizers is associated with clinical improvement. This study investigated whether changes in brain-derived neurotrophic factor (BDNF) levels are associated with the initial antidepressant effects of ketamine, a high-affinity N-methyl-ᴅ-aspartate (NMDA) antagonist.

Method.—Twenty-three subjects aged 18 to 65 years with *DSM-IV* major depressive disorder (treatment resistant) participated in this study, which was conducted between October 2006 and May 2008. The subjects were given an open-label intravenous infusion of ketamine hydrochloride (0.5 mg/kg) and rated using various depression scales at baseline and at 40, 80, 120, and 230 minutes postinfusion. The primary outcome measure was the Montgomery-Asberg Depression Rating Scale score. BDNF levels were obtained at the same time points as depression rating scale scores.

Results.—Despite a significant ($P < .001$) improvement in MADRS scores after subjects received ketamine treatment, no changes in BDNF levels were observed in subjects after they received ketamine compared to baseline. Also, no association was found between antidepressant response and BDNF levels.

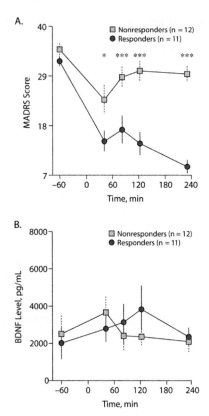

FIGURE 1.—BDNF values and MADRS scores over 230 minutes in subjects with major depressive disorder (treatment resistant) who did and did not respond to ketamine (N = 23). *P < .05, ***P < .001 after Bonferroni correction. Abbreviations: BDNF = brain-derived neurotrophic factor, MADRS = Montgomery-Asberg Depression Rating Scale. (Reprinted from Machado-Vieira R, Yuan P, Brutsche N, et al. Brain-derived neurotrophic factor and initial antidepressant response to an N-methyl-D-aspartate antagonist. *J Clin Psychiatry.* 2009;70:1662-1666, with permission from Physicians Postgraduate Press.)

Conclusions.—This study demonstrates that ketamine's rapid initial antidepressant effects are not mediated by BDNF. Further studies are necessary to shed light on the neurobiological basis of these effects.

Trial Registration.—clinicaltrials.gov Identifiers: NCT00024635 and NCT00088699 (Fig 1, Table 1).

▶ This group of investigators from The National Institute of Mental Health has been examining the potential of ketamine to improve mood in depressed patients. They and others have shown short-term beneficial effects. The authors review succinctly the potential role of brain-derived neurotrophic factor (BDNF) in depression, and they describe the effects of various antidepressant medications on BDNF levels. Surprisingly to us and to the authors, they failed here to find any effect of ketamine infusion on BDNF levels in this chronically

TABLE 1.—Demographic and Clinical Characteristics of Subjects With Major Depressive Disorder (treatment resistant) Receiving Ketamine (N = 23)

Characteristic	Mean	SD
Age, y	43.9	13.9
Age at onset, y	19.2	8.5
Body mass index	30.9	7.6
Illness duration, y	24.8	12.4
Episode duration, mo	80.7	108.5
No. of episodes	31.7	45.3
MADRS score	33.5	4.3
HDRS-17 score	20.8	4.4
BDI score	26.0	7.3
BPRS score	36.9	5.7
YMRS score	5.0	3.1
	N	%
Sex, male	14	61
Education, college	12	63[a]

Abbreviations: BDI = Beck Depression Inventory, BPRS = Brief Psychiatric Rating Scale, HDRS-17 = 17-item Hamilton Depression Rating Scale, MADRS = Montgomery-Asberg Depression Rating Scale, YMRS-Young Mania Rating Scale.
[a]Information was unavailable for a few subjects.

depressed patient sample. This is surprising, given that they did observe clinically an antidepressant effect of ketamine. It is unclear then, why they would advocate for additional studies. This is a useful example of how a study may not always find what it is looking for. This is the process of science!

P. F. Buckley, MD

A Cross-Sectional Evaluation of the Effect of Risperidone and Selective Serotonin Reuptake Inhibitors on Bone Mineral Density in Boys

Calarge CA, Zimmerman B, Xie D, et al (The Univ of Iowa Carver College of Medicine; The Univ of Iowa College of Public Health)
J Clin Psychiatry 71:338-347, 2010

Objective.—The aim of the present study was to investigate the effect of risperidone-induced hyperprolactinemia on trabecular bone mineral density (BMD) in children and adolescents.

Method.—Medically healthy 7- to 17-year-old males chronically treated, in a naturalistic setting, with risperidone were recruited for this cross-sectional study through child psychiatry outpatient clinics between November 2005 and June 2007. Anthropometric measurements and laboratory testing were conducted. The clinical diagnoses were based on chart review, and developmental and treatment history was obtained from the medical record. Volumetric BMD of the ultradistal radius was measured using peripheral quantitative computed tomography, and areal BMD of the lumbar spine was estimated using dual-energy x-ray absorptiometry.

Results.—Hyperprolactinemia was present in 49% of 83 boys (n = 41) treated with risperidone for a mean of 2.9 years. Serum testosterone concentration increased with pubertal status but was not affected by hyperprolactinemia. As expected, bone mineral content and BMD increased with sexual maturity. After adjusting for the stage of sexual development and height and BMI z scores, serum prolactin was negatively associated with trabecular volumetric BMD at the ultradistal radius ($P < .03$). Controlling for relevant covariates, we also found treatment with selective serotonin reuptake inhibitors (SSRIs) to be associated with lower trabecular BMD at the radius ($P = .03$) and BMD z score at the lumbar spine ($P < .05$). These findings became more marked when the analysis was restricted to non-Hispanic white patients. Of 13 documented

TABLE 1.—Demographic and Clinical Characteristics of Subjects With Normal and High Prolactin Concentration

	Normal Prolactin (n = 42)	High Prolactin (n = 41)	Statistical Analysis	P Value[a]
Characteristic				
Race/ethnicity, % non-Hispanic white/African American/Hispanic/other	83/12/2/2	88/7/2/2	Fisher exact	.9
Age, mean ± SD, y	11.8 ± 2.8	11.9 ± 3.0	$t_{81} = .1$	.96
Pubertal status, % at Tanner stage I/II/III/IV/V	44/17/15/22/2	27/24/17/20/12	Wilcoxon = 1858	>.1
Height z score, mean ± SD	0.1 ± 0.9	0.3 ± 0.9	$t_{81} = .1.2$	.2
Weight z score, mean ± SD	0.4 ± 1.0	0.6 ± 1.0	$t_{81} = .9$	.4
Body mass index z score, mean ± SD	0.5 ± 1.0	0.6 ± 1.0	$t_{81} = .6$	.6
Cigarette smoking, n (%)	0	4 (10)	Fisher exact	*.06*
Calcium intake, mean ± SD, mg/d	1024 ± 400	1050 ± 340	$t_{80} = .3$	.8
Vitamin D intake, median (quartiles), IU/d	274 (179–365)	259 (203–373)	Wilcoxon = 1704	.7
Physical activity, median (quartiles)	4.0 (3.0–4.0)	3.0 (2.0–5.0)	Wilcoxon = 1695	.8
Elevated TSH, n (%)[b]	2 (5)	10 (24)	Fisher exact	**<.02**
Prolactin, median (quartiles), ng/mL	12.9 (8.3–16.0)	28.5 (23.2–42.4)	Wilcoxon = 2583	**<.0001**
Testosterone, median (quartiles), ng/dL	57.0 (6.0–313.0)	47.0 (15.0–382.0)	Wilcoxon = 1804	>.3
Pharmacotherapy				
Risperidone dose, mean ± SD, mg/kg/d	0.03 ± 0.01	0.04 ± 0.02	$t_{64} = 3.56$	**.002**
Risperidone treatment duration, median (quartiles), y	2.8 (1.1–3.9)	2.7 (1.7–3.8)	Wilcoxon = 1748	.8
SSRI treatment, n (%)	20 (48)	24 (59)	Fisher exact	.4
SSRI dose, median (quartiles)[c]	1.0 (0.5–1.5)	1.0 (0.8–1.9)	Wilcoxon = 422	.5
SSRI treatment duration, meant ± SD, y	2.9 ± 2.2	3.5 ± 1.6	$t_{42} = 1.03$	.3

Abbreviations: SSRI = selective serotonin reuptake inhibitor, TSH = thyroid-stimulating hormone.
[a]Statistically significant findings are in bold. Findings that are at a trend level are in bolded italics.
[b]The normal range for thyroid-stimulating hormone is 0.27–4.20 μIU/mL In no cases was TSH > 7.0 μIU/mL.
[c]In order to compute a mean SSRI dose across the different medications available, we converted each patient's dally dose into an SSRI-unit equivalent (see text for details).

TABLE 3.—Least Square Means[a] ± SE of pQCT- and DXA-Based Bone Measurements[b] as a Function of Pubertal Stage in Non-Hispanic White Boys and Adolescents Treated With Risperidone

Prolactin Status[c]	Tanner Stage	Total vBMD (mg/cm^3)[d]	Trabecular vBMD (mg/cm^3)[e]	Lumbar Total BMC (g)[f]	Lumbar Total aBMD (g/cm^2)[g]	Lumbar Total aBMD z Score[h]
Normal	I	327.0 ± 12.3	221.4 ± 8.5	26.5 ± 1.6	0.64 ± 0.02	0.25 ± 0.20
Normal	II	351.5 ± 12.6	234.0 ± 9.4	31.7 ± 1.8	0.70 ± 0.02	0.43 ± 0.22
Normal	III	302.7 ± 13.6	213.1 ± 9.5	34.7 ± 2.0	0.71 ± 0.03	−0.31 ± 0.25
Normal	IV	328.9 ± 13.0	225.7 ± 9.5	48.2 ± 1.7	0.86 ± 0.02	−0.16 ± 0.21
Normal	V	427.6 ± 22.1	267.4 ± 16.7	62.6 ± 3.5	0.99 ± 0.04	0.3 ± 0.44
High	I	308.1 ± 11.6	203.2 ± 8.7	24.8 ± 1.6	0.62 ± 0.02	0.32 ± 0.20
High	II	332.6 ± 11.9	215.8 ± 8.7	30.0 ± 1.7	0.67 ± 0.02	0.50 ± 0.21
High	III	283.8 ± 14.8	194.9 ± 10.4	33.0 ± 2.1	0.68 ± 0.03	−0.25 ± 0.26
High	IV	310.0 ± 13.0	207.4 ± 9.8	46.4 ± 1.8	0.84 ± 0.02	−0.09 ± 0.22
High	V	408.7 ± 20.8	249.2 ± 15.4	60.8 ± 3.3	0.97 ± 0.04	0.39 ± 0.42

[a]All least square means were adjusted for stage of sexual development.
[b]vBMD at the radius was generated using pQCT and bone mineral measurements at the lumbar spine were generated using DXA.
[c]The mean prolactin concentration in the group with high (34.4 ng/mL) and normal prolactin (12.2 ng/mL) was used to generate the respective least square means.
[d]Total vBMD at the radius was adjusted for height and weight z scores and physical activity.
[e]Trabecular vBMD was adjusted for height and BMI z scores.
[f]Lumbar spine BMC was adjusted for physical activity, daily intake of vitamin D, and duration of risperidone treatment.
[g]Lumbar spine aBMD was adjusted for physical activity and duration of risperidone treatment.
[h]Lumbar spine aBMD z score was adjusted for height and BMI z scores, daily intake of calcium, and physical activity (see text for details). Abbreviations: aBMD = areal bone mineral density, BMC = bone mineral content, BMI = body mass index, DXA = dual -energy x-ray absorptiometry, pQCT = peripheral quantitative computerized tomography, vBMD = volumetric bone mineral density.

fractures, 3 occurred after risperidone and SSRIs were started, and none occurred in patients with hyperprolactinemia.

Conclusions.—This is the first study to link risperidone-induced hyperprolactinemia and SSRI treatment to lower BMD in children and adolescents. Future research should evaluate the longitudinal course of this adverse event to determine its temporal stability and whether a higher fracture rate ensues (Tables 1 and 3).

▶ Although this study has some obvious methodological limitations, not the least of which is the overall small number of patients who were included in the study, it is an important study and has potentially salutary findings. The methodology of assessing bone density is interesting and impressive (Fig 1 in the original article). The study shows a relationship between hyperprolactinemia and bone loss (Table 1), and this may be related to risperidone (Tables 1 and 3). However, it does not appear to be mediated through hypogonadism as has been found in other studies. The shortcomings include the small patient sample, the cross-sectional evaluation of prolactin and testosterone, the focus only on boys, and the focus only on risperidone as the only antipsychotic. The case made in the study for selective serotonin reuptake inhibitors being contributors to the findings seems weak. Nevertheless, these study findings are salutary and resonate with public concerns about the use of the drugs in developing children and young adolescents.

P. F. Buckley, MD

Functional and Dysfunctional Synaptic Plasticity in Prefrontal Cortex: Roles in Psychiatric Disorders

Goto Y, Yang CR, Otani S (McGill Univ, Montreal, Quebec, Canada; Eli Lilly and Company, Indianapolis, IN; Univ of Paris VI-INSERM/CNRS, France)
Biol Psychiatry 67:199-207, 2010

Prefrontal cortex (PFC) mediates an assortment of cognitive functions including working memory, behavioral flexibility, attention, and future planning. Unlike the hippocampus, where induction of synaptic plasticity in the network is well-documented in relation to long-term memory, cognitive functions mediated by the PFC have been thought to be independent of long-lasting neuronal adaptation of the network. Nonetheless, accumulating evidence suggests that prefrontal cortical neurons possess the cellular machinery of synaptic plasticity and exhibit lasting changes of neural activity associated with various cognitive processes. Moreover, deficits in the mechanisms of synaptic plasticity induction in the PFC might be involved in the pathophysiology of psychiatric and neurological disorders

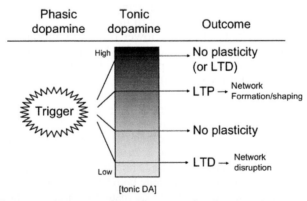

FIGURE 1.—A model of the relationship between dopamine (DA) release and synaptic plasticity induction in the prefrontal cortex (PFC). In the normal condition at a moderate tonic/background DA tone, long-term potentiation (LTP) is induced by high-frequency stimulation of PFC afferent fibers that co-release DA "phasically" from residual DA axon terminals. Slight background increase of DA release facilitates LTP induction, whereas further increase of tonic DA tone impairs LTP induction. In contrast, with reduction of tonic DA tone such as the condition present in the in vitro slice preparation, the "phasic" release of DA preferentially induces long-term depression (LTD) in PFC network. (Reprinted from Goto Y, Yang CR, Otani S. Functional and dysfunctional synaptic plasticity in prefrontal cortex: roles in psychiatric disorders. *Biol Psychiatry.* 2010;67:199-207, with permission from the Society of Biological Psychiatry.)

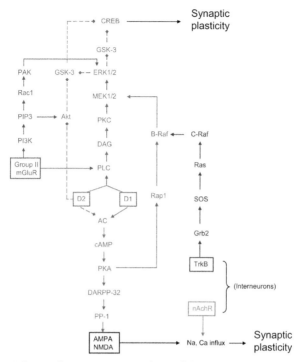

FIGURE 2.—A diagram illustrating receptors and intracellular signaling pathways that are involved in long-term synaptic plasticity induction in the PFC. Receptors and signaling pathways with red, green, blue, and orange indicate those mediated by DA, group II metabotropic glutamate receptor (mGluR), brain-derived neurotrophic factor (BDNF), and nicotinic acetylcholine receptor (nAchR), respectively. Solid lines with arrows indicate activation, whereas dashed lines with arrows indicate inhibition of molecules. Modulation of synaptic plasticity induction in the limbic–PFC pathway with D1 but not D2 receptor stimulation has been shown to involve activation of protein kinase A (PKA) (42), leading to phosphorylation of N-methyl d-aspartate (NMDA) receptors and increase of surface expression of α-amino-3-hydroxy-5-methylisoxazole propionate (AMPA) receptors to increase calcium and sodium influx (44). In contrast, D2 receptor stimulation attenuates this LTP induction (12), which could be achieved through inhibition of this adenylyl cyclase (AC)/cyclic adenosine monophosphate (cAMP)/ PKA signaling cascade. There is also a study showing that coactivation of D1 and D2 receptors activates another signaling cascade consisting of phospholipase C (PLC)/diacylglycerol (DAG)/protein kinase C, which in turn activates mitogen-activated protein (MAP) kinases (e.g., MEK1/2 and ERK1/2) (47). There-fore, LTP induction requiring coactivation of D1 and D2 receptors in PFC local circuitry (22) might involve this signaling pathway, which might involve epigenetic regulation of gene expressions and protein synthesis, as MAP kinases activate cAMP response element-binding protein (CREB), which is a transcription factor regulating gene transcription (96). In addition, D2 receptor stimulation has been shown to inhibit a signaling cascade consisting of Akt/glycogen synthase kinase (GSK)-3/CREB. Group II mGluR stimulation in the PFC has been shown to activate intracellular signaling molecules converging on those activated by DA receptor stimulation such as PLC, Akt, and ERK1/2 (97). The BDNF and its binding receptor TrkB activates signaling pathway converging on those activated by DA through B-ref, which in turn activate MAP kinases. The nAchR is an ionotropic receptor. Therefore, nAchR stimulation expressed on interneurons does not involve activation or inhibition of intracellular signaling molecules but direct change of ion influx. It seems that both BDNF and nAchR modulates synaptic plasticity induction in the PFC through interneurons, facilitating γ-aminobutyric acid (GABA)ergic inhibitory transmission, and suppresses abnormal emergence of LTP induction (16,98). DARPP-32, dopamine and cyclic AMP-regulated phosphoprotein of Mr 32000; Ca, calcium; Na, sodium, other abbreviations as in Figure 1. Editor's Note: Please refer to original journal article for full references. For interpretation of the references to color in this figure legend, the reader is referred to web version of this article. (Reprinted from Goto Y, Yang CR, Otani S. Functional and dysfunctional synaptic plasticity in prefrontal cortex: roles in psychiatric disorders. *Biol Psychiatry*. 2010;67:199-207, with permission from the Society of Biological Psychiatry.)

such as schizophrenia, drug addiction, mood disorders, and Alzheimer's disease (Figs 1 and 2).

▶ This is a comprehensive review of neural networking and long-term potentiation in relation to dopamine and glutamatergic neurotransmission in the prefrontal cortex, with a focus on schizophrenia. The information reviewed is voluminous, and the writing style is terse—both combine to make this a detailed article, highly focused, but not for the fainthearted! There are models and schema that explain the interplay between dopamine synapses and also glutamatergic neurotransmission (Figs 1 and 2). A cascade of signal transduction effects is illustrated. The article concluded—all too briefly—by reviewing the putative pharmacological strategies to enhance cognition in schizophrenia. While the article is slanted toward schizophrenia, it is still evident that the synaptic plasticity and mechanisms described here are also relevant to other psychiatric disorders that could—and do—involve the prefrontal cortex.

P. F. Buckley, MD

Genetic Studies of Drug Response and Side Effects in the STAR*D Study, Part 1
Garriock HA, Hamilton SP (Univ of California, San Francisco)
J Clin Psychiatry 70:1186-1187, 2009

Background.—The Sequenced Treatment Alternatives to Relieve Depression (STAR*D) study sought to identify the best treatment strategy for patients with major depressive disorder (MDD) whose initial pharmacological treatment with citalopram had failed. In the STAR*D study, 4000+ subjects were recruited and 1953 additional subjects donated DNA for use in genetic analysis. Several studies analyzed the serotonin transporter gene (*SLC6A4*) with respect to the phenotype of remission and adverse side effects, such as suicide and sexual dysfunction.

Serotonin Transporter Gene.—*SLC6A4* is the gene studied most in relationship to antidepressant response. The gene product, SERT, transports serotonin back into presynaptic neurons, ending the signaling cycle. The reuptake of serotonin back into the neuron is blocked by selective serotonin reuptake inhibitors (SSRIs). As a result there is more serotonin in the synapse. A promoter insertion/deletion (ins/del) in *SLC6A4* has differential effects, with the inserter allele (long) more active in transcription than the deleter (short) allele. Changing serotonin levels through the action of SSRIs may be the mechanism by which some MDD symptoms can be relieved. Several small studies suggest there may be a DNA variation in this gene related to antidepressant response, but the STAR*D study data indicate this is not true.

Remission.—The STAR*D data were employed by four research groups to study genetic variation and MDD remission links. When all these studies are considered, the genomic coverage is adequate, and the gene

TABLE 1.—Comparison of 3 Studies Investigating the Association Between Remission and 2 Polymorphisms in the *SLC6A4* Gene: Promoter ins/del and rs25531[a]

Study	No. of Remitters vs No. of Controls	Remission Definition	Baseline QIDS Requirement	Adherence/Compliance[b]	Ethnicity	Other Exclusions	Results
Kraft et al,[7] 2007	826 vs 669 nonresponders	QIDS-SR score $\leq$ 5 at study exit	None	None	Caucasian, African American	None	No association in any analysis with remission
Hu et al,[8] 2007	683 vs 664 nonremitters	QIDS-C$_{16}$ score $\leq$ 5 at last treatment visit	QIDS-C$_{16}$, score $\geq$ 10	Excluded nonadherent individuals	Caucasian non-Hispanic, African American	Final QIDS-C$_{16}$ score 6–9; intolerant and "probably intolerant" were excluded from nonremitter group	No association in any analysis with remission
Mrazek et al,[9] 2009	679 vs 815 nonremitters[c]	QIDS-C$_{16}$ score $\leq$ 5 at last treatment visit	QIDS-C$_{16}$ score $\geq$ 10	Excluded nonadherent individuals	Caucasian non-Hispanic, Caucasian Hispanic, African American	None; included temporarily remitters without maintained response as nonremitters	Among Caucasian non-Hispanics only: ins/del: $P_{Corrected} = .024$; no association with SNP; S-A-12 haplotype: $P_{global} = .04$

Abbreviations: QIDS-C$_{16}$ = Quick Inventory of Depressive Symptomatology-Clinician Rated, QIDS-SR = Quick Inventory of Depressive Symptomatology-Self Rated, SNP = single nucleotide polymorphism.
Editor's Note: Please refer to original journal article for full references.
[a]McMahon et al[6] not included, since it did not include 5-HTTLPR or rs25531.
[b]As determined from global rating of compliance.
[c]Numbers determined from data provided in Table 4 of Mrazek et al[9] for promoter insertion/deletion. Numbers are similar for rs25531.

does not appear to be linked to citalopram remission. However, study differences yielded some disparate findings. Two studies used novel single polyneucleotide polymorphism (SNP) detection through direct DNA sequencing, covering more than the promoter area of the gene, and discovered no link between citalopram remission and the gene. In none of the studies were associations found between *SLC6A4* variants and remission when the subjects were African American. However, the small numbers of African Americans included in the STAR*D study make it impossible to form a conclusion as to what this means.

Two polymorphisms, the promoter ins/del and rs25531 A/G SNP, were studied for a relationship with remission status. The three studies varied in terms of phenotype definition and ethnicities included, but were similar in using a 6-week participation in the study and no adjustment for ethnicity besides stratified analysis for each self-reported group. One study found remission linked to 5-HTTLPR in non-Hispanic Caucasians only and links between remission and a haplotype of 5-HTTLPR, rs25531, and a variable number tandem repeat (VNTR) in intron 2. Non-Hispanic Caucasians lacking the 12/12 genotype are more likely to achieve remission. Discordance in these studies may be related to the ethnic composition of the sample, differences in phenotypic definitions, or choice of assessment method.

Conclusions.—Overall, the genetic analyses of the STAR*D data indicate that *SLC6A4* may be an obvious candidate for genetic links to SSRI response, but it is not associated with any efficacy phenotype in MDD patients representative of the North American population who would be seen in a typical psychiatric practice.

▶ This is a brief, yet current, review of pharmacogenetics of treatment response in depression, using the Sequence Treatment Alternative to Relieve Depression (STAR*D) study as a reference point. The results described in this overview are less impressive than one might have considered (Table 1). On the other hand, STAR*D is such a large and robust study of depression treatment that replication of its findings is a challenge for our field. Another more community-based depression treatment study is currently underway, and this might provide a better opportunity for replicating, or not, the pharmacogenetic findings in STAR*D. This is a very important aspect for our field.

P. F. Buckley, MD

A Cytogenetic Abnormality and Rare Coding Variants Identify *ABCA13* as a Candidate Gene in Schizophrenia, Bipolar Disorder, and Depression
Knight HM, Pickard BS, Maclean A, et al (Univ of Edinburgh, UK; et al)
Am J Hum Genet 85:833-846, 2009

Schizophrenia and bipolar disorder are leading causes of morbidity across all populations, with heritability estimates of ~80% indicating a substantial genetic component. Population genetics and genome-wide association studies suggest an overlap of genetic risk factors between these illnesses but it is unclear how this genetic component is divided between common gene polymorphisms, rare genomic copy number variants, and rare gene sequence mutations. We report evidence that the lipid transporter gene *ABCA13* is a susceptibility factor for both schizophrenia and bipolar disorder. After the initial discovery of its disruption by a chromosome abnormality in a person with schizophrenia, we resequenced *ABCA13* exons in 100 cases with schizophrenia and 100 controls. Multiple rare coding variants were identified including one nonsense and nine

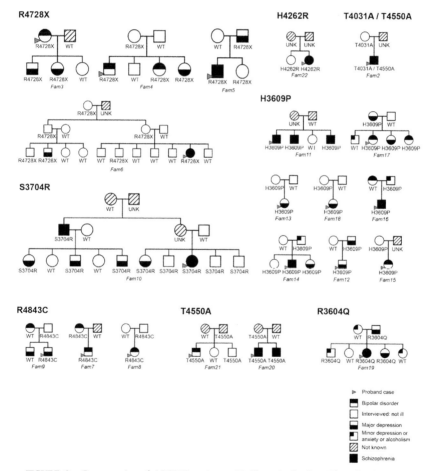

FIGURE 2.—Cosegregation of ABCA13 variants with illness in families. These families were all included in the linkage analysis. Images created with CraneFoot application.[83] Editor's Note: Please refer to original journal article for full references. (Reprinted from Knight HM, Pickard BS, Maclean A, et al. A cytogenetic abnormality and rare coding variants identify *ABCA13* as a candidate gene in schizophrenia, bipolar disorder, and depression. *Am J Hum Genet.* 2009;85:833-846, with permission from The American Society of Human Genetics.)

missense mutations and compound heterozygosity/homozygosity in six cases. Variants were genotyped in additional schizophrenia, bipolar, depression (n > 1600), and control (n > 950) cohorts and the frequency of all rare variants combined was greater than controls in schizophrenia (OR = 1.93, p = 0.0057) and bipolar disorder (OR = 2.71, p = 0.00007). The population attributable risk of these mutations was 2.2% for schizophrenia and 4.0% for bipolar disorder. In a study of 21 families of mutation carriers, we genotyped affected and unaffected relatives and found significant linkage (LOD = 4.3) of rare variants with a phenotype including schizophrenia, bipolar disorder, and major depression. These data identify a candidate gene, highlight the genetic overlap between schizophrenia, bipolar disorder, and depression, and suggest that rare coding variants may contribute significantly to risk of these disorders.

▶ This Scottish genetics group has been the major proponent of the proactive genetic overlap between schizophrenia and mood disorder, especially bipolar disorder. The authors of this article have previously published extensively on this topic. Here, they report very uncommon coding variants that reside in the gene *ABCA13*, a gene known to code for lipid metabolism. In the overall context of voluminous (and all too often irreproducible) genetic findings in schizophrenia, these results appear spurious. However, they do potentially relate to fundamental abnormalities in cell membrane phospholipids that have been reported for decades—now in patients with bipolar disorder. The genetic flow inheritance pattern described here is interesting (Fig 2). The authors indicate that this finding was also evident in the study by the International Schizophrenia Consortium. It is the first time I have heard mention of this anomaly.

P. F. Buckley, MD

Increased neural response to fear in patients recovered from depression: a 3T functional magnetic resonance imaging study
Norbury R, Selvaraj S, Taylor MJ, et al (Univ of Oxford, UK)
Psychol Med 40:425-432, 2010

Background.—Previous imaging studies have revealed that acute major depression is characterized by altered neural responses to negative emotional stimuli. Typically, responses in limbic regions such as the amygdala are increased while activity in cortical regulatory regions such as the dorsolateral prefrontal cortex (DLPFC) is diminished. Whether these changes persist in unmedicated recovered patients is unclear.

Method.—We used functional magnetic resonance imaging to examine neural responses to emotional faces in a facial expression-matching task in 16 unmedicated recovered depressed patients and 21 healthy controls.

Results.—Compared with controls, recovered depressed patients had increased responses bilaterally to fearful faces in the DLPFC and right caudate. Responses in the amygdala did not distinguish the groups.

Conclusions.—Our findings indicate that clinical recovery from depression is associated with increased activity in the DLPFC to negative emotional stimuli. We suggest that this increase may reflect a compensatory cortical control mechanism with the effect of limiting emotional dysregulation in limbic regions such as the amygdala.

▶ The Oxford group has conducted an elegant study of patients' response to fear following treatment for depression. In a high strength (3 T) functional magnetic resonance imaging study, they showed that the integrity to frontal and amygdalar neural networks is (re)established following recovery from depression (Figs 1-3 in the original article). This is a powerful message—and images—for sufferers of depression and for their families. People are often scared that they will remain emotionally blunted and not (re)experience the normal range of emotional responses after being depressed. This study suggests that people who recover from depression reattain their emotional activity. The authors also hint that this approach could even be used as a biomarker of treatment response in depression. This is, however, probably overstretching the conclusions, especially as this is very labor-intensive and complicated research. Nevertheless, there is great interest in seeing whether brain imaging parameters can predict disease progression and/or treatment response in psychiatric conditions. This is a major focus of the current NIMH strategic plan. This approach has also proved successful in other conditions and treatments, the management of (breast) cancer being a good example.

P. F. Buckley, MD

Serotonin Transporter Gene Promoter Polymorphism and Somatoform Symptoms

Hennings A, Zill P, Rief W (Philipps Univ of Marburg, Germany; Ludwig-Maximilian Univ, Munich, Germany)
J Clin Psychiatry 70:1536-1539, 2009

Introduction.—Symptoms of somatoform and affective disorders are thought to be connected to serotonergic neurotransmission because serotonin is known to regulate the functions relevant in these disorders, such as pain and mood. Previous studies have reported associations of these disorders with a functional polymorphism in the promoter region of the serotonin transporter gene, a limiting factor of the serotonergic neuronal system, as its alleles have been associated with differences in levels of synthesized transporter and therefore differences in reuptake efficiency.

Method.—Ninety-one patients with at least 2 unexplained physical symptoms were clinically evaluated and genotyped for the triallelic genotypes of the serotonin transporter gene polymorphism; patients were recruited from 2001 until 2004. *DSM-IV* diagnoses were assessed using the International Checklists for *ICD-10* and *DSM-IV*. Somatic complaints were quantified with an interview version of the Screening for Somatoform Symptoms, persistent symptoms in the last 2 years (SOMS-2) and the SOMS-7 (current symptoms in the last 7 days). Depressive symptoms were quantified with the Beck Depression Inventory (BDI).

Results.—Subjects with higher-expressing allele variants of the serotonin transporter gene (L'L' and L'S') had significantly more somatic symptoms in the last 2 years (trait) than those with lower-expressing variants (S'S') (*P* < .01). No differences could be found in regard to short-term somatic symptoms (ie, in the last 7 days). Neither depressive symptoms nor a comorbid diagnosis of major depression was associated with allelic variants.

Conclusion.—Somatoform symptoms may be associated with a functional polymorphism in the promoter region of the serotonin transporter gene.

▶ The results of this study are surprising. I would have predicted that polymorphism of the serotonin transporter gene would not have been associated with somatoform symptoms—or if the gene was associated—that the proposed relationship would be explained by the confounding presence and/or history of depression. However, this is not what the authors report in this German study. The study reports relationships with somatoform symptoms rather than a DSM-IV diagnosis—the latter is inferred, I guess. Somatoform disorders are often considered as depressive equivalents (ie, the expression of psychic distress/depression in the form of otherwise unexplained somatic complaints). Thus, typically a psychological explanation is invoked to explain the occurrence of these symptoms. The finding here of genetic associations with the serotonin transporter gene—most prominently associated with depression—is unexpected.

P. F. Buckley, MD

Gender Differences in Risk Factors for Aberrant Prescription Opioid Use
Jamison RN, Butler SF, Budman SH, et al (Brigham and Women's Hosp, Boston, MA; Inflexxion, Inc, Newton, MA)
J Pain 11:312-320, 2010

This is a longitudinal predictive study to examine gender differences in the clinical correlates of risk for opioid misuse among chronic pain patients prescribed opioids for pain. Two hundred seventy-five male and 335 female patients prescribed opioids for chronic noncancer pain were asked to complete a series of baseline questionnaires, including the revised Screener and Opioid Assessment for Pain Patients (SOAPP-R). After 5 months, the subjects were administered a structured prescription drug use interview (Prescription Drug Use Questionnaire; PDUQ) and submitted a urine sample for toxicology assessment. Their treating physicians also completed a substance misuse behavior checklist (Prescription Opioid Therapy Questionnaire; POTQ). At 5-month follow-up, women

TABLE 4.—Differences Between Male and Female Patients on Individual Items of the Screener and Opioid Assessment for Pain Patients

Variable	Male (N = 275)	Female (N = 335)	P
Items favoring women SOAPP-R (0-4)*			
Things are too overwhelming	1.65 ±	1.86 ±	$t = 3.55$§
Got into arguments/got hurt	1.25 ±	1.65 ±	$t = 3.21$‡
Impatient with physician	1.55 ±	1.85 ±	$t = 3.12$‡
Sexually abused	.62 ±	.83 ±	$t = 2.56$†
Concerned people judge you	1.98 ±	2.26 ±	$t = 2.42$†
Items favoring men SOAPP-R (0-4)*			
History of being arrested	.59 ±	.37 ±	$t = 3.51$§
Had a bad temper	.91 ±	.69 ±	$t = 2.88$‡
Friends w/ alcohol/drug problems	.98 ±	.78 ±	$t = 2.37$†

*How often are you...
†$P < .05$.
‡$P < .01$.
§$P < .001$.

showed higher scores on the PDUQ ($P < .05$), whereas men had a higher incidence of physician-rated aberrant drug behavior on the POTQ ($P < .05$). An item analysis of the SOAPP-R, PDUQ, and POTQ showed that women tended to score higher on items relating to psychological distress, whereas the male patients tended to report having more legal and behavioral problems. These results suggest that risk factors associated with prescription opioid misuse may differ between men and women.

Perspective.—Understanding gender differences in substance abuse risk among chronic pain patients is important for clinical assessment and treatment. This study suggests that women are at greater risk to misuse opioids because of emotional issues and affective distress, whereas men tend to misuse opioids because of legal and problematic behavioral issues (Table 4).

▶ The results of this study intuitively feel right and resonate well with clinical experience. They may also generalize to other forms of drug abuse, although this should be empirically tested. The researchers excluded cancer patients on pain medications—this is wise because their situation seems unique. It is unfortunate that the study did not include psychiatric diagnostic evaluations, as it is hard when reading this article to get a real feel for who the study subjects are. It is also noteworthy that this component was undertaken as part of a large multicenter study. It may also be relevant that females may be more forthcoming about their abuse and its psychological distress. Nevertheless, this study is useful in giving us a glimpse into gender-specific risk factors for abuse (Table 4) that could help and be incorporated into assessment protocols.

P. F. Buckley, MD

Comparative genomics of autism and schizophrenia

Crespi B, Stead P, Elliot M (Simon Fraser Univ, Burnaby, British Columbia, Canada)

Proc Natl Acad Sci U S A 107:1736-1741, 2010

We used data from studies of copy-number variants (CNVs), single-gene associations, growth-signaling pathways, and intermediate phenotypes associated with brain growth to evaluate four alternative hypotheses for the genomic and developmental relationships between autism and schizophrenia: (*i*) autism subsumed in schizophrenia, (*ii*) independence, (*iii*) diametric, and (*iv*) partial overlap. Data from CNVs provides statistical support for the hypothesis that autism and schizophrenia are associated with reciprocal variants, such that at four loci, deletions predispose to one disorder, whereas duplications predispose to the other. Data from single-gene studies are inconsistent with a hypothesis based on independence, in that autism and schizophrenia share associated genes more often than expected by chance. However, differentiation between the partial overlap and diametric hypotheses using these data is precluded by limited overlap in the specific genetic markers analyzed in both autism and schizophrenia. Evidence from the effects of risk variants on growth-signaling pathways shows that autism-spectrum conditions tend to be associated with upregulation of pathways due to loss of function mutations in negative regulators, whereas schizophrenia is associated with reduced pathway activation. Finally, data from studies of head and brain size phenotypes indicate that autism is commonly associated with developmentally-enhanced brain growth, whereas schizophrenia is characterized, on average, by reduced brain growth. These convergent lines of evidence appear most compatible with the hypothesis that autism and schizophrenia represent diametric conditions with regard to their genomic underpinnings, neurodevelopmental bases, and phenotypic manifestations as reflecting under-development versus dysregulated over-development of the human social brain.

▶ Although to many clinicians autism and schizophrenia may appear radically dissimilar, there is overlap in developmental features and potentially also in genetic attributions between these 2 disparate conditions. This article is comprehensive in its review, spanning from developmental and genetic phenotypic expression to shared clinical manifestations. It appears as if the recent genetic finding of an excess of copy number variants in both autism and schizophrenia has fueled this comparative review. The authors advance—in a compelling manner—the proposition that autism represents a repertoire, whereas schizophrenia represents a dysregulation/overdevelopment of communicative process. For those seeking an understanding of the genetic regulation of brain development, this is an excellent primer. It also has many of the key references in this area, both for schizophrenia and for autism. It is a very useful and informative publication.

P. F. Buckley, MD

Altered gene expression in neural crest cells exposed to ethanol *in vitro*
Wentzel P, Eriksson UJ (Uppsala Univ, Sweden)
Brain Res 1305:S50-S60, 2009

Aim.—To characterize and compare ethanol-induced changes of gene expression in cells from the cranial (cNCC) and trunk (tNCC) portion of the neural crest cell (NCC) population of day-10 rat embryos.

Background.—Previous work has suggested that ethanol-induced embryonic maldevelopment is associated with oxidative stress, and, in particular, that ethanol-induced anomalies of the facial skeleton and heart are associated with disturbed development of the cNCC. We studied alterations of mRNA levels of genes involved in apoptosis, oxidative defense, cellular metabolism, NCC development or inflammation in cNCC and tNCC from rat embryos exposed to ethanol *in vitro*. We specifically evaluated expression differences between cNCC and tNCC genes, possibly reflecting the different teratological susceptibilities of the two cell populations.

Methods.—Neural tube explants from rat embryos were divided in cranial and trunk portions and used for NCC isolation *in vitro* on gestational day 10. The migrating cells from the cranial or trunk explants of the neural tube were subsequently exposed to 0 or 88 mmol/l ethanol concentration with or without addition of 0.5 mM N-acetylcysteine (NAC) for 48 h, harvested, and prepared for gene expression measurement by RT-PCR or immunostaining with either distal-less (DLX) or AP 2-alpha antibodies.

Results.—Evaluation of the immunostained slides showed that approximately 75% of the cNCC and tNCC preparations were of neural crest origin. Exposure to 88 mM ethanol increased the Bax/Bcl-2 ratio in the NCC, and NAC addition diminished this increase. Both cNCC and tNCC upregulated MnSOD and Gpx-1 in response to ethanol, whereas tNCC increased CuZnSOD and EC-SOD after ethanol exposure (cNCC unchanged). Expression of glyceraldehyde-3-phosphate dehydrogenase was downregulated by ethanol in cNCC only. In addition, ethanol exposure caused increased mRNA levels of Pax-3, p53, Vegf-A and decreased expression of Pax-6, Nfe2 in both cNCC and tNCC. Ethanol increased Shh and Bmp-4 and decreased Parp only in cNCC (tNCC unchanged), whereas ethanol exposure increased T box-2 and decreased Gdnf and Ret only in tNCC (cNCC unchanged). In addition, ethanol exposure almost abolished expression of Hox a_1, a_4 and a_5, and left Hox a_2 unchanged in cNCC, whereas all four of these Hox genes were upregulated in tNCC.

Conclusions.—Ethanol causes a shift towards apoptosis in both cNCC and tNCC, a shift, which is diminished by NAC treatment. Oxidative defense genes, and genes involved in neural crest cell development are affected differently in cNCC compared to tNCC upon ethanol exposure. Moreover, ethanol downregulates cNCC Hox genes, whereas tNCC Hox genes are upregulated. These patterns of ethanol-altered gene expression may be of etiological importance for NCC-associated maldevelopment in ethanol-exposed pregnancy.

▶ This is a very interesting study of alcohol-related dysmorphogenesis, perhaps contrary to the prevailing opinion. Alcohol had an effect on the expression of a diverse array of genes. There is also a different pattern of gene expression in cranial versus trunk cells—presumably reflecting site-specific dysmorphogenesis. It is well known that exposure in utero to alcohol can result in the fetal alcohol syndrome (FAS). FAS is associated with both mental and physical retardation, especially of facial and limb regions—so called minor physical anomalies—although in cases of FAS, these are not so minor at all. The methodology of this study is excellent. The authors suggest that the pattern of gene expression reflects apoptosis and oxidative stress changes. However, the widespread changes seem to be more profound than simply confined to 1 pathobiological mechanism. This is always an issue in alcohol research—actually in neurobiological research in psychiatry.

P. F. Buckley, MD

Copy Number Variation in Schizophrenia in the Japanese Population
Ikeda M, Aleksic B, Kirov G, et al (Cardiff Univ, UK; Nagoya Univ Graduate School of Medicine, Japan)
Biol Psychiatry 67:283-286, 2010

Background.—Copy number variants (CNVs) have been shown to increase the risk to develop schizophrenia. The best supported findings are at 1q21.1, 15q11.2, 15q13.3, and 22q11.2 and deletions at the gene neurexin 1 (*NRXN1*).
Methods.—In this study, we used Affymetrix 5.0 arrays to investigate the role of rare CNVs in 575 patients with schizophrenia and 564 control subjects from Japan.
Results.—There was a nonsignificant trend for excess of rare CNVs in schizophrenia ($p = .087$); however, we did not confirm the previously implicated association for very large CNVs (>500 kilobase [kb]) in this population. We provide support for three previous findings in schizophrenia, as we identified one deletion in a case at 1q21.1, one deletion within *NRXN1*, and four duplications in cases and one in a control subject at 16p13.1, a locus first implicated in autism and later in schizophrenia.
Conclusions.—In this population, we support some of the previous findings in schizophrenia but could not find an increased burden of very large (>500 kb) CNVs, which was proposed recently. However, we provide support for the role of CNVs at 16p13.1, 1q21.1, and *NRXN1*.

▶ Last year, we reported on the findings of copy number variants (CNVs) as the major genetics news in schizophrenia research. This study is an attempt to replicate these findings, now in a Japanese sample. However, as the 2 senior authors (Drs Owen and O'Donovan) appreciate, CNVs are rare but important genetic anomalies and their sample size of this patient group (under 600) is just too small to detect findings. It is unclear whether the reported weak signal (P < .087) is relevant or not. This is always a problem in genetics research— failure to replicate earlier findings in subsequent studies that are of small sample size leads to confusion in the field. The original 2 reports of an excess of CNVs in schizophrenia had samples sizes of over 5000 and 3000. This is complicated research that requires large samples. Thus, this kind of analysis of small samples—which results in the inability to find a difference between patients and controls—complicates the picture, in my humble opinion, rather than truly adding to the scientific picture.

P. F. Buckley, MD

Genomewide Association Study of Movement-Related Adverse Antipsychotic Effects
Åberg K, Adkins DE, Bukszár J, et al (Med College of Virginia of Virginia Commonwealth Univ, Richmond; et al)
Biol Psychiatry 67:279-282, 2010

Background.—Understanding individual differences in the development of extrapyramidal side effects (EPS) as a response to antipsychotic therapy is essential to individualize treatment.

Methods.—We performed genomewide association studies to search for genetic susceptibility to EPS. Our sample consisted of 738 schizophrenia patients, genotyped for 492K single nucleotide polymorphisms (SNPs). We studied three quantitative measures of antipsychotic adverse drug reactions—the Simpson-Angus Scale (SAS) for Parkinsonism, the Barnes Akathisia Rating Scale, and the Abnormal Involuntary Movement Scale (AIMS)—as well as a clinical diagnosis of probable tardive dyskinesia.

Results.—Two SNPs for SAS, rs17022444 and rs2126709 with $p = 1.2 \times 10^{-10}$ and $p = 3.8 \times 10^{-7}$, respectively, and one for AIMS, rs7669317 with $p = 7.7 \times 10^{-8}$, reached genomewide significance (Q value < .1). rs17022444 and rs7669317 were located in intergenic regions and rs2126709 was located in *ZNF202* on 11q24. Fourteen additional signals were potentially interesting (Q value < .5). The *ZNF202* is a transcriptional repressor controlling, among other genes, *PLP1*, which is the major protein in myelin. Mutations in *PLP1* cause Pelizaeus-Merzbacher disease, which has Parkinsonism as an occurring symptom. Altered mRNA expression of *PLP1* is associated with schizophrenia.

Conclusions.—Although our findings require replication and validation, this study demonstrates the potential of genomewide association studies to discover genes and pathways that mediate adverse effects of antipsychotics.

▶ It is hard to know what to make of this study. This is a genome-wide association study (GWAS) examining for genetic contributors to antipsychotic-induced movement disorders in patients who participated in the Clinical Antipsychotic Trial of Intervention Effectiveness (CATIE). Some associations are described. However, these relationships appear tenuous and their implications for the pathobiology of movement disorders during the treatment of schizophrenia are uncertain. In part, this likely relates to the extent and measurement of movement abnormalities in CATIE. Most patients did not have tardive dyskinesia. In those patients who exhibited tardive dyskinesia, it was mild. Thus, the capacity of this study is reduced—even given its large sample size that exceeds 700 patients—to evaluate the genetics of movement disorders in schizophrenia. There was a big effort to study pharmacogenetics of schizophrenia and antipsychotic therapy in CATIE. This is such a great opportunity. However, results thus far of pharmacogenetic analyses from CATIE have been pretty marginal.

P. F. Buckley, MD

Lower number of cerebellar Purkinje neurons in psychosis is associated with reduced reelin expression
Maloku E, Covelo IR, Hanbauer I, et al (Univ of Illinois, Chicago)
Proc Natl Acad Sci U S A 107:4407-4411, 2010

Reelin is an extracellular matrix protein synthesized in cerebellar granule cells that plays an important role in Purkinje cell positioning during cerebellar development and in modulating adult synaptic function. In the cerebellum of schizophrenia (SZ) and bipolar (BP) disorder patients, there is a marked decrease ($\approx 50\%$) of reelin expression. In this study we measured Purkinje neuron density in the Purkinje cell layer of cerebella of 13 SZ and 17 BP disorder patients from the McLean 66 Cohort Collection, Harvard Brain Tissue Resource Center. The mean number of Purkinje neurons (linear density, neurons per millimeter) was 20% lower in SZ and BP disorder patients compared with nonpsychiatric subjects (NPS; $n = 24$). This decrease of Purkinje neuron linear density was unrelated to postmortem interval, pH, drugs of abuse, or to the presence, dose, or duration of antipsychotic medications. A comparative study in the cerebella of heterozygous reeler mice (HRM), in which reelin expression is downregulated by $\approx 50\%$, showed a significant loss in the number of Purkinje cells in HRM (10–15%) compared with age-matched (3–9 months) wild-type mice. This finding suggests that lack of reelin impairs GABAergic Purkinje neuron expression and/or positioning during cerebellar development.

▶ The cerebellum has been a real focus for neurobiological research, involving this distinguished group from the University of Chicago. They have also shown abnormalities of reelin, a neurodevelopmental protein that is synthesized in GABAergic interneurons. In one of the very early postmortem studies, Dr Weinberger and colleagues[1] at NIMH showed loss of cerebellar tissue in a postmortem sample of people with chronic schizophrenia. This region was

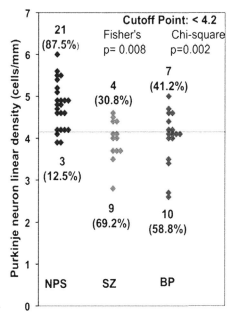

FIGURE 1.—Plot of Purkinje cell number from non-psychiatric subjects (NPS) (*n* = 24), schizophrenia (SZ) (*n* = 13) and bipolar (BP) disorder (*n* = 17) patients. In parentheses is the percentage of subjects with Purkinje cell number above and below cutoff point of 4.2. Note that 30.8% and 41.2% of the SZ and BP disorder patients had Purkinje neuron linear density ≥4.2 neurons/mm vs. 87.5% of NPS. To compare SZ vs. NPS, Fisher's exact test was used (*P* = 0.0008), whereas to compare BP vs. NPS, we used a chi-square test (*P* = 0.002). (Reprinted from Maloku E, Covelo IR, Hanbauer I, et al. Lower number of cerebellar Purkinje neurons in psychosis is associated with reduced reelin expression. *Proc Natl Acad Sci U S A.* 2010;107:4407-4411. Copyright 2010 National Academy of Sciences, USA.)

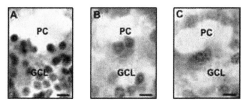

FIGURE 2.—Reelin mRNA in situ hybridization in human cerebellar cortex from an NPS (*A*), a SZ (*B*), and a BP disorder patient (*C*). Note the decrease of reelin mRNA signals in the granular cell layer (GCL) in SZ and BP disorder patients. Purkinje cells (PC) lack a reelin mRNA signal. (Scale bar: 10 μm.). (Reprinted from Maloku E, Covelo IR, Hanbauer I, et al. Lower number of cerebellar Purkinje neurons in psychosis is associated with reduced reelin expression. *Proc Natl Acad Sci U S A.* 2010;107:4407-4411. Copyright 2010 National Academy of Sciences, USA.)

not followed up on as much as other areas (the ventricles and the temporal lobes), and interest in the cerebellum and schizophrenia waned until Dr Andreasen and collegues[2] from the University of Iowa showed that the cerebellum (functioning or a neural relay site) could be part of a widespread functional disconnectivity in schizophrenia. Here, Dr Costa's team from Chicago

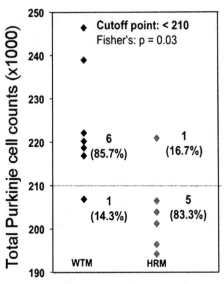

FIGURE 3.—Plot of total Purkinje neuron number from wild-type mice (WTM) ($n = 7$) and heterozygous reeler mice (HRM) ($n = 6$). In parentheses is the percentage of mice with Purkinje cell number above and below cutoff point of 210×10^3. Note that only 16.7% of HRM had Purkinje neuron density $\geq 210 \times 10^3$ vs. 85.7% of WTM. To compare HRM vs. WTM, Fisher's exact test was used ($P = 0.03$). (Reprinted from Maloku E, Covelo IR, Hanbauer I, et al. Lower number of cerebellar Purkinje neurons in psychosis is associated with reduced reelin expression. *Proc Natl Acad Sci U S A.* 2010;107:4407-4411. Copyright 2010 National Academy of Sciences, USA.)

have used the McLean postmortem brain sample to detect a substantial (26%) reduction in Purkinje neurons in the brains of people with schizophrenia and— to a lesser extent—also in people with bipolar disorder (Fig 1). In situ hybridization of messenger RNA from these brains also shows a marked reduction in the expression of reelin (Fig 2). In an analogous study of their mouse model of schizophrenia—the heterozygous reeler mouse—they show similar reductions in Purkinje cells (Fig 3). The methodology in these studies is exemplary. The findings are provocative. This is a great study!

P. F. Buckley, MD

References

1. Kotria KJ, Weinberger DR. Brain imaging in schizophrenia. *Annu Rev Med.* 1995; 46:113-122.
2. Andreasen NC, Pierson R. The role of the cerebellum in schizophrenia. *Biol Psychiatry.* 2008;64:81-88.

Brain-Derived Neurotrophic Factor Signaling Modulates Cocaine Induction of Reward-Associated Ultrasonic Vocalization in Rats

Williams SN, Undieh AS (Univ of Maryland School of Pharmacy, Baltimore; Thomas Jefferson Univ School of Pharmacy, Philadelphia, PA)

J Pharmacol Exp Ther 332:463-468, 2010

Cocaine exhibits high liability for inducing addictive behaviors, but the mechanisms of neuroplasticity underlying the behavioral effects remain unclear. As a crucial mediator of neuroplasticity in diverse functional models, brain-derived neurotrophic factor (BDNF) could contribute to the mechanisms of addiction-related neuroplasticity. Here, we addressed the hypothesis that cocaine increases synaptic dopamine, which induces BDNF protein expression to initiate addiction-related behavior in the rat. An enzyme-linked immunosorbent assay was used to measure BDNF protein expression in rat striatal tissues. For behavioral readout, we used a noninvasive measurement system to measure the emission of 50-kHz ultrasonic vocalization (USV), a response that correlates with electrical brain stimulation and conditioned place preference behavior in rodents. A single injection of cocaine significantly increased BDNF protein expression, but this effect was not further augmented by repeated cocaine administration. A single administration of cocaine elicited significant and dose-related USV responses, and the magnitude of the behavior increased with repeated drug administration. R-(+)-7-Chloro-8-hydroxy-3-methyl-1-phenyl-2,3,4,5-tetrahydro-1H-3-benzazepine (SCH23390), but not raclopride, significantly attenuated cocaine-induced BDNF protein expression, whereas either the D_1-like or D_2-like receptor antagonist blocked cocaine-induced USV behavior. Furthermore, significant USV behavior was elicited by the nonselective dopamine agonist, apomorphine, but not by agonists that are selective for D_1-like or D_2-like receptors. Intracerebroventricular injection of the neurotrophin TrkB receptor inhibitor, K252a, blocked cocaine-induced USV behavior but not locomotor activity. These results suggest that neurotrophin signaling downstream of dopamine receptor function probably constitutes a crucial link in cocaine induction of USV behavior and may contribute to the mechanisms underlying the development of addiction-related behaviors.

▶ This is an elegant series of experiments probing the relationships between brain plasticity, dopamine receptor postsignaling, and cocaine craving in an animal model. It is somewhat unclear, to me at least, just how good a measure of brain activity is ultrasonic vocalization. It is certainly highly technical and while used by these and other authors, it is a technique less known than other electrophysiological measures of brain activity. Notwithstanding that appreciable caveat, this series of studies is informative and well conducted. As illustrated in Figs 2 and 5, cocaine effects on brain-derived neurotrophic factor (BDNF) are evident and inhibitory effects of antagonist agents cause downstream effects on the dopamine-related cellular cascade of signaling events. The authors describe, at least to some extent, how these findings

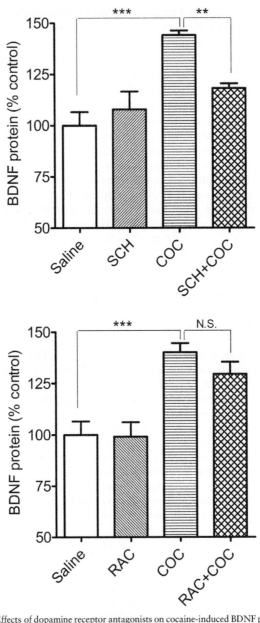

FIGURE 2.—Effects of dopamine receptor antagonists on cocaine-induced BDNF protein expression in vivo. Male Sprague-Dawley rats were pretreated with SCH23390 (SCH) or raclopride (RAC) 20 min before injection of 30 mg/kg cocaine (COC). Animals were killed 24 h later, and BDNF protein levels were assayed in striatal tissues. The data were calculated as percentages relative to saline-treated controls. Each bar is the mean ± S.E.M. ($n = 8$). ***, $p < 0.001$ compared with saline group; #, $p < 0.05$ compared with cocaine group as determined by one-way ANOVA followed by a Tukey post hoc analysis. N.S., not significant. (Reprinted from Williams SN, Undieh AS. Brain-derived neurotrophic factor signaling modulates cocaine induction of reward-associated ultrasonic vocalization in rats. *J Pharmacol Exp Ther.* 2010;332:463-468, with permission from The American Society for Pharmacology and Experimental Therapeutics.)

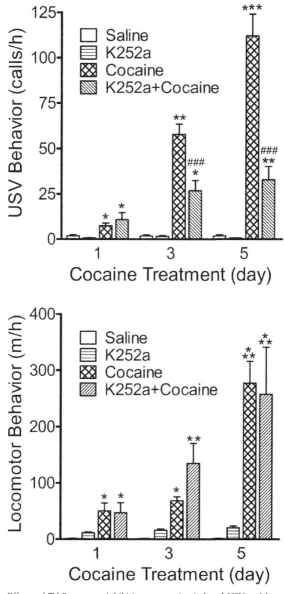

FIGURE 5.—Effects of TrkB receptor inhibition on cocaine-induced USV and locomotor behaviors. Groups of male Sprague-Dawley rats received injections once daily for 5 days of either 20 mg/kg cocaine alone or the same dose of cocaine after pretreatment with an intracerebroventricular injection of the TrkB receptor antagonist K252a (50 µg). After each drug treatment, USV behavior (top) and locomotor activity (bottom) were concurrently measured for 90 min. Each bar is the mean ± S.E.M. ($n = 6$ animals). *, $p < 0.05$; **, $p < 0.01$; ***, $p < 0.001$, compared with the control group, ###, $p < 0.001$ compared with the cocaine group as determined by ANOVA. (Reprinted from Williams SN, Undieh AS. Brain-derived neurotrophic factor signaling modulates cocaine induction of reward-associated ultrasonic vocalization in rats. *J Pharmacol Exp Ther.* 2010;332:463-468, with permission from The American Society for Pharmacology and Experimental Therapeutics.)

might relate to cocaine-related addictive behaviors in humans. It also adds to the growing literature on BDNF in addictions.

P. F. Buckley, MD

Stress hormones in patients with posttraumatic stress disorder caused by myocardial infarction and role of comorbid depression
von Känel R, Schmid J-P, Abbas CC, et al (Univ of Bern, Switzerland)
J Affective Disord 121:73-79, 2010

Background.—Chronic posttraumatic stress disorder (PTSD) has been associated with perturbed hypothalamic-pituitary-adrenal (HPA) axis function and a hyperadrenergic state. We hypothesized that patients with PTSD attributable to myocardial infarction (MI) would show peripheral hypocortisolemia and increased norepinephrine levels, whereby taking into account that depressive symptoms would affect this relationship.

Methods.—We investigated 15 patients with interviewer-rated PTSD caused by myocardial infarction (MI) and 29 post-MI patients with no PTSD. Patients also completed the depression subscale of the Hospital Anxiety and Depression Scale and had blood collected to determine plasma cortisol and norepinephrine levels.

Results.—In bivariate correlation analysis PTSD and depressive symptoms were not significantly associated with cortisol levels. However, patients with PTSD had lower mean ± SEM cortisol levels than patients with no PTSD when controlling for depressive symptoms (77 ± 11 vs. 110 ± 7 ng/ml, $p = .035$). In turn, depressive symptoms correlated with cortisol levels when taking PTSD into account ($r = .36$, $p = .019$). In all patients cortisol levels correlated with total PTSD symptoms ($r = -.43$, $p = .005$) and hyperarousal symptoms ($r = -.45$, $p = .002$) after controlling for depressive symptoms. Depression correlated with cortisol levels after controlling for total PTSD symptoms ($r = .45$, $p = .002$). Posttraumatic stress disorder and depressive symptoms were not significantly associated with norepinephrine levels.

Conclusions.—In post-MI patients we found peripheral hypocortisolemia related to PTSD, respectively hypercortisolemia related to depressive symptoms, when taking joint effects of PTSD and depression into account. No evidence was found for a hyperadrenergic state. Comorbid depressive symptoms ought to be considered to disentangle the unique associations of PTSD with HPA axis dysfunction in cardiac patients.

▶ This study examines the relationship(s) between stress hormones—cortisol and norepinephrine—and posttraumatic stress disorder (PTSD) in patients who have had a heart attack. The relationship to cortisol is clear (Fig 1). No relationship was found between norepinephrine and anxiety or depressive symptoms. There are 2 important methodological issues to take into account when considering these data. First, anxiety and depressive symptoms frequently

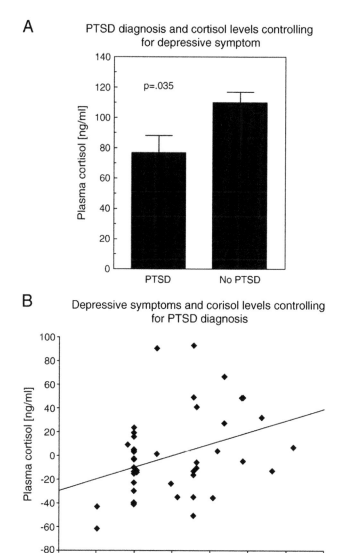

A PTSD diagnosis and cortisol levels controlling for depressive symptom

B Depressive symptoms and corisol levels controlling for PTSD diagnosis

FIGURE 1.—A. Shows lower cortisol levels (mean ± SEM) in 15 patients with PTSD relative to their 29 non-PTSD counterparts after controlling for depressive symptoms (*p* < .04). B. Shows the partial regression plot with fit line for the positive relationship between depressive symptoms and cortisol levels taking categorical diagnosis of PTSD into account (*p* < .02). (Reprinted from von Känel R, Schmid J-P, Abbas CC, et al. Stress hormones in patients with posttraumatic stress disorder caused by myocardial infarction and role of comorbid depression. *J Affective Disord*. 2010;121:73-79, with permission from Elsevier.)

co-occur. Therefore, the authors went to considerable effort statistically to take this into account, repeatedly partially covarying for depression. However, this is still an adjustment, and the likelihood of a strong confound in this study is substantial. Secondly, a percentage of patients (13% in PTSD group, 10% in non-PTSD group) were on antidepressant medications. These do not appear to have been factored into the analyses. Thus, the study is complex as well as the topic itself—not a great surprise!

P. F. Buckley, MD

Brain-derived neurotrophic factor and cocaine addiction
McGinty JF, Whitfield TW Jr, Berglind WJ (Med Univ of South Carolina, Charleston)
Brain Res 1314:183-193, 2010

The effects of brain-derived neurotrophic factor (BDNF) on cocaine-seeking are brain region-specific. Infusion of BDNF into subcortical structures, like the nucleus accumbens and ventral tegmental area, enhances cocaine-induced behavioral sensitization and cocaine-seeking. Conversely, repeated administration of BDNF antiserum into the nucleus accumbens during chronic cocaine self-administration attenuates cocaine-induced reinstatement. In contrast, BDNF infusion into the dorsomedial prefrontal cortex immediately following a final session of cocaine self-administration attenuates relapse to cocaine-seeking after abstinence, as well as cue- and cocaine prime-induced reinstatement of cocaine-seeking following extinction. BDNF-induced alterations in the ERK–MAP kinase cascade and in prefronto-accumbens glutamatergic transmission are implicated in BDNF's ability to alter cocaine-seeking. Within 22 hours after infusion into the prefrontal cortex, BDNF increases BDNF protein in prefrontal cortical targets, including nucleus accumbens, and restores cocaine-mediated decreases in phospho-ERK expression in the nucleus accumbens. Furthermore, 3 weeks after BDNF infusion in animals with a cocaine self-administration history, suppressed basal levels of glutamate are normalized and a cocaine prime-induced increase in extracellular glutamate levels in the nucleus accumbens is prevented. Thus, BDNF may have local effects at the site of infusion and distal effects in target areas that are critical to mediating or preventing cocaine-induced dysfunctional neuroadaptations.

▶ Brain-derived neurotrophic factor (BDNF) is the most studied of the brain neurotrophins. BDNF plays a central role in brain development, especially in synaptogenesis. BDNF can be measured in cerebrospinal fluid and in blood plasma. BDNF can also be measured by immunohistochemical binding analyses in postmortem brain tissue. BDNF has been reported to be reduced in a host of psychiatric conditions, including schizophrenia, depression, and anxiety disorders. It has also been implicated in addiction disorders. This report highlights this relationship. The relationship of BDNF and tropomyosin receptor kinase B (TrkB) receptor to cocaine abuse is described in an elegant series of infusion and in-site hybridization studies of fat brain. The effects of BDNF upon signal

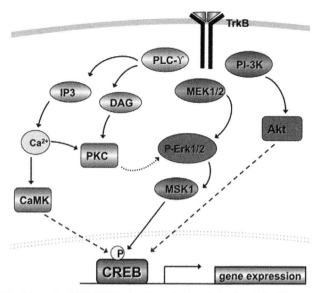

FIGURE 8.—Schematic of BDNF/TrkB signal transduction. Activation of the TrkB receptor initiates downstream changes in CREB-dependent gene transcription via PI3K, ERK/MAPK, and PLC-γ signaling. (Reprinted from McGinty JF, Whitfield TW Jr, Berglind WJ. Brain-derived neurotrophic factor and cocaine addiction. *Brain Res.* 2010;1314:183-193, with permission from Elsevier.)

transduction are also highlighted (Fig 8). This is a complicated series of studies. However, they are extremely well done and the findings are provocative. They also raise the question as to whether BDNF changes are fundamental—process driven or disease specific.

P. F. Buckley, MD

Morphine Use after Combat Injury in Iraq and Post-Traumatic Stress Disorder
Holbrook TL, Galarneau MR, Dye JL, et al (Naval Health Res Ctr, San Diego, CA)
N Engl J Med 362:110-117, 2010

Background.—Post-traumatic stress disorder (PTSD) is a common adverse mental health outcome among seriously injured civilians and military personnel who are survivors of trauma. Pharmacotherapy in the aftermath of serious physical injury or exposure to traumatic events may be effective for the secondary prevention of PTSD.

Methods.—We identified 696 injured U.S. military personnel without serious traumatic brain injury from the Navy–Marine Corps Combat Trauma Registry Expeditionary Medical Encounter Database. Complete data on medications administered were available for all personnel selected.

TABLE 2.—Distribution of Mechanism of Injury among Injured Military Personnel According to PTSD Status*

Mechanism of Injury	PTSD (N = 199)	No PTSD (N = 445)
	no. (%)	
Improvised explosive device	82 (41)	181 (41)
Gunshot	43 (22)	94 (21)
Mortar	17 (9)	38 (9)
Rocket-propelled grenade	8 (4)	36 (8)
Other grenade	12 (6)	30 (7)
Mine	8 (4)	16 (4)
Fragments from blast — NOS	4 (2)	27 (6)
Motor vehicle crash	5 (3)	7 (2)
Fall	8 (4)	4 (1)
Blunt trauma	7 (4)	3 (1)
Crush	0 (0)	4 (1)
Burn	2 (1)	2 (0.5)
Other	3 (2)	3 (1)

Editor's Note: Please refer to original journal article for full references.

*Totals and percentages vary because of missing or unknown mechanisms of injury in 52 patients (8%). Data are from the Navy–Marine Corps Combat Trauma Registry Expeditionary Medical Encounter Database.[29] NOS denotes not otherwise specified.

The diagnosis of PTSD was obtained from the Career History Archival Medical and Personnel System and verified in a review of medical records.

Results.—Among the 696 patients studied, 243 received a diagnosis of PTSD and 453 did not. The use of morphine during early resuscitation and trauma care was significantly associated with a lower risk of PTSD after injury. Among the patients in whom PTSD developed, 61% received morphine; among those in whom PTSD did not develop, 76% received morphine (odds ratio, 0.47; P<0.001). This association remained significant after adjustment for injury severity, age, mechanism of injury, status with respect to amputation, and selected injury-related clinical factors.

Conclusions.—Our findings suggest that the use of morphine during trauma care may reduce the risk of subsequent development of PTSD after serious injury (Table 2).

▶ The recent wars provide an opportunity to advance our understanding of posttraumatic stress disorder (PTSD) both in military and civilian settings. It is observed that there are high rates of mental illness in soldiers returning from Afghanistan and Iraq. Also, rather alarmingly, the rates of mental illness increase more in the months of return to their community. The high rate of suicide in soldiers is also a great concern. Here, the authors examine—the time of onset of trauma—the relationship of morphine use to PTSD. Although the authors are careful in not assigning causality, they report finding the use of morphine is higher in those soldiers without PTSD. This relationship appears in this study to be independent to injury site, severity, and other important factors. It is hard to know what to make of this finding—maybe treating pain most aggressively is a key point, maybe morphine use dulls memory and prevents the onset of PTSD. It is not clear from this study, but this certainly is a provocative study. If taken literally, the results of course could lead to more morphine prescription to injured veterans...then potentially leading to more addiction problems. The causality of effect here is unknown and is the major consideration in understanding these data.

P. F. Buckley, MD

Green tea consumption is associated with depressive symptoms in the elderly
Niu K, Hozawa A, Kuriyama S, et al (Tohoku Univ Graduate School of Biomed Engineering, Sendai, Japan; et al)
Am J Clin Nutr 90:1615-1622, 2009

Background.—Green tea is reported to have various beneficial effects (eg, anti–stress response and antiinflammatory effects) on human health. Although these functions might be associated with the development and progression of depressive symptoms, no studies have investigated the relation between green tea consumption and depressive symptoms in a community-dwelling population.

Objective.—The aim of this study was to investigate the relations between green tea consumption and depressive symptoms in elderly Japanese subjects who widely consumed green tea.

Design.—We conducted a cross-sectional study in 1058 community-dwelling elderly Japanese individuals aged ≥70 y. Green tea consumption was assessed by using a self-administered questionnaire, and depressive symptoms were evaluated by using the 30-item Geriatric Depression Scale with 2 cutoffs: 11 (mild and severe depressive symptoms) and 14 (severe depressive symptoms). If a participant was consuming antidepressants, he or she was considered to have depressive symptoms.

Results.—The prevalence of mild and severe and severe depressive symptoms was 34.1% and 20.2%, respectively. After adjustment for confounding factors, the odds ratios (95% CI) for mild and severe depressive symptoms when higher green tea consumption was compared with green tea consumption of ≤1 cup/d were as follows: 2–3 cups green tea/d (0.96; 95% CI: 0.66, 1.42) and ≥4 cups green tea/d (0.56; 95% CI: 0.39, 0.81) (*P* for trend: 0.001). Similar relations were also observed in the case of severe depressive symptoms.

Conclusion.—A more frequent consumption of green tea was associated with a lower prevalence of depressive symptoms in the community-dwelling older population.

▶ There is overwhelming evidence that patients seek herbal remedies and complementary and alternative medicines (CAMs) as treatments for a host of ailments, including mental disorders. The most noteworthy example is St John's wort for the treatment of depression. Although the original evidence suggested that this herbal compound was an effective treatment for depression, subsequent studies discounted this notion. Nevertheless, patients still seek out

TABLE 1.—Subject Characteristics According to Categories of Green Tea Intake[1]

	Categories of Green Tea Intake			P for Trend[2]
	≤1 cup/d	2–3 cups/d	≥4 cups/d	
n	286	284	488	
Age (y)	75.5 (75.0, 76.1)[3]	76.4 (75.8, 76.9)	75.9 (75.5, 76.3)	0.10
Female sex (%)	48.3	52.8	65.4	<0.0001
BMI (kg/m[2])	23.8 (23.4, 24.2)	23.8 (23.4, 24.2)	24 (23.7, 24.3)	0.80
Serum albumin (g/dL)	4.33 (4.29, 4.36)	4.33 (4.30, 4.36)	4.34 (4.31, 4.36)	0.82
Hypertension (%)	69.6	64.4	70.5	0.61
Diabetes (%)	9.4	8.8	8.8	0.78
History of CVD (%)	19.9	15.9	12.9	<0.01
History of cancer (%)	5.2	4.9	8.8	0.04
History of arthritis (%)	18.5	18.3	17.8	0.80
High CRP (%)[4]	33.9	32.4	31.4	0.46
Smoking status (%)				
Current smoker	16.4	12.7	10.7	0.02
Ex-smoker	39.2	31.0	23.6	<0.0001
Nonsmoker	42.7	55.3	62.9	<0.0001
Drinking status (%)				
Current drinker	41.6	41.2	38.7	0.40
Ex-drinker	14.7	12.0	10.0	0.055
Nondrinker	39.2	44.0	46.3	0.057
PA > level 3 (%)	37.4	41.9	35.3	0.40
Impaired cognitive function (%)				
18 ≤ MMSE < 24	8.4	6.7	7.2	0.58
24 ≤ MMSE < 28	38.5	34.5	34.4	0.29
Impaired IADLs (%)	14.0	15.1	8.4	<0.01
Visiting friends: "yes" (%)	69.6	72.9	81.5	0.0001
Body pain: "yes" (%)	28.0	21.8	20.1	0.01
Lack of perceived social support: total score = 0 (%)	15.7	16.6	10.7	0.03
Educational level ≤12 y (%)	68.2	68.0	71.7	0.26
Living alone: "yes" (%)	22.7	23.9	25.4	0.39
Marital status (%)				
Married	67.1	60.2	59.4	0.04
Widowed or divorced	29.4	34.2	37.5	0.02
Single	3.5	5.6	3.1	0.59
Nutrient intake				
Total energy intake (kcal/d)	1959.9 (1901.3, 2018.5)	2023.9 (1965.2, 2082.7)	1959.6 (1914.8, 2004.4)	0.19
Total protein (g · d⁻¹ · 2000 kcal)	82.8 (81.2, 81.2)	81.7 (80.1, 80.1)	83.2 (81.9, 81.9)	0.34
Folate (μg · d⁻¹ · 2000 kcal)	336.2 (324.6, 347.8)	372.4 (360.7, 384.1)	404.0 (395.1, 412.9)	<0.0001
GDS scores	9.9 (9.3, 10.5)	9.8 (9.1, 10.4)	8.3 (7.8, 8.8)	<0.0001

[1]CVD, cardiovascular disease; CRP, C-reactive protein; PA, physical activity; MMSE, Mini-Mental State Examination score; IADLs, instrumental activities of daily living; GDS, Geriatric Depression Scale.
[2]Obtained by using ANOVA for continuous variables and logistic regression analysis for variables of proportion.
[3]Mean; 95% CI in parentheses (all such values).
[4]Serum CRP concentrations ≥1.0 mg/L.

these CAMs. In this study, green tea consumption was associated with a lower rate of depression in elderly patients (Tables 1 and 2). The causality of this relationship cannot be determined. However, the strength of this observation is quite impressive. This is also the kind of study that gets picked up on CNN

TABLE 2.—Adjusted Relations Between Consumption of Green Tea and Mild and Severe or Severe Depressive Symptoms[1]

	Categories of Green Tea Consumption			P for Trend[2]
	≤1 cup/d	2–3 cups/d	≥4 cups/d	
n	286	284	488	
No. of mild and severe depressive symptoms, defined as GDS ≥11 or use of antidepressants	114	111	136	—
Model 1[3]	1.00	0.95 (0.66, 1.36)[4]	0.56 (0.40, 0.78)[5]	<0.001
Model 2[6]	1.00	0.96 (0.66, 1.40)	0.54 (0.37, 0.78)[5]	<0.001
Model 3[7]	1.00	0.96 (0.66, 1.42)	0.56 (0.39, 0.81)[5]	0.001
No. of severe depressive symptoms, defined as GDS ≥14 or use of antidepressants	75	67	72	—
Model 1[3]	1.00	0.91 (0.60, 1.37)	0.48 (0.33, 0.71)[5]	<0.001
Model 2[6]	1.00	0.92 (0.59, 1.42)	0.46 (0.30, 0.72)[5]	<0.001
Model 3[7]	1.00	0.92 (0.59, 1.44)	0.48 (0.31, 0.75)[5]	<0.001

[1]GDS, Geriatric Depression Scale.
[2]Obtained by using multiple logistic regression analysis.
[3]Adjusted for age; sex; BMI; hypertension; diabetes; history of cardiovascular diseases, cancer, or arthritis; high C-reactive protein (≥1.0 mg/L); history of smoking and drinking habits; physical activity (all 6 levels as a categorical variable); cognitive status; impaired instrumental activities of daily living; selfreported body pain; educational level; living alone; and marital status.
[4]Adjusted odds ratio; 95% CI in parentheses (all such values).
[5]Significantly different from green tea consumption of ≤1 cup/d, P <0.01 (Bonferroni-corrected).
[6]Additionally adjusted for serum albumin concentration, total energy intake, intakes per 2000 kcal of energy intake as protein and folate, black or oolong tea consumption, and coffee consumption.
[7]Additionally adjusted for lack of perceived social support and visiting friends.

and news networks! This study is highly topical and has an interesting message that is of public relevance.

P. F. Buckley, MD

The involuntary nature of conversion disorder
Voon V, Gallea C, Hattori N, et al (Natl Inst of Neurological Disorders and Stroke, NIH, Bethesda, MD)
Neurology 74:223-228, 2010

Background.—What makes a movement feel voluntary, and what might make it feel involuntary? Motor conversion disorders are characterized by movement symptoms without a neurologic cause. Conversion movements use normal voluntary motor pathways, but the symptoms are paradoxically experienced as involuntary, or lacking in self-agency. Self-agency is the experience that one is the cause of one's own actions. The matched comparison between the prediction of the action consequences (feed-forward signal) and actual sensory feedback is believed to give rise to self-agency and has been in part associated with the right inferior parietal cortex. Using fMRI, we assessed the correlates of self-agency during conversion tremor.

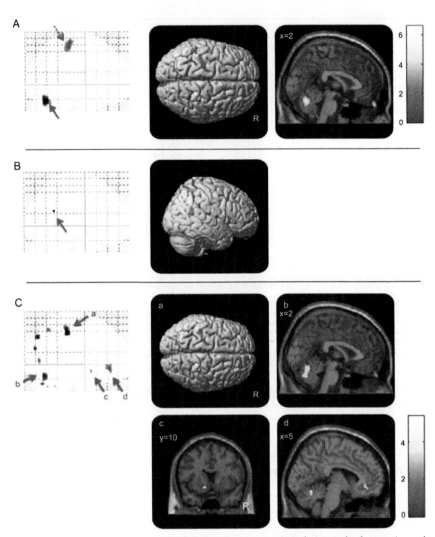

FIGURE.— Conversion tremor and voluntary mimic tremor. (A) Inclusive mask of conversion and voluntary tremor. The glass brain and SPM image show cerebellar vermis hyperactivity (solid arrow) (Montreal Neurological Institute local maximum coordinates reported as x, y, z: 0, −66, −22 mm; Z score: 4.39) and left sensorimotor cortex (dashed arrow) (−26, −26, 58 mm; 3.51) during conversion tremor (C) vs rest (R) and voluntary mimic (V) vs R (2-sample t test). The glass brain and SPM image are shown at $p < 0.001$ uncorrected threshold >5 voxels. (B) Conversion vs voluntary tremor. The glass brain and SPM image show right temporoparietal junction hypoactivity in the contrast of C-R compared with V-R (paired t test). The glass brain is shown at $p < 0.05$ family-wise error whole brain corrected. The SPM image is shown at $p < 0.001$ uncorrected threshold >5 voxels. (C) Temporoparietal junction connectivity map for the contrast of conversion vs voluntary tremor. The glass brain and SPM images show decreased functional connectivity between the right temporoparietal junction (seed) and (a) left and right sensorimotor cortices, (b) bilateral cerebellar vermis, (c) left ventral striatum, and (d) bilateral ventral cingulate/medial prefrontal cortex during conversion vs voluntary tremor. The glass brains and SPM image are shown at $p < 0.001$ uncorrected threshold >5 voxels. (Reprinted from Voon V, Gallea C, Hattori N, et al. The involuntary nature of conversion disorder. *Neurology.* 2010;74:223-228.)

Methods.—We used a within-subject fMRI block design to compare brain activity during conversion tremor and during voluntary mimicked tremor in 8 patients.

Results.—The random effects group analysis showed that conversion tremor compared with voluntary tremor had right temporoparietal junction (TPJ) hypoactivity ($p < 0.05$ family-wise error whole brain corrected) and lower functional connectivity between the right TPJ, sensorimotor regions (sensorimotor cortices and cerebellar vermis), and limbic regions (ventral anterior cingulate and right ventral striatum).

Conclusions.—The right TPJ has been implicated as a general comparator of internal predictions with actual events. We propose that the right TPJ hypoactivity and lower TPJ and sensorimotor cortex interactions may reflect the lack of an appropriate sensory prediction signal. The lack of a match for the proprioceptive feedback would lead to the perception that the conversion movement is not self-generated.

▶ Although this study comprises of a small sample size ($n = 8$), it is nevertheless interesting because of the lack of understanding of the neural or nonneural basis of conversion symptoms. In a within-subject design among patients who presented with a nonneurological tremor, there was evidence of abnormalities on functional magnetic resonance imaging that was subtle and confined to the temporoparietal junction (Fig 1)—the interface between the motor cortex and the parietal sensory associative cortex. The authors elegantly describe the mismatch that they consider is attributable to conversion tremors. This is a huge issue for clinicians in neurology practice and on the general medical floors. Psychiatrists are careful not to ascribe a conversion disorder diagnosis without full evidence of this. This article suggests that even a conversion disorder may have a biological basis; however, I guess this makes sense, as brain activation is required for motor movements. This is a most interesting article.

P. F. Buckley, MD

Neuroinflammation in Alzheimer's Disease and Major Depression

Dobos N, Korf J, Luiten PGM, et al (Univ of Groningen, The Netherlands; Univ Med Ctr Groningen, The Netherlands)
Biol Psychiatry 67:503-504, 2010

Background.—Alzheimer's disease (AD) is the fifth leading cause of death in the world, according to the World Health Organization, and affects 35 million persons worldwide. The core symptom is impaired cognitive function, and currently no cure exists. The brains of AD patients are marked by extracellular deposits of amyloid-β, intracellular aggregates of the protein τ, and loss of cholinergic forebrain innervation. The brain regions most often affected are those involved in cognition, specifically, the cortex, hippocampus, and amygdala. Neuroinflammatory processes contribute to both AD and depression, and the links were investigated.

Inflammatory Contribution.—Microglia comprise 10% to 12% of the cells in the brain. They interact strongly with astrocytes, neurons, and blood vessels and become activated after injury and stress, altering their morphology so they secrete proinflammatory cytokines. These coordinate the local and systemic inflammatory responses to pathogenic challenges, such as the amyloid precipitations of AD. Tumor necrosis factor α (TNF-α) and its receptors are strongly expressed, inducing a neuroprotective signaling cascade. Indoleamine 2,3-dioxygenase (IDO) is induced and reduces tryptophan levels, thereby affecting serotonin (5-HT) synthesis. The end product of the catabolic tryptophan pathway is quinolinic acid, which is a neurotoxic activator of the N-methyl-D-aspartate receptor and contributes to excitotoxic effects in neurodegenerative diseases. Deranged 5-HT levels compromise brain function.

Genetic Factors and Depression.—Depression develops in 28% of patients with chronic viral hepatitis C infection treated with interferon α (IFN-α). Cytokine-induced depression and sickness behavior have been linked to the actions of the enzymes phospholipase A2 (PLA2) and cyclooxygenase 2 (COX2). Genetic variations in the PLA2 and COX2 genes increase the risk of IFN-α-n-induced depression and major depression not related to cytokines. Lower levels of eicosapentaenoic acid resulting from the PLA2 "at risk" genotype are accompanied by an increased risk of major depression and more somatic manifestations of depression. The COX2 "at risk" genotype is linked to lower decosahexaenoic acid levels, which are found in patients with major depression. Specifically in response to IFN-α, these genes raise the risk of having depression. In addition, two genetic variants of the interleukin-1β gene increase the chance of nonremission of major depression after 6 weeks of antidepressant therapy.

Conclusions.—The linkage between brain inflammatory processes and lower levels of tryptophan and 5-HT must be analyzed carefully. Patients with low levels of blood tryptophan as a result of the action of IDO tend to exhibit aggressiveness and lack of impulse control rather than major depression. AD is generally manifest by symptoms of depression, anxiety, irritability, and mood instability. However, evidence seems to suggest a key role for inflammatory processes in both major depression and AD.

▶ Alzheimer disease (AD) has long been associated with inflammatory processes. The presence of gliosis and reactive inflammatory processes are common in AD. This has prompted several studies—largely inconclusive— exploring the role of nonsteroidal analgesic drugs as a potential treatment for AD. Similarly, there is a growing body of literature on depression and inflammation. In part, this might explain—at least from a biological perspective—the substantial comorbidity of depression with many chronic medical illnesses. There are also differences in cytokines in acute phases of depression, compared with arrhythmia or bipolar states. The inflammatory hypothesis is also invoked to explain the epidemiological relationship between depression in late life and a heightened risk of subsequently developing dementia.

P. F. Buckley, MD

Physical and psychosocial functioning following motor vehicle trauma: Relationships with chronic pain, posttraumatic stress, and medication use

Clapp JD, Masci J, Bennett SA, et al (Univ at Buffalo   SUNY, NY; Univ of Memphis, TN)
Eur J Pain 14:418-425, 2010

Chronic pain and PTSD are known to hold substantial comorbidity following traumatic injury. Although pharmacological agents have been examined in the treatment of pain and PTSD individually, little is known regarding the relationship of medication use with functioning in patients with comorbid conditions. This research examined the relationships of pain, PTSD, and medication use across physical and psychosocial functioning in patients with chronic pain following motor vehicle injury ($N = 234$). Separate analyses were conducted for opioids, SSRIs, and sedative/anxiolytics, respectively. Several relevant effects were noted: (1) Pain evidenced strong associations with reduced functioning across both physical and psychosocial domains, (2) Opioid use held interactive relationships with PTSD across both functioning domains. Specifically, opioids were associated with greater physical impairment in patients without comorbid PTSD. Opioids also were related to greater psychosocial impairment in patients without PTSD while PTSD was associated with greater impairment in patients not using opioids, (3) Opioid use evidenced a marginal interaction with pain on psychosocial functioning. Opioids were associated with greater psychosocial impairment among patients with high-pain, and high-pain was associated with greater impairment among opioid users, (4) SSRIs held a marginal interaction with PTSD such that PTSD was related to poorer psychosocial functioning only among individuals not using an SSRI, and (5) Anxiolytic use evidenced a marginal interaction with PTSD on physical functioning although no between-group differences were noted. These data suggest that PTSD symptomology may be an important consideration in determining

TABLE 2.—Means, Standard Deviations, and Intercorrelations for Primary Study Variables

	SIPphys	SIPpsy	Pain	PTSD	Opioid	SSRI	Anxiolytic
SIPphys	–						
SIPpsy	.60**	–					
Pain	.52**	.32**	–				
PTSD	.07	.28**	.16*	–			
Opioid	.27**	.22**	.27**	.05	–		
SSRI	.09	.13*	.13*	.10	.08	–	
Anxiolytic	.10	.06	−.03	.03	.08	.14*	–
M	59.57	27.86	.41	.59	.46	.21	.15
SD	11.34	18.80	.49	.49	.50	.41	.35

Note: SIPphys = SIP physical subscale; SIPpsy = SIP psychosocial subscale; PTSD = posttraumatic stress disorder; SSRI = selective serotonin reuptake inhibitor; Anxiolytic = anxiolytic/sedative-hypnotic medication.
*<.05.
**<.001.

treatment modality for patients experiencing pain subsequent to traumatic injury (Table 2).

▶ This is an ambitious effort to take on the interrelationships between pain, posttraumatic stress disorder (PTSD), psychotropic medications, and overall functioning following a motor vehicle accident. Although the sample size is large and reasonably well characterized, the extent of overlap across the domains of study is extensive. This is especially so with the use of medications where pain medication use and prescription of anxiolytics and/or antidepressants often co-occur. Accordingly, the extent to which these relationships can be teased apart in this study is limited. Moreover, the reported associations make sense—again the study design does not allow us to make any causal inferences. Nevertheless, this is an interesting read (and with challenging statistics) for those who are interested in understanding the murky area of medication, pain, and PTSD.

P. F. Buckley, MD

Fluoxetine Potentiates Methylphenidate-Induced Gene Regulation in Addiction-Related Brain Regions: Concerns for Use of Cognitive Enhancers?
Steiner H, Van Waes V, Marinelli M (Rosalind Franklin Univ of Medicine and Science, North Chicago, IL)
Biol Psychiatry 67:592-594, 2010

Background.—There is growing use of psychostimulant cognitive enhancers such as methylphenidate (Ritalin). Methylphenidate differs from the psychostimulant cocaine because it does not enhance synaptic levels of serotonin. We investigated whether exposure to methylphenidate combined with a serotonin-enhancing medication, the prototypical selective serotonin reuptake inhibitor (SSRI) fluoxetine (Prozac), would produce more "cocaine-like" molecular and behavioral changes.

Methods.—We measured the effects of fluoxetine on gene expression induced by the cognitive enhancer methylphenidate in the striatum and nucleus accumbens of rats, by in situ hybridization histochemistry. We also determined whether fluoxetine modified behavioral effects of methylphenidate.

Results.—Fluoxetine robustly potentiated methylphenidate-induced expression of the transcription factors c-*fos* and *zif* 268 throughout the striatum and to some degree in the nucleus accumbens. Fluoxetine also enhanced methylphenidate-induced stereotypical behavior.

Conclusions.—Both potentiated gene regulation in the striatum and the behavioral effects indicate that combining the SSRI fluoxetine with the cognitive enhancer methylphenidate mimics cocaine effects, consistent with an increased risk for substance use disorder.

▶ There is always concern in the public that we are somehow contributing to a drug seeking culture. The journalists and advocates point out the effects of our medications and the potentially detrimental and even addictive effects of psychotropic medications. To some extent, this is a counterpoint to the earlier Prozac culture of the late 1980s to early 1990s. There are some studies showing that kids who have attention-deficit/hyperactivity disorder (ADHD) are at greater risk of substance abuse when they become adults, with some suggesting that chronic exposure/treatment with stimulants may have sensitized them to drugs and later drug abuse. This study suggests perhaps some rationale for this, in the extent that the observed changes in gene transcription here mimic those that are seen upon chronic exposure to cocaine. This is therefore an interesting and provocative study.

P. F. Buckley, MD

Easy and Low-Cost Identification of Metabolic Syndrome in Patients Treated With Second-Generation Antipsychotics: Artificial Neural Network and Logistic Regression Models

Lin C-C, Bai Y-M, Chen J-Y, et al (Taipei Med Univ, Taiwan; Taipei Veterans General Hosp, Taiwan; Yuli Veterans Hosp, Taiwan; et al)
J Clin Psychiatry 71:225-234, 2010

Objective.—Metabolic syndrome (MetS) is an important side effect of second-generation anti- psychotics (SGAs). However, many SGA-treated patients with MetS remain undetected. In this study, we trained and validated artificial neural network (ANN) and multiple logistic regression models without biochemical parameters to rapidly identify MetS in patients with SGA treatment.

Method.—A total of 383 patients with a diagnosis of schizophrenia or schizoaffective disorder (*DSM-IV* criteria) with SGA treatment for more than 6 months were investigated to determine whether they met the MetS criteria according to the International Diabetes Federation. The data for these patients were collected between March 2005 and September 2005. The input variables of ANN and logistic regression were limited to demographic and anthropometric data only. All models were trained by randomly selecting two-thirds of the patient data and were Internally validated with the remaining one-third of the data. The models were then externally validated with data from 69 patients from another hospital, collected between March 2008 and June 2008. The area under the receiver operating characteristic curve (AUC) was used to measure the performance of all models.

Results.—Both the final ANN and logistic regression models had high accuracy (88.3% vs 83.6%), sensitivity (93.1% vs 86.2%), and specificity

TABLE 2.—Univariate Analyses for Demographic, Clinical, and Metabolic Characteristics of Sample at Yuli Veterans Hospital (N = 383)

Characteristic	MetS (n = 83)		Non-MetS (n = 300)	
	Men (n = 57)	Women (n = 26)	Men (n = 197)	Women (n = 103)
Waist circumference (cm)[a,b]	98.4 ± 8.1[c]	90.1±7.0[c]	81.1 ± 9.0[d]	75.9 ± 9.5[d]
Systolic blood pressure[a,b]	129.4 ± 14.7	125.1 ± 14.9	118.0 ± 14.4[d]	111.7 ± 14.2[d]
Diastolic blood pressure[a,b]	81.4 ± 9.6	81.0 ± 9.6	72.5 ± 9.1	70.9 ± 10.3
Triglycerides[a,b]	189.5 ± 80.3	168.6 ± 65.6	95.7 ± 72.5	83.8 ± 38.7
High-density lipoprotein[a,b]	28.0 ± 7.5[c]	35.3 ± 7.2[c]	38.9 ± 11.3[d]	47.2 ± 12.0[d]
Fasting glucose[a,b]	99.9 ± 41.1	97.4 ± 18.1	90.2 ± 35.6	86.2 ± 14.2
Baseline BMI (kg/m^2)[a,b]	26.6 ± 4.0	27.8 ± 5.8	22.5 ± 3.6[d]	23.7 ± 4.5[d]
Cross-sectional BMI (kg/m^2)[a,b]	28.6 ± 3.4	29.6 ± 3.8	22.5 ± 3.4[d]	23.7 ± 4.6[d]
Baseline weight, kg[a,b]	75.4 ± 13.4[c]	67.5 ± 13.6[c]	62.6 ± 11.1[d]	56.1 ± 10.9[d]
Weight gain, kg[a,b]	5.66 ± 7.44	4.53 ± 11.2	0.02 ± 8.87	−0.03 ± 8.50
Age, y[a]	46.7 ± 12.9	47.3 ± 12.4	48.0 ± 14.6	47.3 ± 12.0
Duration of SGA, mo[a]	47.6 ± 27.0	52.4 ± 29.0	48.0 ± 27.4	45.0 ± 28.2
SGA agent, n (%)				
Risperidone	18 (31.6)	7 (26.9)	91 (46.2)	31 (30.1)
Clozapine	26 (45.6)	15 (57.7)	72 (36.5)	43 (41.7)
Olanzapine	13 (22.8)	4 (15.4)	34 (17.3)	29 (28.2)
Combined mood stabilizer, n (%)[b]				
No = 0	35 (61.4)	19 (73.1)	147 (74.6)	83 (80.6)
Yes = 1	22 (38.6)	7 (26.9)	50 (25.4)	20 (19.4)
Combined antipsychotics, n (%)				
No = 0	53 (93.0)	25 (96.2)	176 (89.3)	91 (88.3)
Yes = 1	4 (7.0)	1 (3.8)	21 (10.7)	12 (11.7)
Antihypertensive medications, n (%)[b]				
No = 0	53 (93.0)	22 (84.6)	194 (98.5)	97 (94.2)
Yes = 1	4 (7.0)	4 (15.4)	3 (1.5)	6 (5.8)

Abbreviations: BMI = body moss index, MetS = metabolic syndrome, SGA = second-generation antipsychotic.
[a]Mean ± SD.
[b]Comparison between MetS and non-MetS patients, t test or κ^2, P value < .05.
[c]Comparison between male and female patients with MetS, t test, P value < .05.
[d]Comparison between male and female patients without MetS, t test, P value < .05.

TABLE 3.—Multiple Logistical Regression Analysis of Metabolic Syndrome on Training Set (n = 225)

Significant Predictor	Odds Ratio (adjusted)	Lower 95% CI	Upper 95% CI	P Value
Waist circumference	9.59[a]	4.31	19.3	<.0005
Diastolic blood pressure	3.04[a]	1.75	5.26	<.0005
Female	4.36	1.62	11.7	.004

[a]Per standard deviation increase.

(86.9% vs 83.8%) to identify MetS in the internal validation set. The mean ± SD AUC was high for both the ANN and logistic regression models (0.934 ± 0.033 vs 0.922 ± 0.035, P =.63). During external validation, high AUC was still obtained for both models. Waist circumference and diastolic blood pressure were the common variables that were left in the final ANN and logistic regression models.

Conclusion.—Our study developed accurate ANN and logistic regression models to detect MetS in patients with SGA treatment. The models are likely to provide a noninvasive tool for large-scale screening of MetS in this group of patients (Tables 2 and 3).

▶ This is a very smart study that addresses a major public health concern in the treatment of schizophrenia metabolic syndrome. This constellation of weight, lipid, and cardiovascular disturbances, which are associated with heightened morbidity and mortality, may be hard to detect accurately without careful and longitudinal screening. Research by our group and several others have shown that many clinicians do not monitor patients as closely as they might for the re-emergence of the metabolic syndrome. Thus, any way to enhance detection would be most welcome. Based upon data collected from a schizophrenia sample (Table 2), the authors here have used complex statistical methods to predict the presence of metabolic syndrome (Fig 1 in the original article). When they look at what aspects of the metabolic syndrome are most telling or predictive, they find that waist circumference and elevated diastolic blood pressure are the most discriminating (Table 3) clinical variables. Ironically, we and others have found that authors are particularly shy at measuring waist circumference in their patients.

P. F. Buckley, MD

Treatment response in major depression: effects of personality dysfunction and prior depression
Gorwood P, Rouillon F, Even C, et al (Paris-Descartes Univ, France; et al)
Br J Psychiatry 196:139-142, 2010

Background.—The impact of personality dysfunction on the outcome of treatment for depression remains debated.

Aims.—To examine the relationship between the number of prior depressive episodes, personality dysfunction and treatment response for depression.

Method.—In a large sample ($n = 8229$) of adult out-patients with a major depressive episode (DSM–IV), personality dysfunction was assessed using the Standardised Assessment of Personality – Abbreviated Scale (SAPAS). Potential predictors of treatment response at 6 weeks were examined via structural equation modelling.

Results.—The amount of personality dysfunction and number of prior episodes of depression were both associated with poor response to treatment. Once personality dysfunction was controlled for, the number of prior episodes of depression was not associated with treatment response.

Conclusions.—Personality dysfunction is associated with impaired short-term response to antidepressant treatment in major depression.

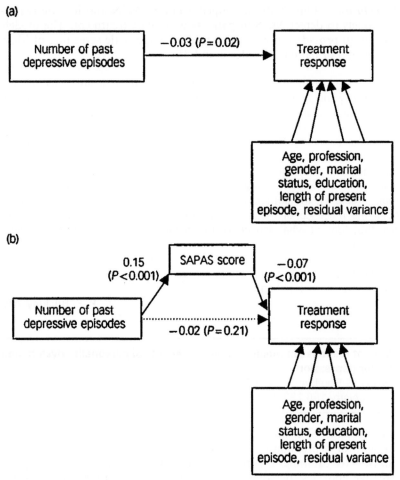

FIGURE 2.—Structural equation model accounting for treatment response in 8229 depressed outpatients, (a) without taking into account the Standardised Assessment of Personality – Abbreviated Scale (SAPAS) score, (b) including the SAPAS score. (Reprinted from Gorwood P, Rouillon F, Even C, et al. Treatment response in major depression: effects of personality dysfunction and prior depression. *Br J Psychiatry*. 2010;196:139-142.)

The apparent detrimental effect of prior depression on treatment response may be accounted for by pre-existing personality dysfunction.

▶ Although many patients who present with acute depression respond to a course of treatment (within 4-6 weeks) with an antidepressant medication, there is ample evidence that for many patients the response to treatment is delayed and/or inadequate. Factors that contribute to an inadequate response include pre-existing organic brain disease, comorbid physical illness, drug-drug interactions with medications that are prescribed for medical conditions, and—of course—social adversity. However, there are also enduring and powerful relationships between previous depression and personality disturbance. As is most evident, the personality disorders of a cyclothymic personality and of a dependent personality illustrate basic traits and emotional styles that predispose to comorbid depression—as well as worsen its outcome. Similarly, there are high rates of depression in patients who have borderline personality disorder—a condition that is known to be associated with poor outcome. Comorbid depression further complicates this situation. In terms of previous depressive episodes, chronic dysthymia is itself a risk factor for subsequent depression. Chronic dysthymia superimposed upon a major depressive episode is often referred to as double depression. These relationships are described in a large (over 8000) sample of patients who were receiving treatment for major depression (Fig 2). The modeling suggests that the effect of a history of depression upon the treatment of a current episode is powerfully influenced by personality disturbance.

P. F. Buckley, MD

A Double-Blind, Randomized Controlled Trial of Ethyl-Eicosapentaenoate for Major Depressive Disorder

Mischoulon D, Papakostas GI, Dording CM, et al (Massachusetts General Hosp, Boston)
J Clin Psychiatry 70:1636-1644, 2009

Objective.—To examine the efficacy and tolerability of ethyl-eicosapentaenoate (EPA-E) monotherapy for major depressive disorder (MDD).

Method.—Fifty-seven adults with *DSM-IV* MDD were randomly assigned from January 2003 until June 2006 to receive 1 g/d of eicosapentaenoic acid (EPA) or placebo for 8 weeks in a double-blind, randomized, controlled pilot study. Response criteria were on the basis of the 17-item Hamilton Depression Rating Scale (HDRS-17). Subjects' plasma lipid profiles were examined by gas chromatography.

Results.—Thirty-five subjects (63% female; mean ± SD age = 45 ± 13 years) were eligible for the intent to treat (ITT) analysis. In the ITT sample, mean ± SD HDRS-17 scores decreased from 21.6 ± 2.7 to 13.9 ± 8.9 for the EPA group (n = 16) and from 20.5 ± 3.6 to 17.5 ± 7.5 for the placebo group (n = 19) ($P = .123$); the effect size for EPA was 0.55. ITT response rates were 38% (6/16) for EPA, and 21% (4/19) for placebo ($P = .45$). Among the 24 study completers, mean ± SD HDRS-17 scores decreased from 21.3 ± 3.0 to 11.1 ± 8.1 for the EPA group and from 20.5 ± 3.8 to 16.3 ± 6.9 for the placebo group ($P = .087$); the effect size for EPA was 0.73. Completer response rates were 45% (5/11) for EPA, and 23% (3/13) for placebo ($P = .39$). Among EPA subjects, baseline n-6/n-3 ratio was associated with decrease in HDRS-17 score ($r = -0.686$, $P = .030$) and with treatment response ($P = .032$); change in n-6/n-3 ratio was associated with change in HDRS-17 score ($r = .784$, $P = .032$). Side effects,

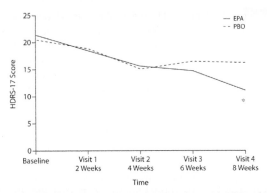

FIGURE 1.—Change in HDRS-17 score over time for 24 patients with MDD taking EPA or placebo (completers). *EPA group had a significant decrease in HDRS-17 score after 8 weeks of treatment ($P = .004$). Abbreviations: EPA = eicosapentaenoic acid, HDRS-17 = 17-item Hamilton Depression Rating Scale, MDD = major depressive disorder, PBO = placebo. (Reprinted from Mischoulon D, Papakostas GI, Dording CM, et al. A double-blind, randomized controlled trial of ethyl-eicosapentaenoate for major depressive disorder. *J Clin Psychiatry.* 2009;70:1636-1644, with permission from Physicians Postgraduate Press, Inc.)

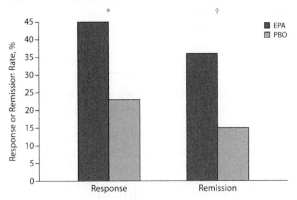

FIGURE 2.—Response and remission rates for 24 patients with MDD taking EPA or placebo (completers). *Fisher $P = .39$ for EPA group vs placebo. †Fisher $P = .36$ for EPA group vs placebo. Abbreviations: EPA = eicosapentaenoic acid, MDD = major depressive disorder, PBO = placebo. (Reprinted from Mischoulon D, Papakostas GI, Dording CM, et al. A double-blind, randomized controlled trial of ethyl-eicosapentaenoate for major depressive disorder. *J Clin Psychiatry.* 2009;70:1636-1644, with permission from Physicians Postgraduate Press, Inc.)

reported in 2 EPA subjects and 5 placebo subjects, were exclusively gastro-intestinal, mild, and not associated with discontinuation.

Conclusions.—EPA demonstrated an advantage over placebo that did not reach statistical significance, possibly due to the small sample and low completer rates, which were the major study limitations.

Trial Registration.—clinicaltrials.gov Identifier: NCT00096798 (Figs 1 and 2).

▶ This is a detailed study report of a placebo-controlled 8 weeks trial of ethyl-eicosapentaenoate (EPA-E) in 57 patients with depression. The study shows a mild difference in reduction in depressive symptoms that favors the use of EPA (Fig 1), although when considered *n* categorical analyses of responder and remitter status these effects are marginal (Fig 2). The study is underpowered to detect significant differences. Moreover, it was clearly a difficult study to recruit for and it took several years to complete—without reaching the intended study sample. However, previous studies had examined the potential of EPA as an adjunctive agent to antidepressant medications, rather than as a primary treatment in this study. The methodology is exemplary. As is clear, the study took a long time to complete and was complex. Recruitment was also difficult, not surprising given the patient sample and the study design.

P. F. Buckley, MD

Sharing and Selling of Prescription Medications in a College Student Sample

Garnier LM, Arria AM, Caldeira KM, et al (Univ of Maryland, College Park)
J Clin Psychiatry 71:262-269, 2010

Objective.—To estimate the prevalence of prescription medication diversion among college students; to compare classes of medications with respect to the likelihood of diversion; to document the most common methods of diversion; and to examine the characteristics of students who diverted medications.

Method.—A cross-sectional analysis of personal interview data collected between August 2006 and August 2007 as part of an ongoing longitudinal study. The cohort of students, who were between the ages of 17 and 19 years at study onset, attended a large public university in the mid-Atlantic region. Information was gathered regarding a wide variety of variables, including demographics, diversion of medically prescribed drugs, illicit drug use, and childhood conduct problems.

Results.—Among 483 students prescribed a medication, 35.8% diverted a medication at least once in their lifetime. The most commonly diverted medication classes were prescription attention-deficit/hyperactivity disorder medication (61.7% diversion rate) and prescription analgesics (35.1% diversion rate). Sharing was the most common method of diversion, with 33.6% of students sharing their medication(s) and 9.3% selling in their lifetime. Comparative analyses revealed that prescription medication diverters had used more illicit drugs in the past year and had more childhood conduct problems than nondiverters.

Conclusion.—If confirmed, these findings have important clinical implications for improved physician-patient communication and vigilance

TABLE 2.—Prescription and Diversion Rates for the Top 3 Most Prescribed Attention-Deficit/Hyperactivity Disorder (ADHD), Analgesic, Other Psychotropic, Asthma/Allergy, and Other Nonpsychotropic Medications Among 483 College Students

Medication	Individuals With a Prescription for This Medication,[a] n	Individuals in the Class Population (N = 2,893[b]) Prescribed This Medication, Weight %	Individuals Who Diverted This Medications,[c] n (%)
ADHD medication	81	5.3%$_{wt}$	50 (61.7)
Amphetamine/ dextroamphetamine	44		31 (70.5)
Methylphenidate	27		10 (37.0)
Methylphenidate extended release	23		9 (39.1)
Other	11		3 (27.3)
Analgesic medication	288	22.0%$_{wt}$	101 (35.1)
Acetaminophen/oxycodone	109		30 (27.5)
Acetaminophen/hydrocodone	100		31 (31.0)
Hydrocodone	38		14 (36.8)
Other	99		37 (37.4)
Other psychotropic medication	145	10.2%$_{wt}$	20 (13.8)
Sertraline	54		3 (5.6)
Escitalopram	30		1 (3.3)
Bupropion	19		0 (0.0)
Other	90		15 (16.7)
Asthma/allergy medication	110	8.2%$_{wt}$	14 (12.7)
Albuterol	32		5 (15.6)
Fexofenadine	28		4 (14.3)
Loratadine	18		1 (5.6)
Other	77		3 (3.9)
Other nonpsychotropic meditation	108	5.7%$_{wt}$	6 (5.6)
Antibiotic	27		1 (3.7)
Anti-inflammatory	16		1 (6.3)
Muscle relaxant	12		2 (16.7)
Other	56		2 (3.6)
Total	483	36.2%$_{wt}$	173 (35.8)

[a]The sum of individuals prescribed each medication within a category may exceed the total number in the category because individuals may be prescribed multiple medications of the same type.
[b]2,893 is the weighted N of the 1,101 who participated in the third annual assessment.
[c]Diversions were measure as prescription medications either shared or sold—if a medication was diverted through both sharing and selling, it was counted only once.

regarding prescribing analgesic and stimulant medications for young adults.

▶ This is quite a fascinating and provocative article. In reality, most kids in the study shared (overwhelmingly more than sold) their medication only once/twice, and habitual misappropriation of licit drugs was particularly uncommon. Moreover, it was basically confined to the prescribed stimulants (Tables 2 and 4). Also, the article reports a high rate of substance use disorder, particularly alcohol misuse. However, the criteria and use of alcohol and other substances reaches the caseness criterion, but this does not appear to be clinically meaningful…that is, it's not describing what a clinician might call an alcoholic. Similarly, the abuse and sharing

TABLE 4.—Bivariate and Multivariate Logistic Regression Examining the Effect of Demographics and Risk Factors of Diversion in a Sample of College Students Prescribed a Medication (n = 483)

Demographic Characteristic	Nondiverters (n = 310), n (%)	Diverters (n = 173), n (%)	Unadjusted Odds Ratio (CI)	Adjusted Odds Ratio (CI)
Sex				
Female[a]	180 (58.1)	81 (46.8)	1.00	1.00
Male	130 (41.9)	92 (53.2)	1.57 (1.08–2.29)*	1.19 (0.78–1.81)
Race				
Nonwhite[a]	77 (24.8)	36 (20.8)	1.00	1.00
White	233 (75.2)	137 (79.2)	1.26 (0.80–1.97)	1.01 (0.62–1.66)
Fraternity/sorority membership				
Nonmember[a]	233 (75.2)	132 (76.3)	1.00	1.00
Member	77 (24.8)	41 (23.7)	0.94 (0.61–1.45)	0.87 (0.47–1.60)
Living situation				
On campus[a]	113 (36.5)	47 (27.2)	1.00	1.00
Off campus	115 (37.1)	83 (48.0)	1.74 (1.11–2.70)*	1.34 (0.83–2.16)
Fraternity/sorority house	40 (12.9)	17 (9.8)	1.02 (0.53–1.98)	1.01 (0.41–2.47)
Relative's home	34 (11.0)	22 (12.7)	1.56 (0.82–2.94)	1.43 (0.71–2.87)
Other	8 (2.6)	4 (2.3)	1.20 (0.35–4.19)	0.97 (0.25–3.79)
Alcohol use disorder				
No *DSM-IV* abuse/dependence[a]	189 (61.0)	72 (41.6)	1.00	1.00
Presence of *DSM-IV* abuse/dependence[b]	121 (39.0)	101 (58.4)	2.19 (1.50–3.20)*	1.33 (0.87–2.05)

Risk Factor	Mean (SD)	Mean (SD)	Unadjusted Odds Ratio (CI)	Adjusted Odds Ratio (CI)
Number of illicit drugs used	0.85 (0.98)	1.50 (1.36)	1.62 (1.57–2.38)*	1.21 (0.97–1.50)
Number of prescription drugs used nonmedically	0.42 (0.78)	0.99 (1.06)	1.93 (1.56–2.38)*	1.52 (1.16–1.99)*
Conduct problems[c]	2.87 (2.18)	3.91 (2.86)	1.19 (1.10–1.29)*	1.13 (1.04–1.23)*

Abbreviation: DSM-IV = Diagnostic and Statistical Manual of Mental Disorders, Fourth Edition.
Editor's Note: Please refer to original journal article for full references.
[a]Reference group.
[b]Meeting *DSM-IV* criteria for abuse or dependence was determined based on modified National Surgery on Drug Use and Health questions regarding *DSM-IV* criteria for alcohol abuse and dependence.[73]
[c]The measurement for conduct problems is the number of conduct problems meeting the criteria for conduct disorder endorsed on Johnson et al,[22] Conduct problem Scale.
*P < .05.

of medications—described as alarming—may not be as egregious as portrayed. However, this is a very serious issue that should be neither trivialized and/or underestimated. This study makes a very interesting read of a really topical issue.

P. F. Buckley, MD

Disrupting the prefrontal cortex diminishes the human ability to build a good reputation

Knoch D, Schneider F, Schunk D, et al (Univ of Basel, Switzerland; Univ of Zurich, Switzerland)
Proc Natl Acad Sci U S A 106:20895-20899, 2009

Reputation formation pervades human social life. In fact, many people go to great lengths to acquire a good reputation, even though building a good reputation is costly in many cases. Little is known about the neural underpinnings of this important social mechanism, however. In the present study, we show that disruption of the right, but not the left, lateral prefrontal cortex (PFC) with low-frequency repetitive transcranial magnetic stimulation (rTMS) diminishes subjects' ability to build a favorable reputation. This effect occurs even though subjects' ability to behave altruistically in the absence of reputation incentives remains intact, and even though they are still able to recognize both the fairness standards necessary for acquiring and the future benefits of a good reputation. Thus, subjects with a disrupted right lateral PFC no longer seem to be able to resist the temptation to defect, even though they know that this has detrimental effects on their future reputation. This suggests an important dissociation between the knowledge about one's own best interests and the ability to act accordingly in social contexts. These results link findings on the neural underpinnings of self-control and temptation with the study of human social behavior, and they may help explain why reputation formation remains less prominent in most other species with less developed prefrontal cortices.

▶ This is a fascinating and elegant study examining a higher order human attribute—reputation. It has implications for neuropsychology and forensic psychology. It should be a must read for politicians and lawyers!! It suggests that the lateral aspect of the dorsolateral prefrontal cortex is responsible for the integrity of reputation. The study is very well conducted and combines nicely neurobiological, psychological, and attributional behaviors. However, it does feel a little reductionist to propose a reputation lesion. Also these kinds of studies, although very well done, are difficult to replicate. Obviously, this is an important consideration in this case.

P. F. Buckley, MD

Are Gold Standard Depression Measures Appropriate for Use in Geriatric Cancer Patients? A Systematic Evaluation of Self-Report Depression Instruments Used With Geriatric, Cancer, and Geriatric Cancer Samples
Nelson CJ, Cho C, Berk AR, et al (Memorial Sloan-Kettering Cancer Ctr, NY; Columbia College of Physicians and Surgeons, NY)
J Clin Oncol 28:348-356, 2010

Purpose.—Geriatric issues in cancer are becoming prominent. Depression is a significant concern for both the elderly and patients with cancer, yet identifying depression in these patients is difficult and often leads to under-recognition. We conducted a systematic review to determine which depression instruments are appropriate for use in geriatric patients with cancer.

Methods.—We identified the most commonly used self-report depression instruments. We then used the criteria established in the US Food and Drug Administration Draft Guidance on Patient-Reported Outcome Measures to determine the extent of validation evidence of these measures in geriatric cancer populations. Finally, we determined which instruments captured depressive symptoms that are common among elderly patients with cancer.

Results.—Eight measures were selected as the most commonly used instruments. These were the Beck Depression Inventory-II, Brief Symptom Inventory-18, Center for Epidemiologic Studies–Depression Scale, Geriatric Depression Scale-15, Hospital Anxiety and Depression Scale, Patient Health Questionnaire-9, Profile of Mood States–Short Form, and Zung Self-Rating Depression Scale. Many have been validated for use with geriatric adults and patients with cancer; however, data addressing content validity and responder definition were lacking. To date, there is no validation information for geriatric patients with cancer. Furthermore, symptom profile analysis revealed that these measures do not identify many symptoms signaling depression in geriatric patients with cancer.

Conclusion.—The validation evidence for use of common depression instruments in geriatric patients with cancer is lacking. This, and the possibility that these measures may not assess common depressive symptoms in geriatric patients with cancer, questions the adequacy of these scales in this population (Tables 3 and 4).

▶ Depression clearly is common in patients who have cancer, perhaps particularly so in those patients who are more elderly. However, for clinical management purposes, distinguishing between psychic and somatic symptoms that are the expression of comorbid depression instead of being aspects of cancer itself is important and complex. Moreover, grieving is an aspect of awareness of coming to terms with cancer, especially in the elderly where the likelihood that the cancer could be life shortening is greater. Thus, the use of psychiatric rating scales for depression could help distinguish between both causes, assuming the scales are valid in this patient population. The review of self-report scales (Tables 3 and 4) reveals that these scales are likely not sensitive

TABLE 3.—Reported Validation and Psychometric Properties of Eight Self-Report Instruments to Measure Depression in Geriatric, Cancer, and Geriatric Cancer Populations

Property	BDI-II	BSI-18	CES-D	GDS-15	HADS	PHQ-9	POMS-SF	Zung SDS
Validation in geriatric population								
Extent of validation								
Validation study conducted	●	○	●	●	●		○	●
Age ranges of geriatric populations in validation study conducted, years	≥ 55	56-88	60-96	65-100	60-92	≥ 60	55-94	60-97
Validation in sample representative of US population	●		●	○				●
Validation in specific ethnic minority sample			●	●				
Validity statistics								
Test-retest reliability	○			○		●	○*	
Internal consistency	●		●	●			○	●
Content validity								
Convergent validity	●	○	●	●	●		○	●
Discriminant validity	●	○		○	●		○	●
Known-groups validity	●		●	○			○	●
Predictive validity								
Ability to detect change					●			
Interpretability statistics								
Recommended cut-off scores	●	●		●	●	●		
Minimum important difference						●		
Responder definition								
Validation in cancer population								
Extent of validation								
Validation study conducted	●	●	●	●	●	●†	●	●
Age ranges of cancer populations in validation study conducted	n/p	30 to ≥ 80	n/p	n/p	16-86	n/p	18-65	n/p
Validation in sample representative of US population			●					
Validation in specific ethnic minority sample		●‡	●					
Validity statistics								
Test-retest reliability			●§	●				
Internal consistency	●	●	●	●	●		●	●
Content validity								
Convergent validity	●	●	●	●	●	●†	●	●
Discriminant validity	●	○	●	●	●	●†	●	●
Known-groups validity	●	●	●	●	●		●	●
Predictive validity								
Ability to detect change								
Interpretability statistics								
Recommended cut-off scores	●	●	●	●				
Minimum important difference								

(Continued)

TABLE 3. (*continued*)

Property	BDI-II	BSI-18	CES-D	GDS-15	HADS	PHQ-9	POMS-SF	Zung SDS
Responder definition								
Validation in geriatric cancer population								
Validation study conducted								

NOTE: Filled circle indicates that data found for listed instrument met guidelines for acceptability (as defined in Methods section).

Open circle indicates that data were not found for listed instrument; however, data were found for parent instrument that met guidelines for acceptability (as defined in Methods section).

Abbreviations: BDI-II, Beck Depression Inventory-II; BSI-18, Brief Symptom Inventory-18; CES-D, Center for Epidemiologic Studies–Depression Scale; GDS-15, Geriatric Depression Scale-15; HADS, Hospital Anxiety and Depression Scale; PHQ-9, Patient Health Questionnaire-9; POMS-SF, Profile of Mood States–Short Form; Zung SDS, Zung Self-Rating Depression Scale; n/p, not published.

*One of the subscales for the POMS showed a test-retest reliability coefficent of only 0.68 in a geriatric population; however, the majority of its subscales demonstrated coefficients greater than 0.7.

†Data found for a computer-based administration of the PHQ-9 only.

‡The study sample comprised only 27 patients.

§For the CES-D, the reported test-retest reliability coefficient in a cancer population was 0.57, which was below the minimum threshold of 0.7 that we established for inclusion.

TABLE 4.—Symptom Profile Analysis of Eight Self-Report Instruments to Measure Depression: Inclusion of Symptoms Commonly Reported in Geriatric Patients with Cancer

Symptom	BDI-II	BSI-18	CES-D	GDS-15	HADS	PHQ-9	POMS-SF	Zung SDS
Physical functioning								
General aches and pains/stomachaches		●						
Diffuse somatic complaints		●						
Late insomnia	●							
Psychological functioning								
General malaise		●	●	●	●		●	●
Hopelessness	●	●	●	●		●	●	●
Mood variation*	●							
Sexual functioning								
Change/loss of sexual interest	●							●

NOTE: Filled circle indicates that data found for listed instrument met guidelines for acceptability (as defined in Methods section).

Abbreviations: BDI-II, Beck Depression Inventory-II; BSI-18, Brief Symptom Inventory-18; CES-D, Center for Epidemiologic Studies–Depression Scale; GDS-15, Geriatric Depression Scale-15; HADS, Hospital Anxiety and Depression Scale; PHQ-9, Patient Health Questionnaire-9; POMS-SF, Profile of Mood States–Short Form; Zung SDS, Zung Self-Rating Depression Scale.

*Zung SDS mood variation reported as follows: "Morning is when I feel best."

enough to distinguish depression versus cancer in this population. This is a very specific report, although it is still a very useful constitution for those who work in this field.

P. F. Buckley, MD

Deep brain stimulation of the subcallosal cingulate gyrus for depression: anatomical location of active contacts in clinical responders and a suggested guideline for targeting

Hamani C, Mayberg H, Snyder B, et al (Toronto Western Hosp, Ontario, Canada; Emory Univ School of Medicine, Atlanta, Ga; et al)
J Neurosurg 111:1209-1215, 2009

Object.—Deep brain stimulation (DBS) of the subcallosal cingulate gyrus (SCG), including Brodmann area 25, is currently being investigated for the treatment of major depressive disorder (MDD). As a potential emerging therapy, optimal target selection within the SCG has still to be determined. The authors compared the location of the electrode contacts in responders and nonresponders to DBS of the SCG and correlated the results with clinical outcome to help in identifying the optimal target within the region. Based on the location of the active contacts used for long-term stimulation in responders, the authors suggest a standardized method of targeting the SCG in patients with MDD.

Methods.—Postoperative MR imaging studies of 20 patients with MDD treated with DBS of the SCG were analyzed. The authors assessed the location of the active contacts relative to the midcommissural point and in relation to anatomical landmarks within the medial aspect of the frontal lobe. For this, a grid with 2 main lines was designed, with 1 line in the anterior-posterior and 1 line in the dorsal-ventral axis. Each of these lines was divided into 100 units, and data were converted into percentages. The anterior-posterior line extended from the anterior commissure (AC) to the projection of the anterior aspect of the corpus callosum (CCa). The dorsal-ventral line extended from the inferior portion of the CC (CCi) to the most ventral aspect of the frontal lobe (abbreviated "Fr" for the formula).

Results.—Because the surgical technique did not vary across patients, differences in stereotactic coordinates between responders and nonresponders did not exceed 1.5 mm in any axis (x, y, or z). In patients who responded to the procedure, contacts used for long-term stimulation were in close approximation within the SCG. In the anteriorposterior line, these contacts were located within a 73.2 ± 7.7 percentile distance from the AC (with the AC center being 0% and the line crossing the CCa being 100%). In the dorsal-ventral line, active contacts in responders were located within a 26.2 ± 13.8 percentile distance from the CCi (with the CCi edge being 0% and the Fr inferior limit being 100%). In the medial-lateral plane, most electrode tips were in the transition between the gray and white matter of SCG.

Conclusions.—Active contacts in patients who responded to DBS were relatively clustered within the SCG. Because of the anatomical variability

TABLE 1.—Clinical Outcome in Patients with Major Depression who Responded or did not Respond to DBS of the SCG*

Subgroup	No. of Patients	HAMD-17 Score Preop	HAMD-17 Score Postop (1-yr FU)	% Improvement
Responders	11	24.3 ± 3.7	8.2 ± 2.5	66.4 ± 9.0
Nonresponders	9	24.1 ± 3.2	18.0 ± 4.8	26.1 ± 13.8
All	20	24.2 ± 3.4	12.6 ± 6.2	48.2 ± 23.2

*Results are expressed as the mean ± SD. Abbreviation: FU = follow-up.

in the size and shape of the SCG, the authors developed a method to standardize the targeting of this region.

▶ Dr Mayberg, who is now at Emory University but was at the University of Toronto when this pioneering work was undertaken, has been a world leader in deep brain stimulation for patients who have intractable depression. This work has received worldwide attention. This report describes, in considerable detail, the selection of the distinct areas of the brain that are the focus of deep brain stimulation. Although the study is small, the results are impressive (Table 1). In the responder group, they achieved a 66% decrease in symptoms. The nonresponder group achieved on average a 26% reduction in symptoms. The subcallosal cingulate gurus appears to be the preferred and most effective target site for deep brain stimulation for depression. This work has been featured on TV, in newspapers, and in magazines. It has grabbed the public's attention. This is very good. It is also, however, methodologically very sound work and exemplary science—as this article demonstrates!

P. F. Buckley, MD

Article Index

Chapter 1: Child and Adolescent Psychiatry

Chapter 2: Psychotherapy

Chapter 3: Alcohol and Substance Abuse

Chapter 4: Psychiatry and the Law

Chapter 5: Hospital and Community Psychiatry

Chapter 6: Clinical Psychiatry

Chapter 7: Biological Psychiatry

Author Index

Printed and bound by CPI Group (UK) Ltd, Croydon, CR0 4YY

08/05/2025

01864677-0015